Psychology for Nurses and Health Visitors

John Hall

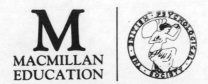

MACMILLAN
EDUCATION

Published by THE BRITISH PSYCHOLOGICAL SOCIETY and
MACMILLAN PUBLISHERS LIMITED.

Distributed by Higher and Further Education Division
MACMILLAN PUBLISHERS LTD., London and Basingstoke.
Associated companies and representatives throughout the
world.

ISBN 0 333 31876 5 (paper cover)

Printed in Hong Kong

H & H   44084 (2) 7.99 6 90

Note: throughout these texts, the masculine pronouns have
been used for succinctness and are intended to refer to both
females and males.

The conclusions drawn and opinions expressed are those of
the authors. They should not be taken to represent the
views of the publishers.

Contents

(v)

Foreword

This book is one of a series, the principal aims of which
are to illustrate how psychology can be applied in particular professional contexts, how it can improve the skills
of practitioners, and how it can increase the practitioners'
and students' understanding of themselves.

Psychology is taught to many groups of students and is
now integrated within prescribed syllabuses for an increasing number of professions. The existing texts which teachers
have been obliged to recommend are typically designed for
broad and disparate purposes, and consequently they fail to
reflect the special needs of students in professional
training. The starting point for the series was the
systematic distillation of views expressed in professional
journals by those psychologists whose teaching specialisms
relate to the applications of psychology. It soon became
apparent that many fundamental topics were common to a
number of syllabuses and courses; yet in general introductory textbooks these topics tend to be embedded amongst
much superfluous material. Therefore, from within the
British Psychological Society, we invited experienced
teachers and authorities in their field to write review
chapters on key topics. Forty-seven chapters covering 23
topics were then available for selection by the series'
Volume Editors. The Volume Editors are also psychologists
and they have had many years of involvement with their
respective professions. In preparing their books, they have
consulted formally with colleagues in those professions.
Each of their books has its own combination of the
specially-prepared chapters, set in the context of the
specific professional practice.

Because psychology is only one component of the various
training curricula, and because students generally have
limited access to learned journals and specialist texts, our
contributors to the series have restricted their use of
references, while at the same time providing short lists of
annotated readings. In addition, they have provided review
questions to help students organize their learning and
prepare for examinations. Further teaching materials, in the
form of additional references, projects, exercises and class
notes, are available in Tutor Manuals prepared for each
book. A comprehensive tutorial text ('Psychology and
People'), prepared by the Series Editors, combines in a

single volume all the key topics, together with their associated teaching materials.

It is intended that volumes will be revised in the light of changing requirements. Evaluative and constructive comments, bearing on any aspect of the series, are most welcome and should be addressed to us at the BPS in Leicester.

In devising and developing the series we have had the good fortune to benefit from the advice and support of Dr Halla Beloff, Professor Philip Levy, Mr Allan Sakne and Mr John Winckler. A great burden has been borne by Mrs Gail Sheffield, who with skill, tact and courtesy, has managed the production of the series: to her and her colleagues at the BPS headquarters and at the Macmillan Press, we express our thanks.

Antony J. Chapman
Leeds

Anthony Gale
University of Southampton

January 1982

Tutor Manuals, price £1 each, are only available from
The British Psychological Society
St Andrews House
48 Princess Road East
Leicester
LE1 7DR

Introduction
John Hall

Introduction

Definition of nursing

One of the most widely used British textbooks of general nursing is introduced with the following definition of nursing:

> The unique function of the nurse is to assist the individual, sick or well, in the performance of those activities contributing to health or its recovery (or to a peaceful death) that he would perform unaided if he had the necessary strength, will or knowledge. And to do this in such a way as to help him gain independence as rapidly as possible. This aspect of her work, this part of her function, she initiates and controls; of this she is master. In addition she helps the patient to carry out the therapeutic plan as initiated by the physician. She also, as a member of a medical team, helps other members, as they in turn help her, to plan and carry out the total programme whether it be for the improvement of health, or the recovery from illness or support in death.

This piece, by Virginia Henderson (Harmer and Henderson, 1955), subsequently appeared in the International Council of Nurses book (1972) and in the twentieth edition of Pearce (1980).

As a definition of nursing, it is significant from a psychological viewpoint, in that it underlines the nurse's involvement with normal as well as sick people, and stresses the nurse's role in motivating and informing the patient. It emphasizes the need to maintain the patient's psychological independence, while supporting the patient who is co-operating with the therapeutic regime. It speaks of the need for nurses to work closely with others, and the importance of positive health care and the process of rehabilitation. In short, it recognizes the key psychological role of the nurse for both patient and colleague.

Structure of the book

The purpose of this book is to introduce the trainee and trained nurse to a wide range of topics in psychology of relevance to nursing. The topics have been chosen to be relevant to nurses working in general and in psychiatric nursing, in hospitals and in the community, in supervising and teaching posts as well as at the bedside.

The book is planned as seven separate but related parts. Each has an introductory chapter, and two or three other chapters. The introductory chapter to each part is written to highlight the relevance to nurses and nursing practice of the topics concerned, and to indicate any important topics not covered in the other chapters in that part. Each introductory chapter is illustrated by reference to recent clinical or experimental studies or accounts, all of which have been written by hospital and community nurses or published in nursing journals. The subsequent chapters in each part review the state of current psychological knowledge in each particular topic area, and refer to the most relevant recent research studies and reviews of those topics. The separate parts need not be read in consecutive order, but may be studied as needed, although it is recommended that all readers look at Part I, 'Psychology and Nursing', before reading any others.

Each part of the book thus brings together several areas of psychological knowledge and their application in nursing, and each concludes with a series of questions to help readers organize their learning, to stimulate them to think further about the topics covered, and to prepare for examinations. Each set of questions includes some which are designed to reflect the content of recent questions set in General Nursing Council examinations for Registered Nurses, and in examinations for the Diploma in Nursing of London University. Depending on the level of nursing qualifications for which readers may be preparing, additional information can be gleaned from the references and annotated reading which are given for each chapter.

A glance at the contents page at the front of the book shows how the sections are organized. Part I introduces the main concepts and assumptions made by psychologists. Parts II and III look at the whole span of life, dividing the span into two consecutive periods. Part II starts with a look at pregnancy - a period of special interest to midwives and health visitors - and examines development up to adolescence. Part III covers family life, and human development from adulthood to death, paying attention to the period of bereavement.

Part IV deals with the way in which we understand people, particularly by looking at how we understand ourselves, and how we come to terms with abnormal or strange behaviour. Part V describes the range of assessment methods developed by psychologists, many of which can be used by nurses in either ordinary nursing practice or in research. Part VI outlines some of the principal psychological methods of producing change in thoughts, feelings and behaviour of both healthy people - including nurses themselves - and patients. Part VII is the last part and deals with a range of nursing issues where psychology is helpful in either understanding the problem or leading to change, and looks in detail at topics of immense importance: for example, pain.

The book does not pretend to offer a comprehensive introduction to psychology as a scientific discipline: such a task would lead to a much longer book than this one, and in any case would not meet the needs of most nurses.

Reference material

A special feature of the book is the use made of research and descriptive material published in nursing journals. Many nursing students have difficulty in obtaining access to libraries with adequate psychology sections, or may not wish to buy a more academic psychological textbook of limited relevance to their interests. A number of nursing journals and nursing research monographs now contain articles and information highly relevant to the psychology of nursing. References to these sources and to the sources in other chapters are not provided in order to show how erudite the authors are. They are given to provide the source of a particular set of results or conclusions; to give an example of some particular point; or to indicate further reading on a topic.

References appear in the text as the name of a person or group of people, followed by a year. Each reference is amplified at the end of each chapter, at which point a reference list, arranged in alphabetical order, give additional information. Where a reference is to a book, the title of the book, the name of the publisher and place of publication are provided. This full reference will enable a library to obtain a copy of the book for you. Where a reference is to a journal or magazine, the volume number of the journal, or date of issue of the journal, are given, together with the page numbers on which the article is printed. With this information you can trace the original article yourself from back numbers of the journal, or again ask a library to obtain it for you. At the end of the volume you will find further recommended reading lists to enable you to study any topics that have interested you in greater depth.

The nursing journals which have been referred to are likely to be available or obtainable in many schools or nursing, so it should be possible for you to read at least some of the references in the original. There is no substitute for reading research studies in their original form. You will be able to decide for yourself how carefully the study was conducted, and whether the conclusions were justified. You will be able to appreciate the practical steps which are involved in research, and so perhaps be encouraged to carry out a study or experimental investigation yourself. Furthermore, original books or articles themselves give further references, so that looking at a single recent publication will often assist you considerably in following up those topics which especially interest you.

There are a number of ways of checking what information is available on interesting topics. One way is to look at a guide to the various nursing journals which are published, to see which journals are likely to cover the topics of concern to you. One such guide is that written by Binger and Jensen (1980).

Another way is to go through the various indexing and abstracting publications which are available and which enable you to find out what articles have been published on a particular topic over the previous few months. The major psychological example of such a publication is 'Psychological Abstracts', which is published every month and gives very full coverage of the large majority of recently published psychological research, complete with a good cross-indexing system to help you identify articles of interest. There are several similar medical indexing publications, and the British Department of Health and Social Security now regularly publishes abstracts of recent nursing research articles in 'Nursing Research and Abstracts' which started in 1979.

A word of advice and encouragement
Many of the ideas and terms used in this book will be new to you. You need to think about them carefully, and about your day-to-day work, before applying them. But the psychological ideas, information and techniques presented in the book will give you an opportunity to improve the standard of care your patients receive, to understand better the people around you, and maybe to go on to contribute to nursing and psychological knowledge yourself.

Acknowledgements

I would like to thank those people who have advised me on the content and layout of this volume, especially Isabel Speight, who is currently Professional Officer with the English National Board for Nursing, Midwifery, and Health Visiting (and previously was Professional Officer with the Joint Board of Clinical Nursing Studies); also P. J. Farrell, Director of Nurse Education, Gwynedd School of Nursing, Bangor. In addition, I would like to thank two former colleagues with a particular commitment to teaching nurses: Joe Beswick, Senior Clinical Psychologist, Aston Hall Hospital, nr Derby, and Sue Llewellyn, Senior Clinical Psychologist, Middlewood Hospital, Sheffield.

References

Binger, J.L. and Jensen, L.M. (1980)
Lippincotts Guide to Nursing Literature. Philadelphia: J.B. Lippincott.
Harmer, B. and Henderson, V. (1955)
Textbook of the Principles and Practice of Nursing. New York: Macmillan Inc.
Henderson, V. (1972)
ICN Basic Principles of Nursing Care. Geneva: International Council of Nursing.
Pearce, E. (1980)
A General Textbook of Nursing. London: Faber & Faber.

Part one
Psychology and Nursing

1

Psychology and nursing
John Hall

What is psychology?

Psychology is typically defined as the scientific study of
behaviour and experience. This raises the question of what
is meant by 'scientific', 'behaviour', and 'experience'.
The significance of each of these terms has varied in the
relatively short history of psychology.

While contemporary psychology uses many technical procedures and items of equipment, and while sophisticated
experimental design and statistical analysis are commonplace, the aspiration or even desirability of psychology to
be a true 'science' has been challenged. From the earliest
days of psychology as a separate discipline, there have been
disputes about the extent to which inner experience is a
valid subject of psychological enquiry. For example, at the
turn of the century, a group of psychologists working in
Wurzburg introduced the notion of 'systematic experimental
introspection', but it was later questioned by the early
behaviourist J. B. Watson who denied that the study of
experience had any value whatsoever.

Arguments continue, but for our purposes psychology can
be taken as the systematic study of the behaviour of people
and animals; and the word 'behaviour' should then be interpreted to cover thoughts, emotions and utterances, as well
as acts. Psychological investigations are usually designed
to indicate clearly the relationship between several factors, or to generalize beyond the sample of people (or
animals) studied to a greater population from which the
experimental sample was drawn. Psychologists are concerned
to establish general principles of behaviour and general
relationships, in the expectation that these general findings will enable useful predictions and explanations to be
made about the behaviour of individual people. Psychology
usually starts from everyday behaviour and experience; and
abnormal or unusual behaviour is explained first of all in
terms of the concepts and words used to describe normality.

**Psychology and common
sense**

Psychology is sometimes dismissed as plain common sense.
Yet common sense is often not very common, and often cannot take us beyond our own limited experiences and opinions.
Proverbs and old wives' tales give a picture of distilled
folk wisdom that can meet most human dilemmas. But psychological enquiry can go beyond unaided common sense. For

example, 'surprising' results have been obtained from psychological studies of pain, sleep and hypnosis. Then again, the effects of being put in a warm environment without everyday noises, and in diffuse lighting, might be thought to be entirely positive. But the effects of unusual types of environment cannot be predicted by common sense alone. Experiments have been conducted with volunteers who were placed in baths of water at blood heat, with cuffs over their hands to minimize tactile stimulation, with 'white noise' (or random sounds) fed to their ears through headphones, and with translucent goggles over their eyes. The volunteer subjects were grossly disorientated by this procedure, and chose not to continue the experiments despite the offer of a high rate of payment.

Psychology and other disciplines

Psychological explanations of behaviour do not exclude other explanations. For example, the act of eating can be examined nutritionally in terms of the dietary and calorific value of food, physiologically in terms of muscle activity in the mouth and throat, and psychologically in terms of the observable behaviour of the person. No one system of explanation takes account of all the ways in which people live. For many practical purposes a psychological explanation can be highly valuable especially when considering either the behaviour of people who are ill, or the behaviour of those who care for them.

The social sciences
Psychology is increasingly seen as one of the 'behavioural sciences', 'life sciences', or 'human sciences'. These terms refer to groupings of psychology, sociology, economics and other subjects, and they imply that aspects of these subjects are relevant to caring professions. There are uncertain boundaries between psychology and some of these other disciplines, and overlaps with them have become identified as separate 'sub-subjects' in themselves. For example, the area of overlap between psychology and physiology is psychophysiology. While no practical purpose is served by a demarcation dispute about areas of overlap, there are sometimes important differences in method between psychology and other disciplines and these differences should be fully recognized. It is especially important for nurses to distinguish clearly between psychology and other disciplines with which it is commonly confused.

Thus patients may say they have seen a psychologist when in fact they have seen a psychiatrist. Clarifying who a patient has actually seen can clarify the sort of treatment the patient has probably been receiving.

Psychiatry
Psychiatry is that branch of medicine concerned with the diagnosis and treatment of mental disorder. The very notion of 'mental illness' has been disputed, and certainly differs

conceptually and sometimes legally from one country to another. In some European countries neurology and psychiatry are practised as one specialty. The way in which schizophrenia is diagnosed in the United States differs from in Britain. Hence the boundaries between psychiatry and other medical fields vary, and consequently so does the way in which psychiatric practice is organized, although all psychiatrists are medically qualified.

Psychoanalysis

Psychoanalysis is the system of understanding and treating mental conflicts and disorders developed by Sigmund Freud. Freud modified his views considerably during his own lifetime, and since his death in 1939 there have been further major modifications to classic psychoanalytic thought from other analysts such as Adler, Jung and Klein. Psychoanalytic theory assumes that there is subconscious or unconscious motivation underlying behaviour, and that access to subconscious feelings is essential to produce insight. The method of free-association, and the examination of transference phenomena (feelings between therapist and patient), are characteristics of analytic treatment methods. Psychoanalytic ideas have had an impact far beyond the treatment of neurotic problems, extending to the fields of religion, art and literature. Psychoanalysts need not be medically qualified, but they have all received a lengthy and thorough training, of which the analysis of the trainee analyst is an important part.

Psychotherapy

Psychotherapy is a term used to describe any method of psychological treatment which relies primarily on talking. There are several different approaches to psychotherapy apart from those influenced by psychoanalytic ideas. Ellis has developed a 'rational-emotive' therapy which is fairly directive, while the 'client-centred' approach of Rogers is typically non-directive. There is an increasing interest in group psychotherapy, where small groups of clients or patients analyse their problems with a therapist. Hybrid terms such as 'behavioural psychotherapy' have been developed to indicate that there is a strong verbal component to behaviour therapy techniques.

Why study animals?

As already noted, psychology is concerned not only with the behaviour of people, but with the behaviour of animals. Psychologists believe that the principles governing many functions such as perception, motivation and learning are similar for several species. If different species share similar types of central nervous system and similar types of sense organs, then the principles may be transferable to an appreciable degree from one species to another. Sometimes considerable 'jumps' are made when explaining human behaviour in terms of results from animal experiments. For example, it has been suggested that the behaviour of rats in densely crowded cages may give us some understanding of how people react to the crowded conditions of modern urban living. Nevertheless, experiments can be useful in explaining behaviour when research with people would be impossibly impractical or expensive. Some experiments would be unethical, such as investigations into the effects of early separation between child and mother. Experiments with monkeys, for example, help us understand this process under conditions that are still humane to the animals concerned. There is obviously a limit to the extent to which such animal experiments, although they may be of interest in themselves, adequately explain human behaviour. None the less, at the very least they have given valuable direction to many areas of psychological investigation, and in some fields of psychology - such as learning theory - it would have been impossible to achieve the present body of psychological knowledge without animal experiments.

Ethical problems in psychological research
There are some human functions, such as thinking, which certainly cannot be studied through animals, as well as other areas of functioning, such as group behaviour, which rely so much on the use of developed language that animal experiments are of little or no value. For some of these areas of functioning it is possible for psychological questions to be posed in such a way that they cannot be researched in any acceptable fashion. One question might be, 'What would be the effect on a child of total separation from any adult figures during, say, the first five years of life?' There have been a few individual studies of wild or 'feral' children, but it would be ethically quite inappropriate to mount an experiment on such effects in a planned way. Similarly, it would be unacceptable to carry out an experiment which investigated, to the limit, the extent to which people are willing to inflict pain on others. In a classic series of experiments Milgram (1964) investigated this type of behaviour, in one study examining the willingness of a 'naive' subject in the experiment to give very high levels of electric shock to a supposed 'learner' in the experiment. Two confederates of the experimenter acted in such a way that the naive subject was induced to go on giving shocks up to 450 volts, despite hearing shouts and cries from the learner. The equipment was arranged so that no shock was actually delivered to the learner subject, but it illustrates how group influence in experimental situations could lead to unacceptable treatments being given. The study also illustrates the need to think through the ethical implications of some experiments. Thus there may be some behavioural questions which cannot be answered through systematic research, since it is not possible to design or carry out a rigorous study or experiment. In most countries, to ensure that agreed ethical criteria are met, there is some form of review for any proposed research on patients.

Where clear answers are impossible to provide, speculation may begin. Speculation may be informed, trying to proceed from established knowledge, or merely guesswork. When guesswork takes over, then psychology as a systematic discipline disappears. This does not prevent the appearance in some popular magazines of articles purporting to be 'psychological', but typically these contain nothing more than the guesses or opinions of the writer. While many of these articles may be fun, they are not psychology.

What is a psychologist?

A 'psychologist' is simply a person who studies or applies psychology. As yet there is in Britain no law which registers the title 'psychologist'. However, some other western countries have passed legislation which protects at least some uses of the term psychologist, especially if the people covered by the legislation offer some service direct to the public.

The usual use of the term implies that the person concerned has at least obtained a university degree in psychology. There is an increasing number of people who may hold a degree of which psychology is a major part, but who work as members of another profession. A growing number of doctors, nurses, health visitors, therapists and social workers possess such degrees, and they may well be interested in integrating their psychological knowledge with their other professional knowledge and skills.

Graduates in psychology may choose to use their knowledge in a non-specialized way, by entering some field like personnel work, the probation service or business management. Those people who continue to be identified as psychologists work in one of two major fields: either teaching or applying psychology professionally. Many teachers of psychology are found in universities, mostly in departments of psychology, teaching post-graduate and undergraduate students. Many other teachers work in polytechnics or colleges. In addition to teaching psychology to undergraduates, they may be teaching people who are training for such professions as social work and teaching, as well as post-basic nursing courses such as those for tutors and community nurses. A high proportion of teachers of psychology are also involved in research, both basic and applied, and in a number of countries there are opportunities to be a full-time research psychologist; in Britain they are employed by bodies like the Medical Research Council.

Psychologists in health and education services
As far as nurses and health visitors are concerned the two types of professional applied psychologist that they are most likely to meet are educational psychologists and clinical or medical psychologists. Both types of psychologist have pursued a specialized post-graduate training, leading to a diploma or a post-graduate degree. Clinical or medical psychologists work in close collaboration with doctors and

other health care staff, assessing and treating a wide range
of mental, behavioural and physical problems. In Britain
most clinical psychologists are employed in the National
Health Service and work with the psychiatrically disturbed
(adults and children) as well as with the mentally handicapped, the elderly, the neurologically impaired, and
others. Educational psychologists work in collaboration with
teachers and colleagues in School Psychological Services.
They are mostly employed by local authority education departments, working with children with educational problems,
or children with conduct or emotional disorders. Apart from
these two types of applied psychologist, some psychologists
work with offenders in prisons. Occupational psychologists
may undertake work in collaboration with training centres
and rehabilitation assessment centres; and some provide a
vocational guidance service.

What is nursing?

This book is for nurses and health visitors, so a question
such as 'What is nursing?' may seem unnecessary. But 'nursing' has two main meanings. The first is the care of the
sick in their own homes, usually by members of their family
or by friends, when they are suffering from a temporary
illness: this sort of nursing is usually not very technical,
and requires few, if any, specific skills from the people
who are doing it. The second, nursing as a professional
activity, is carried out by specially qualified people,
often in a special setting. This is a relatively recent
development.

While nursing is older than psychology as a professional
activity, it was precisely the absence of any professional
approach to nursing by the British Army in the Crimean War
of 1854-1856 that set Florence Nightingale on her pioneering
course. Thus nursing as an activity which requires special
knowledge and formal skills is about 125 years old. Nursing
has now become clearly identified as a key link between,
first, sophisticated and sometimes stressful medical decisions and procedures and, second, maintenance of normal
bodily and psychological functioning. A development beyond
simply caring for the sick is the growth of interest in
positive maintenance of health, as illustrated by the edu-
cative work of the health visitor and public health nurse.
Every new development in medicine, surgery and community
medicine has led in turn to changes in the type of nursing
necessary to transmit those developments to patients, their
families and the general public.

This means that the practice of nursing has become
increasingly complex. In order to integrate the knowledge
possessed by the nurse, and the practical skills required,
interest is growing in what is known as the 'nursing process'. This term describes a four-stage cycle of assessment,
planning, implementation and education which goes on whenever a patient presents with an illness, or with some
interest in maintenance of health.

The analysis of the nursing process in terms of these four stages makes it clear that nursing today is much more than the provision of a hygienic and comfortable environment and provision of hotel and personal services connected with, for example, feeding and urination. Just considering assessment alone, a whole range of complex decisions may be required. Is a wound healing? Is the correct site being used for an intramuscular injection? Are the bruises on a young child likely to be accidental, or have they been caused deliberately? Has the patient been applying an ointment correctly? Is an old lady likely to be mobile enough to return home on her own? For some of these decisions there will be other staff and other family members involved, but often it is the nurse's task to initiate action (because of doubt or concern) or to make a rapid decision, because no one else is there.

Psychology and nursing

Aspects of psychology relevant to nursing vary from one task to another. Taking the hypothetical assessment decisions mentioned in the previous paragraph, assessment of whether a wound is healing depends on sight, and on the response of the wound to carefully applied pressure and to the touch of the hands: perceptual skills are important in such a decision. Choice of an injection site depends upon knowledge of underlying bone structure, muscle structure and the distribution of nerves and blood vessels: specific recall or visual memory of an illustration or model is therefore required. Assessment of the probability of non-accidental injury requires both knowledge of the probable cause of bruising or scarring on particular body sites and also knowledge of the past history of the child and family.

Some individual nursing decisions have a high degree of psychological relevance. Others, such as those in operating theatre nursing, have less psychological relevance. However, whatever the individual decision or task, there is a person at the centre of the illness or health problem. Patients have to be spoken to and understood. They have to be persuaded, cajoled and informed about many matters. The personal relationships between patients and those who care for them are not only the main instrument of keeping them as happy and well informed as possible, but affect their willingness to co-operate as well as their rates of recovery. A major source of variation (and interest) in the work of nurses is the variety of people with whom they have to interact. Quite apart from the medical problems that each patient presents, all patients are unique in terms of their combinations of age, abilities, attainments, interests, sexuality and social background. Each one of these attributes may be important in determining their response to an individual nurse, and to a particular regime of nursing care.

What is a nurse?

While the nursing process can be used to analyse a wide range of nursing activities, in most developed countries it is easy to define 'a nurse', since there is in most such countries a statutory form of training, and some degree of legal protection of the title 'nurse'. There are important national differences in the ways in which nurses have been trained but, in Europe at least, these differences have been diminishing in recent years. A set of 'EEC Nursing Directives' was signed in 1977, and training of nurses is now being modified stage by stage in all European countries. The directives stipulate a basic training programme of three years, with a programme of theoretical instruction yoked to a programme of clinical instruction in specified areas of care.

Apart from people who can thus be recognized as registered or qualified nurses there are those people who work as assistant or auxiliary nurses: they work within a nursing management structure and are supervised by trained nurses. They may not perhaps call themselves nurses, but the patients may call them nurses and regard them as such. Assistant nurses often carry out a major proportion of the 'bedside' nursing, and, especially in long-term care hospitals, they may considerably outnumber the trained nurses. This book is not intended for assistant nurses, but their role in the nursing process cannot be overlooked, nor should the psychological problems of supervising and training them be overlooked.

In Britain there is a well-differentiated set of nursing qualifications. The current system of basic nurse training is related to four different client groups:

* the physically ill adult; SRN (State Registered Nurse: England, Wales and Northern Ireland) or RGN (Registered General Nurse in Scotland);
* the physically ill child; RSCN (Registered Sick Children's Nurse);
* the mentally ill; RMN (Registered Mental Nurse);
* the mentally handicapped; RNMS (Registered Nurse for the Mentally Subnormal in England, Wales and Northern Ireland) or RNMD (Registered Nurse for Mental Defectives in Scotland).

A small number of nurses enter by other routes, training as orthopaedic, dental or nursery nurses. Thus the initial attitudes and expectations of nurses can be established in a wide variety of different settings, with sometimes no overlap at all. This process of initial training also serves to socialize the nurse into a particular role. It can affect the willingness of nurses to move to other types of nursing, and can even affect attitudes to patients from other diagnostic groups who may stray into their particular ward. Some nurses in general hospital work, for example, find difficulty in relating to patients who have a psychiatric difficulty as well as a physical difficulty. In some countries the initial training of all nurses is generic, so this problem does not arise. After initial training a range of additional types of qualification can be obtained, including the Certificate in Health Visiting, which is the qualification for British public health nurses. Health visitors are familiar figures to new mothers, as well as to other people living at home who may be quite markedly handicapped or at risk of some particular disease or condition.

Apart from variations in patient-related skills and knowledge, nurses vary in the extent to which they can utilize psychological expertise in their professional contacts. Ward charge nurses and sisters are effectively the managers of their wards. They supervise and co-ordinate the work of perhaps a score of people. Senior nurse managers have to recruit, interview and appoint staff, and they may have to contribute to major service planning and expenditure decisions. Trainee nurses are taught by nurse educators who themselves have to learn how to become effective teachers and how to organize schools of nursing. The word 'nurse' is thus used to describe a group of people initially trained as nurses, possibly additionally trained as health visitors, midwives or tutors, working in a wide range of settings and using a wide range of skills and knowledge. Hence being a 'good' nurse in some settings demands knowledge and skills that are not primarily patient-centred, but which may have considerable psychological relevance.

The aims of this book

A useful psychology of nursing should achieve two goals:

* relate psychology as a discipline to the process of nursing;
* relate psychologists as people to nurses as people.

Much psychological research is not immediately applicable to nursing. Even when it is applicable, its relevance may be obscured by difficulties of terminology, or by the problems in conveying to nurses the essential concepts underlying the research. Some nursing syllabuses try to overcome this difficulty by providing an introduction to basic psychology which includes topics such as perception and motivation. While well-meaning, this type of syllabus leads to teaching of a watered-down academic psychology which has little appeal to nursing students and often little appeal to psychologists or nurse tutors teaching it. On the other hand it is helpful to see how basic psychological concepts are relevant to nursing practice. Crow (1976) has carried out such an examination, looking at the contribution of psychology to the steps of the nursing process outlined earlier in this chapter. She picks out the potential contribution of a knowledge of perception to planning the ward environment; she looks at the literature on motor skills and its relevance to performing everyday activities such as dressing; and she analyses the possible contribution of psychological work on motivation. An opposing approach is to make all teaching theme-related, so that, for example, normal child development is taught in the paediatrics and child care section of a nursing course. A totally theme-related presentation of psychology does not overcome the problem that there is a specifically psychological way of looking at people, and this viewpoint or framework should be understood before the nurse gets into too much detail in any one specific aspect of psychology.

One touchstone of a psychological approach is the degree of reliance upon controlled observation of behaviour. Controlled observation is not the same as experimentation: the latter implies some manipulation of events so that the relationship between sets of events can be more clearly understood. The contribution of a psychological perspective to nursing research has been reviewed by Hayward (1977). He has looked at the value of 'psychological indicators' in nursing research, seeing how psychological measures and methods can highlight those phenomena relevant to nursing knowledge and nursing research. Clinical medicine owes many of its major discoveries not to experimentation, but to careful observation, often of many cases. Each observation requires the existence of some system for classifying events which can then be recorded and analysed.

Psychology has its origins in several other sciences. A number of early psychologists were very interested in physiology and genetics. The Russian physiologist Pavlov conducted the earliest experiments on what is now called classical (or Pavlovian) conditioning. Sir Francis Galton explored a surprisingly large number of psychological topics but is especially known for his books 'Hereditary Genius' (1869) and 'Natural Inheritance' (1889). Hence from its earliest days psychology has been concerned with topics such as brain function, genetics and the relationship between inner or mental events and possible bodily consequences.

Much of psychology is concerned with the behaviour of individuals, but nurses often encounter patients in groups. Nurses will be concerned with groups of patients as they repeat procedures from one patient to another in adjacent beds, or manage a group at one time. Sometimes they will be involved in seeing a patient with relatives or visitors. Ward staff themselves form a group, and issues of collaboration with other staff members, and of possible differences in priorities between different shifts on a ward, can prompt disagreement and discussion between nurses.

Thus the psychology of nursing has to cover the basic concepts of scientific method and observation. It has to cover key concepts in biological aspects of psychology and psychophysiology. It has to cover the psychology of individuals and the psychology of groups. It has to present psychological findings and ideas clearly, and it has immediately to relate them to the nursing process and nursing care.

If psychology is a new subject to nurses, their acceptance of it in their practice will be coloured by the psychologists whom they meet. Increasingly there are psychologists working in fields of health care, such as neurology and general practice, as well as in the more familiar fields of adult psychiatry, child psychiatry and mental handicap. So nurses will have an opportunity to see psychology in practice in the health services and, of course, to learn from what they see.

In increasing numbers nurses are studying psychology to a relatively high level, perhaps for a Diploma in Nursing or for a degree. The assumptions underlying such study need to be carefully examined. Smith and Todd (1978) described the way in which they structured the contribution of social science teaching to a degree course in nursing, after realizing from students' comments that a traditional approach was not sustaining their interest:

> Our approach rested on an unexamined belief that there was only one way in which to introduce the language and perspectives of the social sciences, namely, the way in which they had been introduced to us who were to become practising social scientists.

This article shows the need to think carefully about how to integrate psychological and nursing concepts so that this increased demand for teaching is met appropriately. Similar trends are developing among physiotherapists, occupational therapists and others, so that there is a steady increase in the number of people in health care services who, while perhaps not calling themselves psychologists or considering themselves as such, have a considerable amount of psychological knowledge and skill. This increase in knowledge promises a considerable growth in the application of psychology to nursing, with benefit both for the patient and the profession.

References

Crow, R.A. (1976)
A fresh look at psychology in nursing. Journal of Advanced Nursing, 1, 51-62.

Galton, F. (1869)
Hereditary Genius. London: Macmillan.

Galton, F. (1889)
Natural Inheritance. London: Macmillan.

Hayward, J.C. (1977)
Psychological indicators in nursing research. Journal of Advanced Nursing, 2, 251-259.

Milgram, S. (1964)
Group pressure and action against a person. Journal of Abnormal and Social Psychology, 69, 137-143.

Official Journal of the European Communities (1977)
Legislation 20: L176. London: HMSO.

Smith, G. and Todd, F. (1978)
Inter-relating nursing care and the social sciences: specialist disciplines in an applied course. International Journal of Nursing Studies, 15, 143-151.

2

How do you know? Psychology and scientific method
D. Legge

How do you know?

Of all the lessons that one might learn at school, probably the most important is how to find out. Systematic changes in the school curriculum and in methods of teaching have given pupils today arguably the soundest preparation they have ever had and the best foundation for intellectual independence.

There is a basic dilemma in education: on the one hand there is the plethora of facts unearthed and polished by our predecessors, and on the other is the need to prepare pupils to find out for themselves and to develop sufficient confidence to question academic authority. It would be a denial of the principal benefits of a literate culture to withhold the hard-won knowledge received from earlier generations: we have the advantage of standing on the shoulders of those who have gone before. But too great a dependence on received wisdom could over-emphasize the value of current knowledge, hiding the real possibility that it is wrong, misunderstood or out of its relevant context.

The introduction of discovery learning methods in schools has tended to strike a better balance between these two sources of knowledge than faced earlier generations of pupils. In a previous time 'experiment' was used loosely as a label to refer to a wide variety of practical demonstrations and enquiries. At the worst it was used about practical work that was designed to bring about a particular specified outcome. If that outcome was not achieved the 'experiment' might even be said to have failed. This is a travesty. An experiment cannot fail. It may give rise to unexpected results, it may be poorly designed and the desired experimental conditions may not be achieved, but it cannot fail. In contrast, an attempt to demonstrate a phenomenon can fail. The difference is that the experiment is a special procedure for finding out. It gives rise to knowledge. What the knowledge is about depends upon the design of the experiment.

Discovery learning is a rather slow way of becoming better informed. It would be many thousands of times quicker to learn chemistry from textbooks than by repeating centuries of experimentation and building up the same body of knowledge from one's own painstaking experimentation. Didactic instruction is undoubtedly quicker, but knowledge acquired from an authority may be received as if impressed on tablets of stone. It may be depended upon as if it were inviolable and unquestionably reliable. Few scientists have such a view about the original knowledge that they have personally discovered. Truth is a relative concept and the 'facts' of today may be exploded as myths tomorrow. It is important to be just a little sceptical of received wisdom lest it be elevated to the status of dogma. It is important to find out, and it is important to know how you know.

Making a mental model of the world

Few of our school experiences prepare us for a view of science that identifies a reality outside ourselves which we seek to describe by our scientific theories. That reality is not open to us. We have to build a model of it for ourselves, and that model is our scientific knowledge. In general, the model is simpler than reality, and it has the massive advantage that since we have built the model, we can understand it. Reality is a different order of problem. If the model is a sufficiently good one, it will behave like reality. It will give us a way of understanding reality because we understand our model.

For example, Newton developed his celebrated laws of motion. They describe how bodies move in space as a function of the forces bearing upon them. They are precisely formulated as mathematical equations and offer a basis for predicting the movements of physical bodies. They are not, however, correct under all circumstances. In particular they break down at extremes of velocity and distance. But on an earthly and human scale Newton's model is immensely valuable because it works. The model describes closely enough how certain aspects of the world work.

Acquiring knowledge

How do you know? The simplest way is by deduction from a set of assumptions or premises. Provided the assumptions are true and the logic is sound, knowledge flows unremittingly. This is knowledge that depends upon the existence of a developed model that is relevant to the issue. Sometimes such models relate to only part of the real world and we then extend them beyond their domain of relevance and validity at our peril. Scale models offer some assistance to design engineers but only as analogies. It could be disastrous to assume that the load-bearing characteristics of a model bridge would be reflected in comparable scale in the full-grown version.

Another way of finding out is to ask. Asking another person, or his writings, is a way of seeking human authority. The success of this approach depends upon the question being well phrased so that it is understood; and likewise the answer. It also depends upon the questioner choosing an authority who knows the answer! The main problem with this approach is that a critical evaluation of answers can only be attempted where several authorities can be approached.

Several versions of the same basic authority should not mislead us into believing that such consensus guarantees truth. Reference to an authority does have one cardinal virtue, however, and that is its convenience and speed. No other way of getting answers can be accomplished so quickly.

Empirical enquiries

The best way of finding out about the real world, however, is to ask a question directly of that world rather than of its interpreters. If you have a question about the motion of moving bodies (like billiard balls) the best way of finding an answer is to study the motion of, say, billiard balls. It is more direct and less likely to be distorted than asking a snooker-player his opinion. It may even be better than asking a physicist. This reference of questions to the world to which they refer is the essence of empiricism. It is the foundation upon which all science is based. Science has as its principal aim the description of the world in sufficient detail that at least it will be possible to predict its behaviour.

The physical sciences were the first to break away from natural philosophy as a methodology developed that allowed these empirical questions to be posed. Chemistry and physics were born. Somewhat later biology established itself as well. At the same time it became clear that there were relatively good ways of asking empirical questions that led to unambiguous answers, and there were also less satisfactory ways.

Causal explanations

A prominent feature of the physical sciences was the success of explanations couched in causal terms. The concept was that a particular act or condition would unerringly be followed by another, much as a billiard ball will move predictably (by Newton's Laws more or less!) when struck by another. The causational concept is a very attractive one because it offers a very compact basis for description, but even more so because it provides an obvious basis for prediction. It also identifies strongly the sort of observation that should be made in order to test the prediction, and hence to test that particular model of the world.

Once a phenomenon of some kind has been identified an obvious first question is 'What causes it?' What set of conditions willl guarantee its occurrence? For example, what are the critical factors which determine photosynthesis? It is fairly obvious that one way of getting an answer to this sort of question is to vary conditions and observe what happens. It would quite quickly become clear that one of the main features of an efficient procedure is the unambiguous determination of the relation between the factor being manipulated (the independent variable) and the factor being observed (the dependent variable).

Attributing effects

Perhaps the strongest, and therefore most sought after,

evidence in science is the kind that leads to 'unequivocal attribution of effect': in simpler language, 'we know what caused it'. It establishes that two variables should be considered and connected, perhaps by a causal chain. It may also establish the nature of that connection, perhaps in sufficient detail to admit a mathematical definition of the relationship.

The simplest way of achieving this desirable unequivocal attribution is to demonstrate that introduction of a factor is associated with the appearance of a phenomenon and removal of that factor with its disappearance. If no other factor affects the phenomenon, one would be likely to feel confident in asserting that the factor caused the phenomenon. An investigation in which a factor is carefully manipulated and the effects of such manipulation are carefully monitored is an experiment. The key feature of the experiment is the manipulation of some factor, which must not be left to vary by chance or by association with some other uncontrolled factor. Sometimes the term controlled experiment is used to stress the fact that close control of the conditions of observation is essential. The controlled experiment produces the best evidence there can be, leading to unequivocal attribution of effect.

The importance of the experiment as a method of finding out becomes more obvious when one compares it with other techniques that might be used instead. For example, let us consider the problem of isolating factors that lead to the development of lung cancer. A number of studies of the incidence of lung cancer (and also bronchitis and other chest diseases) revealed that cigarette smokers seemed to be more likely to develop lung cancer than non-smokers. The data were not absolute, of course, so that many smokers died of 'natural causes' without ever developing cancer and some lung cancer victims had never smoked. The next problem is to discover just what this statistical association between smoking and cancer means.

A number of substances are known to be carcinogenic. For example, certain coal tar compounds applied to the skin of mice have been shown to produce tumours. Though in much reduced concentrations, similar compounds are produced in burning tobacco, so the suggestion that tobacco smoke might produce tumours in the respiratory tract is not a far-fetched one. At least some of the intermediate links in a causal chain already exist. On the other hand, the fact that many smokers manage to avoid lung cancer shows that the story is not a very simple one. Smoking is clearly not the only factor and, indeed, it may very well not be the most significant one.

More sophisticated studies have contrasted the morbidity of smokers in rural and urban areas, of different ages and socio-economic groups. There have also been national comparisons. One of the most interesting findings is that smokers who give up the habit have a smaller chance of developing lung cancer than those who do not, though a higher chance than abstainers. This sort of study focusses on smoking and cancer rather than on the general problem of the aetiology of cancer. Decades of studies searching for a single cause have left researchers sceptical of finding such a solution and, instead, the prevailing expectation is that a cluster of factors will together determine the onset of the disease. At most, smoking could be identified as one of those causal factors. Its status might be a major factor, or subsidiary; it might have a primary or a contextual role to play. Either way, if causal, its influence would be relatively direct.

The principal limitation of the studies of associated incidence such as that described above is that one cannot be sure how whatever was observed happened. The effect cannot be unequivocally attributed to particular prior events and conditions. In the case of smoking and cancer the group of smokers differs from the group of non-smokers by more than just the breathing in of tobacco smoke. For instance, they comprise different individuals. This might not be a serious difficulty, provided that the people in one group do not share a common feature other than smoking. Unfortunately, they probably do. Why do the smokers smoke? Is it perhaps because they have some characteristic, no matter whether it be psychological (such as anxiety) or physiological (such as nicotine dependence)? If so, then smokers differ from non-smokers, not only in what they do (that is, smoke) but also in their constitution. Logically we are now incapable of separating two hypotheses about where the association between smoking and cancer comes from. On the one hand is the causal relationship, on the other the possibility that a tendency to smoke is due to some internal characteristic which is also a predetermining factor influencing the development of cancer.

One might argue that this confusion would be removed by observing that smokers who become abstainers have a reduced morbidity. Unfortunately, and this is borne out by the experiences of smokers who attempt to give up, some smokers find it relatively easy to give up, some difficult, and some try but never succeed. This variation between individuals could reflect a variation in the power of the internal factor. A weak factor would allow a smoker to give up easily but would also mean a relatively weak tendency to develop cancer. Studying the morbidity of smokers who become non-smokers voluntarily would tell nothing about the directness of the link between smoking and cancer. Smoking might still be no more than an index of an individual's morbidity.

The only way of settling this question is to gain control of the main variable that has hitherto been left uncontrolled: that is, the question of who smokes. If the experimenter chooses who smokes instead of allowing the subjects to choose, he can effectively separate the act of smoking from the predilection to smoke. In practice this means either forcing non-smokers to smoke and smokers to stop smoking or both. The decision of who is treated in this way has to be unrelated to any other relevant factor and a random decision is usually found to be the best way of achieving this.

Ethical considerations make it unthinkable to carry out this experiment on human beings. Clearly it would be unacceptable to force on people a treatment - smoking - that was thought might very well induce a fatal disease. Forcing people to give up a potentially dangerous habit is less of an ethical problem than a problem of practicability. It is doubtful whether sufficient control over other people's lives can be exerted outside a prison or similar institution. Animals have, however, been subjected to enforced smoking and a sufficient proportion have developed tumours to lend very powerful weight to the hypothesis that tobacco smoking is a primary causative agent in the development of lung cancer. It is not a necessary cause, since non-smokers may also develop cancer. Nor is it a sufficient cause because by no means all smokers will succumb. It is, however, a very significant factor, and a very substantial improvement in health could be achieved if tobacco smoking were to become an extinct behaviour pattern.

When experiments may not be used

The logical preference for using experiments to ask questions is, perhaps, an obvious one. The reasons for not using experiments are less obvious in the abstract, although when one is plunged into the actuality of doing research they become overwhelmingly real. We have mentioned one or two reasons in discussing the cancer example above. There are some things that it is generally agreed one should not do to one's fellow man. There are ethical constraints to our research. This difficulty is an intrinsic feature of social science or medical research, but it very seldom impinges upon research in the physical sciences. In general, we have little compunction about subjecting concrete beams to sufficient forces to destroy them, or stretching wires to the point that they cannot recover their previous form. Inanimate subject matter does not require much, if any, consideration. We see below that there are other advantages, too, that physical scientists enjoy and, perhaps, sometimes take for granted.

In the cancer example we saw how the ethical boundaries which would have prevented an experiment being carried out were circumvented by using animal subjects in place of the ethically unacceptable human ones. This is a partial solution in some instances. The limiting circumstances are, first, that there are ethical reservations about using animals (and there is increasing concern about the extent to which Man exploits sub-human species who have generally no way of lodging their objections) and, second, whether they really possess those essential characteristics which would permit the results of the experiment to be generalized to human beings. Animals may be invaluable in testing new drugs and pharmaceutical preparations that are intended for use with humans. The bulk of animal experiments are toxicity studies on new chemicals. It is reasonable to expect that substances which poison animals will probably poison Man, and vice versa. On the other hand, an experiment concerning feelings will inevitably have to be conducted on human subjects. Even if animals have feelings, they do not have the power to communicate them and this severely limits their usefulness. In consequence, it may be that no experiment could be done at all, in which case the only source of knowledge would be non-experimental.

In practice, surrendering the use of the experiment is seldom the result of ethical constraints. More often it is simply because the control necessary to do an experiment is not available. The resources required may exceed those that can be afforded. In some cases control is lacking on logical grounds. The missing resource may be knowledge rather than cash.

The classic example of resource limitations prohibiting experimentation is in astronomy. Observing the heavens from earth can lead to a plethora of hypotheses about the universe, its contents and how they relate to one another. Theories of planetary motion would be easiest to test if one could carry out experiments by, for example, moving planets about, extracting them from their orbits and so on. Failing the power to do that, astronomers have had to use other means of finding out. A considerable portion of social science research is like astronomy. The researcher lacks the power necessary to manipulate variables to the extent necessary to carry out an experiment.

The third main reason for not carrying out an experiment stems from the conclusions one would want to draw from its results. In order to effect the degree of control necessary to achieve experimental manipulations and make precise, preferably quantifiable, measurements, laboratory conditions are often preferred. In the physical sciences this is nothing but an advantage. It is of no concern to a concrete beam whether it is subjected to forces in a laboratory or in a tower block of flats. It is the forces, its composition and age, the prevailing temperature, humidity and to some extent, its past history that determines its behaviour.

Human subjects play a rather more active role in experiments than do concrete beams and they tend to be very well aware of the difference between the reality of their normal life and the unreality of the 'games' which they are invited to play in laboratories. Even without that awareness of context, it may be that the version of a task which is devised and enacted in the laboratory is critically different from the real-life situation it was designed to simulate. For example, one cannot be absolutely certain that the speed of reaction in a real-life emergency which arrives without warning will be accurately mimicked by a reaction-time experiment conducted in a laboratory where the 'unexpectedness' of the emergency is at best relative. The problem is to determine the 'ecological validity' of the simulation. It is really the old problem of what degree of generalization is permissible from the observations that have been made. Essentially the same questions have to be asked about the concrete beam. Its characteristics in a warm, dry laboratory might be radically different at the bottom of the North Sea. But it is generally true that there is more likely to be limited generalization in the social sciences.

This problem has led many researchers to maximize the reality value of their research situations and to minimize the use of laboratory-based research. They feel that the potentially misleading quality of laboratory research is so serious a problem that they prefer to make their observations in more realistic circumstances, accepting the severe restrictions placed on the manipulation and control of experimental variables. It is a dilemma. Should one conduct relatively well-controlled experiments (which allow quite precise attribution of experimental effects) but which have limited relevance to natural behaviour, or use real-life (ecologically valid) situations which frequently leave considerable uncertainty about what induced whatever was observed? There is likely to be room for both kinds of research, and there are probably persisting differences in preference between researchers. This underlines the importance of discovering the strengths and weaknesses of the non-experimental and quasi-experimental methods that have been devised as alternatives to experiments.

Alternatives to experimentation

One of the great advantages in doing experiments is that the conditions under which the observations are made are very carefully designed to provide information about particular questions. In other circumstances one has to make the most of whatever information is available. Returning for a moment to the example of astronomy, the researcher has available to him only the options of looking in different directions at different times. His difficulty is to relate the information he gathers to his developing model of the universe. In these circumstances, since there is no way of knowing what particular aspects of what could be recorded might be relevant at some time and from some particular perspective, there is considerable pressure to record observations in as objective a way as possible. There is also a premium on precise description.

Non-experimental studies are usually either descriptive or correlational. In the former an attempt is made to record what is or what happens, without (necessarily) giving reasons or accounts of what causes what. Studies of this kind are potentially of immense value since they can define the general arena in which detailed accounts of what leads to what must be placed. They are also useful in relating the development of theoretical models to the reality of a life-situation. They are, however, very difficult to do because of the virtually infinite variety of things that could be relevant to record, so that even the most objective recorder would find it necessary to make some selection. The appropriateness of that selection is what makes the results of such a study valuable or worthless.

Correlational studies come in various forms, varying as to the restrictiveness of the set of variables that can be intercorrelated after the data have been collected. In essence, correlation is a statistical technique which measures the closeness of an association between two or more variables. Associations may vary from perfect correlation in which any change in one variable is reflected by a change in the other, to a much looser relationship marked by a mere tendency for changes in the two variables to go together. Correlational studies may involve selecting what to observe, and that is certainly the case when specialized instruments are used to make the observations (mental tests, for example), but they do not intervene in ways that are necessary in an experiment which depends upon manipulating and controlling variables, as well as accurate observation and recording. Studies of this kind can reveal what variables tend to change together, but they cannot reveal why. As we saw above, statistical studies of the incidence of lung cancer and smoking reveal that the disease is significantly correlated with the behaviour. They cannot lead to the inescapable conclusion that the one causes the other. If two variables are causally related there must be a correlation between them, but the reverse is not true.

One-subject studies

A particularly difficult set of problems surrounds asking questions about a particular individual. For example, if a young man visits a hypnotist before taking a driving test and subseqently passes it, what can be said about the effect of the hypnotist's treatment on his success? The answer is very little, with confidence. Clearly the hypnotist may have helped: there are several reports available of people believing that their test anxiety was reduced in this way. But our particular young man may not be exactly the same as other people so grouping him together with them may not be appropriate. One basic difficulty is that we cannot set up a control. We cannot discover how our examinee would have fared without hypnotism. Once he has taken the test and passed it, no fair comparison could be made by subsequently testing him again without a visit to his hypnotist. Though in some studies it makes sense to use a subject as his own control, in many others it does not. The subject is likely to be affected to a significant extent by one experience, so that he is not going to behave in a comparable manner if that experience is repeated. From the research point of view this raises almost insurmountable problems. There is no way in which one can achieve an unequivocal picture of what causes a particular individual to behave in a particular way, without either assuming that his behaviour patterns will be very similar to those of other people, or that he will be unaffected by his experience. Neither assumption will ever be wholly true, and the advances that can be made in understanding him will depend upon how true these assumptions are for particular aspects of his behaviour.

On theories and data

One of the reasons why it is important to be careful about collecting data in attempting to find out why something happens is that of the difficulty in spotting when an answer is a true one.

Many people have been taught that one of the most important aspects of science is that its theories are disciplined by data. They are kept in touch with the real world they seek to describe. If the theory says one thing and the data say something else, then the theory must change to accommodate the data.

Two schemes of investigation have been described as representing two distinct ideals. Inductive research involves making unselected observations of phenomena followed by ordering and categorizing them, from which a theoretical structure may emerge. Linnaeus' development of a taxonomy of plants is often held up as an example of inductive research. The alternative scheme is hypothetico-deductive research which progresses by a series of two-phase investigations. The first step involves establishing an hypothesis. Following that, a prediction is derived which can be tested directly against data collected for the purpose.

It is most unlikely that either of these schemes is actually used in its pure form. It is inconceivable that Linnaeus never developed any ideas about relevant dimensions of his taxonomy until all the observations had been made, and that his later observations were uninfluenced by his earlier ones. Likewise, the hypothetico-deductive method cannot be used unless there is a pre-existing theory, which is likely to have benefitted at some stage from random, if not comprehensive, unselected observations of phenomena under investigation.

This contrast focusses on the relative roles of theory and data. Ideally theory suggests relevant observations. Data indicate how satisfactory existing theories are and may point to how they should be modified to become more satisfactory. Having got an enquiry off the ground, progress ought to be orderly. In fact it very seldom is. The most basic problem is that human nature seems to abhor a theoretical vacuum. Almost any theory is better than none at all. Perhaps this explains why magical explanations are preferred to a simple state of ignorance. It is almost as if man needs to have the sense of power that 'knowing how it works' confers. Whatever the reason, however, an embarrassing piece of data is unlikely to result in the only available theory being jettisoned. If there are two or more competing theories, however, data appear to be more powerful and the relative credibility of different theories may very well be adjusted accordingly.

The unexpected weakness of data is not completely accounted for by the need to maintain at least one theory. No theory is likely to survive when faced with strong data that are incompatible with it. The problem is that many data are just not that strong. There is residual doubt about just what the observations from a particular study really mean for that particular theory.

This undesirable state of affairs can arise most easily if the theory has been only poorly defined and, especially, if the rules of correspondence between the elements of the theory and observable aspects of the real world have been omitted or only ambiguously specified. But even when the rules of correspondence are clear, the status of data can be diminished if the data collection scheme has been a rather haphazard one, and particularly if the attribution of any effects observed remains equivocal. A fair conclusion is that a poorly defined theory that seems to explain phenomena which otherwise defy explanation, and an area of enquiry that precludes, or makes very difficult, experimental research, has a very good chance of surviving for a long time irrespective of its actual validity.

Progress without experiment

Much of the foregoing might seem to be pointing in a rather unpromising direction. In order to establish unambiguously that a particular variable reliably produces a particular effect, the experiment is not only the best available research design, it is also irreplaceable. As the advertisements used to say, 'accept no imitations'. However, it would be wrong to conclude that experiments are inevitably effective, as our brief consideration of the relationship between theory and data reveals.

Research is basically a slow business in which researchers inch towards some better appreciation of the world they study. They develop their models, making them increasingly sophisticated as they make progress. The barriers to progress are many and varied including their own mental limitations and the pressures upon them from the prevailing intellectual atmosphere. Experiments can be done which shed no light at all on the question at issue. Many experiments promise more than they deliver once the post mortem has been completed. In this climate of imperfection the fact that experiment may be precluded is disappointing but not, relatively speaking, a disaster.

The development of models of the world is not as neat and tidy a process as, perhaps, we should wish. The prevailing model is the one that seems best able to cope with all that is known (or, better, all that we believe) to be true about the phenomenon we seek to understand. Provided that enough different snapshots from different vantage points can be correlated it is quite possible that ultimately the same model will arise as would have come from direct experimentation. It will almost certainly take longer, but the same end-point may well be reached. This optimism is supported by the progress made in astronomy where experimentation is virtually prohibited. Since the system under investigation is in motion, successive observations provided different but complementary information. As a result Man has managed to navigate unmanned space ships to the outer parts of the solar system and successfully explore the moon.

In many areas of social science, experimentation is either very difficult or unlikely to provide what is needed. In such circumstances correlational studies and descriptive studies of one kind or another are the only sources of information available. Perhaps this will mean slow progress, but there is little doubt that our curiosity about ourselves will be a sufficient motive for the questions to be pressed, and eventually useful answers will emerge. It matters not at all that they should emerge untidily, only that they turn out to be effective aids to our understanding.

Research and common sense

Doing research is essentially detective work, but often with an all-important difference. Police detectives cannot ask questions in the same way that the experimental scientist can. Instead they have to hope that the (probably incomplete) set of data which they collect will distinguish between the competing theories they hold about the crime under investigation. Some science is also like that, and social science especially. Maybe scientists have one major advantage in that their antagonist is nature, which may not be co-operative but is most unlikely deliberately to confuse and deceive.

Just as police detective work has a list of dos and don'ts to guide it into a successful path, so there are good and bad ways of doing science. Most of this chapter is about using common sense in finding out. There are no magical methods and the main thing to remember is to avoid ambiguity. Before starting an investigation, be absolutely clear about what the question is. It will only get more confused later if it is not clear at the start. The study itself needs to yield data that can be interpreted. Ideally, any effect observed should be unequivocally attributable to a particular variable or set or variables. Whatever scheme seems likely to achieve these goals will be worth using. A scheme that will not may well not be worth the effort of putting into practice.

Unfortunately, while much of the physical sciences allow these guidelines to be followed closely, the social sciences are more difficult to tame. Unequivocal attribution is difficult to ensure, and easiest when dealing with laboratory behaviour: a version of behaviour which may not be identical with that in real life. Often compromise is necessary, and progress is painfully slow.

Statistics

There are relatively few special tools available to the researcher corresponding to the finger-print kit of the detective. One of the principal ones, however, is statistics, a branch of mathematics concerned with the determination of the likelihood of events occurring. It is a particularly useful tool in those areas of study which are not very clearly determinate. It was originally developed to help analyse various questions in agriculture which are made difficult by the fact that plant growth is affected by a vast number of factors, some intrinsic to the plant, some extrinsic. This situation is not unlike that in human behaviour and it is no surprise that psychologists have taken up statistics enthusiastically and developed specialized procedures for their own use.

The main advantages that statistics confer are schemes for summarizing data and making them easier to remember and communicate, schemes for measuring the relatedness of two or more variables (correlation) and schemes for aiding decision making. They are important for deciding whether any effects have been netted in the data, and that is a precondition for determining what caused them. In conjunction with experiments, statistics make it possible to face psychological research with some confidence. However, the techniques, though not particularly difficulty to use, are specialist and study in some depth is recommended before trying to use them. It is best to practise under the guidance of an expert first, before launching oneself into research.

Further study

It has only been possible to mention a few basic ideas in this brief introduction to psychological discovery. The interested reader will, we hope, feel an urge to plunge deeper into the jungle. There are an ever-increasing number of texts to guide the way. The next stage in that journey may be aided by three slim volumes out of the Essential Psychology series published by Methuen. They are:

Gardiner, J.M. and Kaminska, K. (1975)
First Experiments in Psychology. London: Methuen.
Legge, D. (1975)
An Introduction to Psychological Science. London: Methuen.
Miller, S.H. (1976)
Experimental Design and Statistics. London: Methuen.

3

Biological bases of behaviour
Irene Martin

Effective human survival on this earth is achieved by adaptive behaviour, made possible by the evolution of a brain and nervous system which bear the imprint of solutions to survival over millions of evolutionary years. For man, some large part of his knowledge has been acquired during his lifetime, but for him as for all living creatures there are innate programmes which regulate many functions. Whatever we do, my writing, your reading, our sitting, breathing and wakefulness involve countless electrical and chemical events within us, most quite beyond conscious awareness.

A biological approach focusses on the adaptiveness of behaviour in relation to events in the environment, on the role of brain functions in behaviour, and on psychophysiological aspects of emotionality, arousal, motivation and mechanisms of coping with stress. It is concerned with individual differences, since there are marked variations between individuals in memory, learning, intelligence, and in the general ability to cope with life events, and these are attributable in part to genetic and physiological mechanisms. The question of maladaptive behaviour is relevant and is considered in such contexts as excessive anxiety, stress and psychosomatic reactions. Finally, modes of investigation are described in which psychological and physiological principles interact.

The first task is to determine which kinds and classes of behaviour interest us, what their importance is, and what theories can account for them.

What is behaviour?

To begin with human behaviour at its most accessible level we can watch the individual in action, speaking, socializing, playing games, and going to work: that is, performing the usual range of human activities and interactions with the world around. Suppose we begin like modern ethologists - those who study the behaviour of animals in natural settings - and extend the study to man so that we become man-watchers. Suppose, further, that just like the study of animals we cannot ask the people we are watching why they do certain things or what they are feeling; we simply observe. We would see how people greet one another, dress, flirt, fight and demonstrate. It might be useful to use some classification such as 'parental behaviour', 'work behaviour', 'social behaviour' or 'illness behaviour'.

But 'parental behaviour' is very broad. It includes reproduction, home-making, maternal/paternal roles, feeding, education and development of the young. For purposes of analysis it needs to be broken down, and when this is done we quickly arrive at hundreds of small 'units' of behaviour: feeding the baby, cuddling and contact, organizing a daily schedule, and so on. If we ask one simple question such as how does a baby's perception of the mother's face develop, we need to take careful measurements in a laboratory-type setting, comparing and measuring reactions to 'mother's face' with reactions to other faces and objects in the environment. In this way psychologists are led from the straightforward observation of the stream of life to much more detailed aspects of activities and behaviour, and the breaking down of what is observed into manageable segments is essential for understanding and measurement, as all sciences have recognized.

Rapid advances in a science often follow the identification of a meaningful and measurable 'unit': for example, the cell in physiology, the neurone in neurophysiology, the gene in genetics. It may be that psychology has not yet found the most appropriate 'unit' for describing behaviour, and at present it deals with both narrow (e.g. reflexes) and broad (e.g. 'play') types of responses. Once a meaningful and measurable unit of behaviour has been identified, ways of measuring and interpreting it must be developed. The analysis of behaviour therefore requires the development of appropriate units, measurement (which typically involves norms and variation), the abstraction of certain concepts, and theories which try to explain and predict behaviour.

Evolution

A biological approach emphasizes the role of the brain. It is possible for evolutionary development to follow many routes, each of which offers a specific adaptive advantage. Some animals survive better in their environments because of their strength, speed or camouflage. The story of man's evolutionary development centres on the brain and nervous system, in conjunction with developing manual dexterity. Lowly organisms do not possess a recognizable brain, but gradually it develops to become the complex structure we know.

Certain consequences follow from this evolutionary approach. One is to view man's behaviour as continuous with that of other animals so that explanations of motivation, emotion and learning can be applied across species. Another is to examine the inheritance of response patterns which are built into the nervous system as part of its inherited structure, and to consider the role of genetics in behaviour. These, however, are controversial issues. Some writers maintain that intelligence (and personality and illness) are inherited, others that they result from environmental influences; some that man's emotionality is

powered by physiological urges, and others that it arises
from the way life events are perceived and interpreted. It
has also been proposed that human social organizations
represent a new stage of evolution, a viewpoint which has
been vigorously attacked by those who object to the 'bio-
logizing' of human society because of ethical and political
implications.

It is useful for a biologically-based psychology to make
assumptions about the working organization of the brain, and
a typical classification refers to: (i) an input sensory
system which provides information about the world through
eyes, ears, touch, taste, smell; (ii) a central processing
unit which stores, codes and interprets the input; and (iii)
an output muscular system through which we move and act in
the world. It is also a useful assumption that an organism
cannot survive unless it has an innate mechanism that tells
it when it is favourably correlated with its environment.
This carries the implication that there must be some form of
subjective awareness of welfare and comfort, including the
machinery for not liking to be uncomfortable.

welfare system

Detection of the positive and negative in the world is an
innate feature of all forms of life. A plant turns towards
the sun and light; it absorbs water and minerals as
required. For animals, positive or negative evaluations are
accompanied by a pattern of physiological changes organized
towards approach or withdrawal. Most animals move towards
those events which are good and promote welfare, and move
away from those which are dangerous and destructive of
life.

These positive and negative evaluations and perceptions
of beneficial and harmful factors can be generalized to
other environmental events through processes of conditioning, and in this way many likes and dislikes can be
acquired. Experiments with humans have shown that if neutral
stimuli are paired closely in time with a pleasant event
such as a good lunch or with unpleasant putrid odours, the
neutral stimuli will subsequently be rated as more pleasant
or more unpleasant.

It is a common experience that tastes which were once
pleasant become disagreeable or even revolting when they
have been associated with discomfort or nausea. In this way
new evaluations allow the anticipation of favourable or
unfavourable events, thus diminishing harmful effects and
enabling the organism to ensure a better adjustment to its
environment.

concepts of behaviour

There are a number of concepts which link the study of
behaviour and the brain and these include arousal, emotion,
motivation, learning and memory. One of the most striking
and easily observable features of human activity is the
shift along a dimension of arousal, from deep sleep to
intense wakefulness. Another is the episodic occurrence of

emotion, especially love, fear and anger; and, of course, those motivated states relating to hunger, thirst and sex.

Arousal

Humans, in line with many animals, show phases of sleep, wakefulness and high energy output. At high levels of arousal, many cognitive functions such as speed of reaction, memorizing, learning, etc., improve. The spur of high arousal when writing examination papers must be a common experience; extreme agitation, on the other hand, can exert an unpleasant handicapping effect. It seems that up to a certain optimal point arousal acts as a spur to do well, but when it becomes too intense and spills over into anxiety behaviour is disorganized and people are unable to perform efficiently. Although the concept of general arousal was initially described from observation of behaviour, its status has been made more plausible by the discovery of a structure within the brain, the reticular formation, which seems to serve as a general arousal system for the cortex.

Emotion

Many observations indicate that emotionality is related to the activity of the autonomic nervous system, and internal bodily upheaval is one of the surest signs we have that we are emotionally disturbed. This physiological disturbance is believed to have a biological utility in the preparation for action. Under emotional arousal the heart beats faster, hormones are released, and blood is diverted to the brain and skeletal muscles to mobilize the body for prompt and efficient fight or flight.

Action in the jungle often means escape from predators. Man is a highly socialized and domesticated animal, whose emotionality is more likely to be triggered by social factors such as evaluation by other people, threat of failure, meeting strangers and so on. In adult humans, social interactions at work and in the family, and the means of smoothing social relationships, assume great importance.

In all these situations extensive psychophysiological changes occur, although largely below conscious awareness. Many people do not judge their internal states very precisely, even with physiological events which might seem obvious, like an increased heart rate or high level of muscle tension. The evidence suggests rather that perception of bodily activity and actual bodily activity are not very highly related.

The significance of concepts of arousal and motivation lies not only in their linkage with the brain and nervous system but also in relation to stress, health and well-being. Man no longer lives in a jungle, but the 'emergency' services he has inherited still act as though he did; the signs of danger are not from predators but become conditioned to stimuli, events and people in the course of everyday interaction with the environment. These events can trigger excessive physiological arousal which may be felt as psychological states like anxiety and judged to be highly unpleasant.

Motivation

One popular conception of motivation is that of 'drives' which energize behaviour in specific directions: that is, towards food, water and sexual partners and away from pain and punishment. Animals deprived of fundamental biological needs become restless and active, cross obstructions and learn different responses in order to achieve their goals. It is therefore implied in many theories of motivation that organisms act mainly to reduce basic drives, and that many forms of responding are learned because the reduction of drives (by eating, drinking, etc.) is rewarding.

In a general biological sense both motivation and emotion can be viewed as a complex integration of behaviour involving selective attention to certain events, a heightened physiological state of excitement, and certain probable patterns of action. These patterns of action are common to most higher species of animals and have a clear biological utility in coping with the environment and with survival. However, it has always seemed evident that biological theories of motivation are thinly stretched when it comes to human experience. Various social needs relating to achievement, power, affiliation, etc., have been postulated which do not readily fit into existing drive theories, and to date no single satisfactory theory of motivation has been formulated in human psychology.

Conditioning

We learn to do certain things and learn not to do others. Of the skills we learn, some of the most dramatic involve muscular co-ordination, as in tennis, skating or swimming. Another set involves mental skills, such as extensive memorizing and the development of concepts about the world. There is another category of responses - evaluations, perceptions, feelings and emotions, many of which occur outside normal conscious awareness - which are believed to be learned through the process of conditioning.

The process of conditioning relates to the pairing of a 'neutral' with a 'significant' stimulus. Most people are familiar with the outline of Pavlov's conditioning methods with dogs in which a quiet tone (neutral conditioned stimulus, CS) is followed by food (a significant unconditioned stimulus, UCS). Pavlov recorded the salivation which occurred as a natural response (unconditioned response, UCR) to the food, and demonstrated that the salivary response gradually comes to be given to the tone CS. Though the outline may be familiar, however, the connection between salivating dogs and human behaviour, personality and illness is not self-evident.

Suppose we replace the terms CS and UCS with life events and the CR and UCR with widespread physiological responses related to emotionality and pain. The implications become clearer. If one has ever been in a car crash, the general constellation of events - sounds, place, people, shouting - act as a significant and traumatic UCS, arousing great fear and widespread bodily reactions (UCRs). Return, even many years later, to the place where the accident occurred and the once neutral cues of the road and surrounding terrain will probably re-evoke the previous sensations and emotions (as CRs) quite powerfully. The significant aspects of conditioning are that two events have become associated in such a way that feelings and bodily reactions can be activated by certain stimuli, once of themselves 'neutral' but having preceded important events, and thus coming to exert strong and lasting effects on our feelings and reactions.

The development of conditioned fears has obvious biological utility in preparing for and avoiding dangerous situations which might lead to pain and death. However, many human fears become attached to a variety of relatively harmless objects such as birds and insects, high places, and aeroplanes, having injections, walking in the streets; that is to say, situations in which it is inappropriate to have anything more than a mild anxiety response. Certain individuals seem to acquire conditioned phobias and fears very rapidly, but they can sometimes be effectively treated using a variety of 'deconditioning' techniques.

Problems with concepts in psychology

Terms like arousal, emotion and conditioning have been derived from the analysis of behaviour and are related to underlying physiological mechanisms. There are several difficulties with these concepts. In the first place, psychologists are divided as to whether (i) they want to relate psychological concepts to physiology and the brain, and (ii) even if they want to whether this is always a feasible thing to do. Could we not obtain information which is just as (or more) useful by asking individuals how they feel or see a particular event? After all, most clinicians have to rely on the patient's answers to such questions as 'How do you feel?' or 'Where is the pain?'

Information provided solely by a person's self-report unfortunately has its limitations. Quite simply, what people say of their behaviour and what they actually do are often not very highly related. We have a surprisingly limited conscious access to our own feelings and motivations, and asking how a person feels may not provide an adequate answer for various reasons. An important one relates to the use of words such as anger, anxiety, pain and depression: there is no way we can be sure that your use of words to describe subjective experience is the same as mine. A major difficulty with many psychological terms is that of definition, and a much-valued aim is the use of terms with minimal ambiguity: that is, to make the language of psychology more precise.

Individual differences

There are many ways of considering variations in human

behaviour. Not all of them relate to the brain and nervous system, but in this section we concentrate on those theories which relate personality to arousal and emotion systems of the brain.

Eysenck, for example, postulates that individuals range along a continuum of arousal, extraverts having a chronically lower level of cortical arousal than introverts, who have a relatively high level. Because of this, introverts have a reduced need for external stimulation to attain their optimal levels of arousal. Thus a high level of internal arousal accounts for the introvert's relative aversion to stimulating activities, exciting events and social contacts. By contrast, the extravert's low level of internal arousal leads to a search for external stimuli - noise, excitement, new experiences and many social contacts - in order to achieve an optimum level of arousal. If prevented from seeking these kinds of varied stimuli the extravert may become bored and readily distractable.

Eysenck's scheme also includes the dimension of neuroticism. This has been related to excessive activity of the autonomic nervous system; people who are high on the neuroticism dimension are described as having strong and labile emotions, while those at the other end experience less strong and more stable emotions. Taken together, the two dimensions of extraversion-introversion and neuroticism form four quadrants: those people who are both introverted and unstable tend to be moody, anxious, reserved, unsociable; those both introverted and stable tend to be calm, even-tempered, careful and thoughtful. People who are both extraverted and unstable tend to be touchy, restless, aggressive, excitable and impulsive; those who are both extraverted and stable are lively, easy-going, outgoing, carefree people. Further descriptions refer to the introvert as reacting to low levels of sensory stimuli, and as being sensitive and reactive to frustration.

Other personality scales measure such traits as impulsiveness (e.g. the tendency to act on the spur of the moment without planning), and sensation-seeking, which refers to unusual activities such as sky-diving, speed-racing, taking drugs, etc. Attempts have been made by many investigators to relate personality measures derived from such questionnaires to general autonomic reactivity, cortical excitability, adrenalin/noradrenaline output, and, more recently, to a number of biochemical variables.

Intelligence is another source of variation between individuals which is believed to have a biological/genetic basis. Conventional tests of intelligence (IQ) usually measure cognitive tasks similar to those involved in scholastic examinations, and might give disadvantageous results for members of minority groups from different cultural and educational backgrounds. This has stimulated a search for alternatives to the usual IQ test and in recent years measurements of small electrical changes obtained from surface scalp electrodes have been made as indices of 'neural efficiency', the hypothesis being that when a stimulus occurs, neurones which are fast and efficient generate characteristic waves of evoked potential.

Several studies have reported correlations between these measures and intelligence, but it is too early to say whether this approach will have any practical value in the intelligence issue.

Environmental stressors

Conditions on which life and health depend are found both within and without the living organism. Inside there is the whole complex machinery which regulates the internal 'environment'; that is, the circulating organic liquid which surrounds and bathes all of the body tissues. Outside are all the changing features of the environment which require powers of adaptation and learning to cope with change.

Most animals are innately equipped to deal with the specific changes of importance they are likely to encounter; most, too, learn to react more efficiently as a result of experience. One important mechanism, for example, is that of habituation; learning not to respond when a response is no longer necessary. Thus animals once alarmed by the irregular rattle of passing trains soon learn that they can safely graze in adjacent fields without generating endless fear responses.

There are several theories of stress which involve the concept of individuals being driven beyond their powers of coping or adaptation, such that equilibrium is not easily restored.

The psychobiological use of the term 'stress' has its origins in the work of Selye in Canada, who sees stress as the state of the organism following failure of the normal mechanisms of adaptation. If stressor agents (Selye's work was mainly with rats and involved such stressors as intense heat, cold, virus infections, intoxicants, haemorrhage, muscular exercise, drugs, injury and surgical trauma) are applied intensely or long enough, they produce certain general systemic changes which represent the animal's attempt to cope with the situation. These common changes constitute the response pattern of systemic stress. They include autonomic excitability, adrenalin discharge, and such symptoms as an increased heart rate, decreased body temperature and muscle tone, blood sugar changes and gastrointestinal ulcerations. These changes occur in an initial reaction to the stressor agent, which Selye labelled the alarm reaction. If noxious stimulation continues but is not too severe, a second phase occurs, which he labelled the stage of resistance, and in which the adaptive powers of the body act to counteract the stressor. If noxious stimulation persists, this stage gives way to the final stage of exhaustion, which may ultimately lead to death.

It is important to know whether psychological stimuli can also induce a systemic stress syndrome, with similar physiological response patterns occurring in similar stages. Men in stressful situations such as paratroopers,

submariners, pilots and combat infantrymen, have demonstrated that life-threat and social-status-threat situations
can induce symptoms of systemic stress, the degree of stress
depending on the type, intensity and duration of the threat
and on certain pre-stress sensitizing factors such as personality and previous conditioning experiences. However, the
attempt to extend Selye's idea of general systemic stress to
include psychological aspects has met with many problems.
Psychological stress factors are less easy to define,
measurements of the physiological changes are less easy to
make and there are obvious ethical limitations on laboratory
research with human volunteers.

Certain issues in psychological stress are amenable to
laboratory-type investigations with both human and animal
subjects, and one theme relates to general 'coping behaviour', particularly with reference to the control which an
individual feels he has over frustrating situations. These
studies indicate that stress reactions to unavoidable and
uncontrollable aversive stimuli are much more severe than
those resulting from exposure to situations over which the
individual can develop control. It seems to be not only the
exposure to, say, painful and unpleasant stimuli which leads
to distress, but the knowledge of not being 'in control' of
them which leads to feelings of helplessness in susceptible
individuals. Contemporary life provides many frustrating
situations over which we have little or no control, for
example, bureaucratic decisions, cancellation of scheduled
trains, being treated rudely when no retaliation is possible, traffic disruptions, and so on: situations in which
there may be few successful methods of coping. One speculation is that persistent exposure to such conditions can
generate feelings of hopelessness and helplessness, which
may contribute towards lack of motivation and possibly even
to depression.

Relations between physiology and behaviour

A fundamental assumption is that the unique character of
human beings, their ability to think, feel, learn and
remember, lies in the brain and in the pattern and chemistry
of inter-connections between neurones. Exactly how information is received about the world, how it is processed,
interpreted, learned and stored are questions being pursued
with an enormous range of sophisticated techniques.

Brain research
Under this heading come those studies which use brain imp-
lantation techniques, that is, the placing of electrical or
chemical stimulation devices in the brain, and these have
provided many illustrations of how brain stimulation affects
motivational and emotional behaviour. In some experiments,
animals have been provided with a lever which triggers
electrical stimulation of their own brains and when electrodes are placed in parts of the limbic system (a phylo-
genetically old part of the brain, the functions of which

are obscure but believed to relate to emotionality) these animals press the lever almost continuously, as if there were something very positive about this experience. This work often refers to the 'pleasure' areas of the brain.

Dramatic effects have also been produced through destroying localized regions of the brain: wild, unmanageable animals have been transformed into gentle creatures that could be fed by hand, while other procedures have produced a state of violent rage even in very tame laboratory rats.

As a result of the development of surgical techniques and the powerful effects of brain intervention observed on behaviour, it has been thought that brain surgery might alleviate severe and intractable behaviour problems such as hyperexcitability and violent, destructive and uncontrollably aggressive behaviour, and some exploratory attempts have been made in this direction. It is not easy to evaluate the results of these operations: on the whole, there is always a cost-benefit factor in neurosurgery. No miraculous recovery is ever accomplished with the kinds of very severe behavioural problems which have been referred, and although relief from disabling symptoms may be obtained, there is always the chance that it will create other difficulties.

There are also ethical problems associated with brain surgery. Some people have argued that violent prisoners, for example, should be treated by surgical means rather than spend a lifetime in prison. Others feel that because the brain is the reservoir of creativity and individuality it should never be disturbed unless it is clearly diseased or injured.

Many brain-behaviour studies arise from accidental brain lesions, following which a variety of disorders have been noted in speech, motor behaviour, memory and perception. These vary in extent and quality as a function of the nature and place of injury, and detailed mapping of the disability will hopefully lead to a better understanding of how speech, memory, etc., are organized within the brain. Assessment of this type of deficit can be assisted by the use of appropriate psychological tests; in the case of emotional deficits, however, no tests are available and assessment is more difficult. As a result, much less is known about the effects of brain and central nervous system damage on normal human feelings. Reports on the emotional life of those suffering from accidental spinal lesions suggest a reduction in the intensity of feeling, and an awareness of a more 'mental' kind of emotional response than of a powerful physiological drive.

Recent work has highlighted the psychological importance of brain chemistry, which seems to be involved in processes such as attention and sensitivity to pain, mood and emotionality. One theory, for example, is that certain chemicals in the brain determine mood shifts as seen in mania and depression, from which it might follow that corrections for chemical imbalance could be achieved by drug administration.

There are, however, many complications when human beings are involved in treatment of this kind, for as well as direct pharmacological effects, psychological factors such as expectancies of both the therapist and patient, and aspects of the therapeutic setting, also play a part. A related observation is that some patients claim satisfactory pain relief from placebos (i.e. completely inactive, 'dummy' tablets) for many kinds of symptoms, and attempts have been made, so far without clear resolution, to identify who these people are and what the mechanism is by which the effect is produced.

Physiological psychology

Topics frequently studied under this heading include motivation, memory and learning, and this kind of research usually involves animal subjects. A traditional method of study is to lesion specific regions of the brain to examine the effect on behaviour. Another approach is to correlate electrical events within the brain with the course of learning and performance.

A major unresolved question is whether there is a single anatomical site or physiological process responsible for memory, learning, and motivated behaviour. Several theories concentrate on the synaptic connections between the neurones of the brain, long thought to relate to learning and memory. In recent years there has been an interest in the role of the hippocampus in learning and the storage of short-term memories. This is a structure tucked within the very old part of the cerebral cortex. In humans, bilateral lesions associated with this area have been shown to cause a severe and lasting memory deficit characterized by the inability to learn new information. Patients with such lesions appear to have undiminished powers of perception but they are largely incapable of incorporating new information into their long-term store.

A topic of profound importance is how we register and record the events of the world about us. Research in the past decade has revealed the existence of cells within the brain which appear to react quite specifically to different aspects of a sensory stimulus. They have been termed 'feature detectors' in that some cells will fire at the onset of a stimulus, others to its colour, others again to its duration, intensity and localization in space. Some neurones are specially tuned to respond to complex stimuli, to time characteristics and to novelty. Thus incoming stimuli leave traces of their characteristics within the nervous system. These traces or 'neuronal models' preserve information about the intensity, quality, duration, etc., of past stimuli and it is against these stored models that new events are compared. Several theorists have proposed that there is an analysing mechanism within the brain which assesses the novelty and significance of incoming events in such terms as: is this event new or has it happened before? Is it significant or irrelevant? It then activates the appropriate response or damps down responding (as in habituation) if the event has occurred many times before and is unimportant. In this way we build up an internal picture of the external world, and act on that information.

The brain appears to have two halves (hemispheres) which were once assumed to be similar in function, as are the two kidneys and two lungs. Actually, there are some specialized functions which are found only in one or other of the two sides. The best example is that of language: damage to a particular region of the cortex on the left side of the brain leads to aphasia; damage to the corresponding area on the right side leaves the faculty of speech intact. This asymmetry is also reflected in memory defects arising from damage to the temporal region of the brain. Injury to the left side can impair the ability to retain verbal material but leave intact the ability to remember spatial locations, faces, melodies and abstract visual patterns.

One of the most interesting recent findings is that different emotional reactions follow damage to the right and left sides of the brain. Comprehension of the affective components of speech is impaired with right but not with left lesions, and the comprehension of humorous material is different in patients with left and right hemisphere lesions. While this specialization of the hemispheres should not be over-exaggerated, it does suggest a unique kind of specialization within the human brain.

Psychosomatic medicine

One of the most striking features of psychosomatic illness is the marked individual difference in susceptibility to illness, and in the patterning of symptoms. Why one patient should develop gastric ulcers while another develops high blood pressure is a question that has often been asked and not yet satisfactorily answered.

There is reasonably general agreement that prolonged emotional disturbance associated with deleterious physiological effects can arise from conflict, stress and certain life changes and that these may lead to tissue change and organic disease.

There have been many theories concerning the psychophysiological specificity, or patterning of response, which is a feature of psychosomatic disorders. One possibility is a genetic component which determines the organ system involved, another that this combines with a learning process such as classical conditioning. Conditioned visceral responses can occur to all sorts of stimuli and can be remarkably persistent over time. They are of particular interest in that while visceral organs have cortical representation, the activity of visceral organs is not easily discriminated and is generally below normal conscious awareness. This suggests that an individual might become conditioned to respond to inappropriate internal or external stimuli over long periods of time during which he would have no knowledge of the progressive disturbance of function.

As just mentioned, it is believed that the recent occurrence of conflict, emotional upheaval or environmental stress is implicated in the precipitation of symptoms. Several researchers have attempted to assess the recent changes in individuals' lives prior to illness onset, and an association between them has been repeatedly documented. However, even the highest of these correlations is relatively modest, suggesting that recent life changes alone do not exert a strong primary effect on illness onset. What effect they do exert seems to be influenced by the way in which an individual perceives them, as well as by the individual's coping capabilities and illness behaviour characteristics.

Investigations into coronary heart disease both in the USA and Europe have reported a constellation of personality traits, attitudes and life styles alleged to characterize this illness. A 'Type A' behaviour pattern comprising ambitious, driving and competitive work behaviour with a sense of urgency towards deadlines and associated with more intense cardio-vascular reactions has been compared with the more placid, less reactive 'Type B' individual who is less inclined to develop coronary heart disease. However, no clear-cut method of dividing people into 'Type A' or 'Type B' categories is available, and correlations between behaviour patterns and illness are still at a preliminary stage.

A fully satisfactory explanation of psychosomatic illness must account for the continuity, chronicity and specificity of symptoms, and explanations are likely to be multifactorial in nature. Undoubtedly progress will follow better diagnosis. Psychosomatic disorders traditionally include asthma, gastric ulcers, some cardio-vascular disorders, hypertension, and tension headaches. These are very globally defined illness categories, within each of which specific subforms of the illness can probably be delineated.

Psychophysiology

Attention, interest, thinking and feelings are accompanied by generalized changes throughout the brain and nervous system. Against this background, specific excitation occurs in the performance of specific tasks: looking at a picture entails a complex mosaic of eye movements, playing tennis involves the patterning of muscle action potentials and attending to a speaker requires the inhibition of other inputs.

How the psychological constructs of attention, thinking, and feeling interact with physiological changes, and what the nature of their interaction is, remains a complex and fascinating research problem. The direction of causality is uncertain: is it the perception of a threatening situation which arouses the physiological concomitants of anxiety, or does the physiological arousal come first and determine the nature of the perception?

Psychophysiology is an area of study which concentrates on human behaviour, and tries to analyse the cognitive, verbal and psychological aspects of behaviour in relation to the physiological. The term physiological in this context refers to those variables which can be recorded by means of small disk electrodes which can be attached to the surface of the skin. The range of variables which can be recorded in this way is very wide and includes heart rate, palmar skin resistance (attributable to palmar sweating), skin temperature, blood flow, respiration, and cortical potentials recorded from the surface of the brain.

Most of these variables show constant on-going activity: the heart, lungs and cortical potentials show rhythmic changes and also quite striking changes in response to simple stimuli such as lights and tones. More complex situations - verbal instructions, conversation, calling the individual by name, mental arithmetic tasks, and so on - can produce larger changes of long duration.

When the individual is left quietly to relax this activity shows a steady decline. If now an unexpected stimulus is given, a startle or orientating ('what is it?') response occurs. When the same stimulus is repeated, the response becomes smaller on each subsequent occasion until it no longer occurs: that is, it has habituated. Among psychophysiologists there is substantial interest in the physiological changes which occur in habituation, in conditioned autonomic responses, and in the patterning of reactivity to mild stressors which occurs in different individuals.

Useful information concerning the neurophysiology of cognitive processes in humans can be obtained from recording cortical potentials in response to stimuli. The combined electrical activity of millions of neurones in the brain is recorded in electro-encephalographic recordings. There is evidence that certain components of the cortical response are related to the physical attributes of the stimulus (its sensory modality, intensity), while other components reflect the individual's evaluation of the significance or meaning of the stimulus. Selective attention to one stimulus and not to another can be demonstrated in that components of the cortical response to the monitored stimulus are enhanced, as compared with those to an irrelevant stimulus.

Psychophysiological responsivity has often been considered in relation to clinical anxiety. Anxious patients frequently report trembling, sweating, shortness of breath, palpitations and muscular tension, and these have been recorded in situations where the patient is at rest, trying to relax, and also in response to different stimuli. There are several reports of anxious people typically responding more readily, habituating more slowly, and taking longer to recover from stimulation.

Psychophysiological measures can provide useful indicators of autonomic and cortical reactivity in different situations. They are helpful in their demonstration of individuals' idiosyncratic response profiles, in the study of habituation, relationship to task performance, processing of information, and in their indication of the variety of changes which occur along the sleep-wakefulness continuum. Perhaps the future may also see further links between psychophysiological research and the problems of psychosomatic medicine and psychiatry.

Concluding comments

If the aim of psychology is to clarify man's behaviour in this world it must accord a central position to biology, since this of all disciplines is the most directly linked to the understanding of living beings. The biological basis of behaviour refers to evolutionary, genetic, physiological and brain-behaviour mechanisms, and more recently has been extended to human social behaviour. Such an approach does not deny the importance of environmental factors or their capacity to modify the organism's behaviour; indeed, it strives towards methods of studying and assessing their contribution.

The biological approach has gained in impetus from the massive technological and theoretical advances of recent decades. The discovery within molecular biology of deoxyribonucleic acid (DNA) and the theory of the genetic code tell us how the information is coded which determines that a new life will inherit the characteristics of its parents. Other developments make it possible to record electrical events from single neurones within the brain, and to measure minute traces of brain chemicals. Studies by ethologists have made us all familiar with the behavioural repertoire of animals in their natural habitat.

Yet there remain many challenges to the understanding of human nature. The work which psychologists have to do centres on the analysis of behaviour into useful segments, and the derivation of meaningful concepts such as attention and arousal, emotion, memory and stress. It must contend with individual variation, possibly along dimensions such as extraversion, neuroticism and impulsiveness, and elucidate the psychophysiology of neurosis and stress reactions. The goal which lies ahead in the biological context is the fitting together of these psychological concepts with the mechanisms of bodily activity which underlie human individuality and welfare.

Psychology and nursing:
Part I questions

1. What aspects of psychology are most relevant to working with colleagues of other professions?
2. Is it useful to consider health education as part of nursing?
3. What topics in psychology are most closely related to the concept of 'the nursing process'?
4. Is a nursing training the most appropriate preparation for caring for the mentally handicapped?
5. Is a psychology degree necessary to apply the findings of psychological research in clinical practice?
6. Evaluate any ONE research study you know of that applies psychological principles to the care of patients, and discuss the limitations of the study.
7. Write a short essay on the function of theory in psychological research.
8. Is it useful to consider psychology as a discipline to be clearly distinct from other disciplines?
9. How could you investigate the claims of astrology or palmistry to be scientific?
10. What aspects of psychology are likely to be most relevant to patient care?
11. How might research findings on sensory deprivation be relevant to nursing in an intensive care unit?
12. Is it psychologically useful to talk of a good memory or a bad memory?
13. What ethical problems can arise in conducting research with patients?
14. Are the physical sciences an adequate basis for the development of psychology as a science?
15. When is there value in carrying out a purely descriptive study?
16. Is it always necessary to study a group of people to demonstrate a theoretical point, or can one person suffice?
17. What are the different methods of drawing a sample of subjects from a wider population of potential subjects?
18. What are the main advantages of experimental enquiries? Are there any disadvantages?
19. Statistics were originally developed to clarify the results of agricultural research. Why have they been so enthusiastically applied to psychological research?

20. What are the relative advantages and disadvantages of the cross-sectional and longitudinal approaches to obtaining data?
21. 'There are lies, damned lies, and statistics.' Are there?
22. Discuss the limitations of research which relies solely on correlational methods.
23. How can theoretical generalizations inform your thinking about particular patients?
24. Discuss, with particular reference to intelligence, the use of psychological tests to explore personal characteristics.
25. What explanation can you offer for the fact that some people are more anxious than others?
26. Describe some of the bodily symptoms thought to be related to stress.
27. Why do you think it is generally ineffective to 'tell' someone not to be afraid or to be angry?
28. Describe some forms of brain research which might be relevant to your clinical work.
29. What is meant by the nature versus nurture controversy?
30. How relevant are psychoanalytic concepts to the current developments in psychology?

Part two

Understanding Yourself and Other People

Part Two

4

Understanding people
John Hall

In the course of a single day most nurses will probably meet several dozen different people. Some of these people will be patients, some will be visitors to the hospital, others will be folk met at a local shop or on the bus, and some will be colleagues at work.

Each one of these people will be different: they have been through different experiences in their lives which now influence the way they view the world, and therefore how they relate to other people. When one of those people becomes a patient we have to understand them if we are going to help them as much as we can; or, if they are a member of our particular clinical team, we have to understand them if we are to work with them as effectively as possible.

The relationship between a nurse and patient is essentially an individual one. Apart from the differences between individual patients, individual nurses bring to the relationship their own personal background and skills, with their own sets of attitudes and expectations. Some of those skills and attitudes are modified by training, but others remain unchanged by experience. Thus an important determinant of nurse-patient relationships is the nurse's awareness of his or her own individuality and abilities, and how that affects the capacity to care for people in a varying range of circumstances.

Patients and nurses do not necessarily interpret the same activities and events in the same way. Macilwaine (1981) was interested in the differing perceptions of nursing activities in five different psychiatric units in general hospitals. She conducted 25 interviews with patients and 25 with nursing staff of the units. While the nurses saw their activities in terms of specific therapeutic functions, the patients did not view nurses as the main formal therapists. To take another example, the patients interpreted as 'aloofness' those qualities which the nurses perceived as being 'emotionally detached' and 'objective'. Overall, it appeared that both nurses and patients identified the same activities, but construed them quite differently.

The involvement of a nurse in any one relationship does not occur by choice, but because the nurse happens to work on a particular ward or in a particular community when the patient needs help. To this relationship the nurse is expected to bring a compassion and concern for the other person, yet most of us have at least occasional days when we find it difficult to make that concern apparent, and when we care for others in a rather routine way. Ideally, nurses are expected to be emotionally mature so that their own legitimate emotional needs are not met at the expense of the patient; yet inevitably we look to our work to meet some of our emotional needs, and some of our needs will be met by patients through our relating to them in ways which are not wholly designed for the patient's benefit.

In a perfect world nurses should be able to tolerate frustrations such as seeing a patient deteriorate when every rational treatment has been tried, or the frustration of being unable to modify all the environmental factors which might alleviate the pressure on a harassed young mother. Many nurses have to cope with death and grief, not only by physically being in contact with the dying and grieving but through their own private grief at the death of patients of whom they have grown fond.

A public stereotype of nurses often portrays them as female, single, and dedicated and able to tolerate these pressures. Chapman (1977) discussed the way in which this image has tended to persist, although it is no longer accurate in view of the increasing number of male nurses, the increase in the proportion of married nurses, and the emergence of more aggressive professional attitudes among nurses. Her discussion examines ways in which the image of the nurse can be brought closer to reality. This can be achieved by nurses themselves correcting misrepresentations in local and national media, both 'mass' and professional. Recruitment literature needs to be more realistic, and nurses may need to demonstrate more positively their unique function, which remains complementary to the treatment function of the medical profession.

Stress in nursing

There are two major implications of these stereotyped views of nursing. First, nurses need to understand themselves as part and parcel of understanding their patients. Second, emotional and personal stress is an important part of both initial adjustment to many fields of nursing, and in continuing adaptation during the course of a nursing career.

Stress is not confined to nurses: physical or mental illnesses have consequences which arise not only from the illness itself, but also from the associated stress. Stress can arise from a range of 'stressors', such as unexpected events, or loneliness. Wilson-Barnett (1980) described the general problems of stress in patient management, and the various strategies which can be adopted to alleviate stress, such as the provision of appropriate information. She had looked at ways of reducing the stress produced by undergoing a barium enema, and her article is illustrated by the type of information given to patients undergoing this procedure in order to show the benefits of adequate information provision. The article was one of a series in a journal issue solely concerned with looking at stress from several viewpoints.

Work in most health care professions requires the individual professional to deal with events and people in ways that the 'man-in-the-street' would find difficult technically and personally. Not only is the professional sometimes required to respond immediately and effectively to entirely unanticipated emergencies, but to do so in a way which ensures that the normal emotional response to such emergencies will not interfere with the 'professional' task concerned.

There are a number of responses to such pressures: one response is to deny the pressure and press on regardless. But one symptom of such disregard is, for example, the high rate of smoking among nurses. Interestingly, the rate of smoking is highest among hospital nurses when compared with a number of other health workers. They also show the lowest rate of stopping smoking amongst all those groups.

Problems of staffing intensive care units are another example of the way in which stress is manifested. Such units have become common in general hospitals over the last 20 or so years, but along with benefits to the patients have come problems for the nurses. It is common in such units to find high staff turnover levels, and more frequent periods of sick-leave in comparison with other wards.

Bishop (1981) carried out a simple questionnaire study among the nurses of two intensive care units: she had only a 50 per cent response rate to her questionnaire, indicating the care which has to be taken to obtain reasonable return rates in such studies. The returned questionnaires did, however, indicate the problems encountered by working in such a unit, the pressures imposed by the isolation procedures, and the rage and frustration produced by misuse of medical and technical skills. Psychological stress was specifically identified and was produced by such factors as working with seriously ill patients who may be unconscious or delirious, as well as by overstimulation produced by the high levels of patient turnover. The feelings of failure produced by the loss of a patient need to be recognized, and nurses may need to be supported through their initial feelings of inadequacy and fear.

Another response is for individual nurses to identify what is for them the field of nursing which both maximizes personal interest and minimizes stress. Nursing is unusual in the wide range of activities and settings it encompasses, and there are many opportunities to change from a type of nursing which is not enjoyed. Nonetheless there are likely to be some areas of nursing which are generally unpopular, but where skilled nursing is still required. It then becomes the responsibility of both nurse managers and colleagues to support and guide those who are, perhaps, taking a lot of sick leave as a consequence of such pressures, without necessarily implying any criticism of the capacity of the individual nurse so affected.

One way of finding out about the main skills required of nurses in different settings is to conduct a large-scale survey among them: for example, of the main activities they perform. Moses and Roth reported in 1979 the results of such a survey, conducted on about 20,000 of the 1.4 million registered nurses in America. The survey provided detailed information on the training of the nurses, the settings in which they worked, and their mobility. The study paid particular attention to the tasks carried out by nurses: over 57 per cent of the nurses spent the majority of their time during a usual work week in direct care activities. The following were among the activities listed:

* 83.6 per cent administered medicines;
* 58.9 per cent obtained health histories;
* 31.6 per cent performed some part of physical examinations;
* 5.6 per cent had primary responsibility for management and delivery of normal mothers.

Apart from the information yielded by the study, the report gives interesting information on the way in which the 20,000 subjects of the survey were selected.

Social motives

One aspect of understanding people is understanding what they want from social relationships, and what they have to offer. There are differing social motives, just as there are differing biological motives such as the wish to satisfy hunger or to maintain body warmth. Social motives may not be so easy to identify clearly, but an understanding of social motives can help both in understanding ourselves and others.

Our motives are not always conscious. Sometimes we know exactly what we hope for from a relationship, whereas at other times we are not ourselves aware of our motives, though they may be apparent to someone else who knows us well. Additionally we may have fantasies about other people which we admit to no one else, not even to a wife or husband. There may be conflict between our motives: it is not unusual to encounter people who simultaneously fascinate and repel. The social motives of patients may be unclear or confused, especially if they are apprehensive about being in hospital, or worried about their condition.

One goal of a patient in establishing a relationship may be to create a dependent relationship. In these, close and submissive relationships are sought with people who will provide help and protection. Conversely, dominant people seek to control others. Some dominant people are authoritarian in that they are systematically dominant towards those whom they perceive as inferior in status or power to themselves. Paradoxically, authoritarian people tend to be submissive to those whom they perceive are superior to them in status. People who behave in a culturally narrow way are termed 'ethnocentric', and similarly tend to be rigid in their adherence to the culturally 'alike' and in their rejection of the culturally 'unlike'.

Ruiz (1981) looked at the relationship between the ethnocentrism of 163 nurse teachers from 19 American schools of nursing, and their attitude towards culturally different patients (meaning Spanish, Jewish or Black patients). She was interested in the attitudes of staff, because students are likely to pick up their attitudes to patients from the people who teach and supervise them. The study showed that the staff members who were dogmatic or close-minded saw all patient groups as more annoying and more superstitious than staff members, who were more open-minded. It was also found that the more ethnocentric staff members had less favourable attitudes towards culturally different patients, with the implication that such staff members would find it difficult to convey a positive attitude to students who were caring for culturally different patients.

Another motive in creating a relationship is affiliation. It is found in both experimental and everyday settings that some people spend more time 'getting on with' other people than getting on with the job in a task-centred way. This search for affiliation is often associated with achieving physical closeness to the other person, perhaps involving more body-contact, and a more 'personal' choice of conversational topic.

Most people want to feel wanted and valued for themselves, because they believe they are of some worth. The wide relevance of this concept of self-esteem is growing in acceptance, and it is of interest that the provision of even quite simple knowledge of people's level of performance can act as an extremely strong reinforcer of behaviour. On the other hand, people do not want to receive unfavourable information about themselves. Despite the effort which most people take to avoid negative feedback about themselves, a clinically significant proportion of people consider they are worthless and inferior even in the absence of information supporting that idea.

It is relatively easy to understand people who search for affiliative relationships, or who behave in order to maintain their self-esteem. The role of aggression in social motivation is more complex, but none the less real. Many people find explicit aggressive behaviour very difficult to tolerate, and may respond by becoming aggressive themselves when rationally they know that such a response is inappropriate. While there is a strong social sanction on the overt expression of aggression, only a superficial survey is needed of the aggressive content of some sports (such as boxing) and many popular films and television series, to indicate that aggression cannot be ignored as a strong social motive for at least part of the population.

Understanding abnormality   As well as understanding ourselves, our patients, and colleagues by normal criteria, at least a proportion of our patients may be abnormal psychologically. Part of this abnormality may be explicable in terms of their physical illness, or a legitimate response to it. Other parts of their unusual behaviour may not be so explicable, and this raises the question of how normality - and abnormality - is defined.

'Abnormality' does not necessarily imply any central psychological malfunctioning. A person may be considered abnormal by virtue of some unusual skill or aptitude, such as those very few people who retain eidetic imagery beyond their youth and then display what is known as photographic memory. Similarly, some personality attributes may be highly unusual, and hence statistically 'abnormal', but are associated with unusual achievements. Thus those people who can tolerate the very long periods of social isolation implied by long single-handed sailing voyages may have very 'introverted' personalities, in that they have a very low need for social contact. What is considered abnormal is a function of many factors, including the age, sex and race of the person being labelled, and the power and professional status of the person making the designation.

The concept of psychological abnormality thus has a much wider application than to those phenomena labelled 'psychopathological'. Psychopathology is extremely important to many nurses, and from a psychological perspective it is important to consider the varying ways in which disturbed, deviant, or socially distressing behaviour can be analysed. It is equally important to see how different analyses can also be made of conditions and behaviour which are not usually considered psychological.

A number of types of abnormality are simply exacerbations of what we all feel from time to time. Periodic mood change is a very common experience, associated perhaps with the time of day, or with the menstrual cycle for women. With such mild swings from 'normality', it is often difficult to ascribe a clear label. For example, family doctors in Britain see about 90 per cent of all cases of mild anxiety or depression without referring them on for specialist help. With these mild cases, it is difficult to assign a clear diagnosis. There is, particularly in America, interest in what are known as 'borderline' states, where it is difficult to decide whether an individual is schizophrenic or more properly belongs to another diagnostic category. Thus there may be agreement that something is wrong psychologically, without necessarily agreement about the nature of the abnormality. Generally, the greater the degree of abnormality the easier it is to label or diagnose.

Eating and drinking are very familiar acts. Disorders of drinking may be associated with glandular disturbance, or in a colloquial way may refer to alcoholism. Until recently little attention was paid to eating disorders, yet it is now clear that there are a number of abnormal forms of eating. Anorexia nervosa is fairly well known as a disorder, occurring most frequently in adolescent girls, involving marked reduction in food intake and associated loss of body weight and symptoms such as amenorrhoea. Other aspects of eating which affect nursing care are the effect of altered meal times in hospital, since the expectation of food is determined as much by normal routine as by physiological hunger, and the difficulty which some patients have in adapting to special long-term diets, such as those without gluten for people with coeliac disease.

Less well known than anorexia is bulimia nervosa, a related condition but one not so physically conspicuous. Bulimics vomit or regurgitate their food after eating it, so that they may eat considerable quantities of food, yet maintain normal body weight. Bulimics may further indulge in 'binge' eating, where they walk down a street, buying and eating two or three cream buns from each baker's or confectioner's, or eating whole loaves of bread at a sitting. Although their body weight remains normal, they are at risk physically because the repeated vomiting alters the electrolyte balance in the body to dangerous proportions.

Another problem associated with eating is obesity. Obesity can be defined in various ways, such as relative weight compared to a standard for a given age and height, or skinfold thickness at certain standard sites on the body. Rates of obesity appear to be increasing. A number of attempts have been made to understand obesity psychologically, by looking at relationships with personality and by examining the levels of arousal of obese people. Obesity is not a socially acceptable condition, and can lead to other medical complications. Since it results from an inability to modify patterns of eating, and since it can be modified by psychological means, obesity, as with bulimia, offers a good example of a medical problem which can be redefined as a psychological abnormality.

Patterns of sexuality give another example of the way in which behaviour may be defined as abnormal, and where definitions of abnormality change over time. Several aspects of sexuality may be approached in this way. Surveys of the sexual behaviour of married couples suggest that about half of such couples have persistent difficulties in their relationship, such as premature ejaculation and failure to experience orgasm. While sexual deviations, such as fetishism (desire to have intercourse in the presence of, or while wearing, a special 'fetish' object or garment) are generally thought to be unsatisfactory substitutes for 'normal' intercourse, a significant proportion of partners accept and condone such deviations.

Masturbation used to be thought to be a harmful and morally dangerous practice. It is now clear that masturbation by males in western societies is virtually universal and very much more common by females than had previously been thought. Also there is no contemporary evidence that the practice is, by itself, dangerous. Similarly, more recent information on homosexuality, following changes in legislation in Britain, suggests that a higher proportion of people have some homosexual experience than was commonly believed.

The person most often quoted in popular accounts of sexual behaviour is Kinsey, on account of his widely read surveys published about 30 years ago (Kinsey, Pomeroy and Martin, 1948; Kinsey, Pomeroy, Martin and Gebhard, 1953). Kinsey's work suffered from a number of methodological problems, such as a bias towards better educated people in his sample, and any work in this field poses a number of ethical and technical difficulties, quite apart from the embarrassment which open discussion of the topic can still cause. However, sexual difficulties confront many physically handicapped people, and psychological research in this field both offers them an opportunity for help, and reveals how mistaken public attitudes about 'normal' sexuality have been.

A third area of 'abnormal' behaviour of relevance to nursing is violence. Many nurses are in the 'front-line' of violence in the health service when dealing with patients under the influence of drugs or alcohol or delinquent adolescents or adults. There is no doubt that physical violence in health care settings can be very dangerous, especially when elderly or immobile patients may be the victims. However, violence also occurs in some unexpected sections of the health care services, and may be tolerated to a considerable degree by some nursing staff. Ambulance staff, for example, are commonly called to homes where domestic strife has escalated to violence, and not infrequently have to deal with brawls between drivers of vehicles involved in accidents. Nursing staff in mental handicap hospitals often accept punches and minor assaults from their patients as part of the job. Health visitors may be assaulted on a home visit, or subjected to provocative verbal abuse from an unemployed spouse. Thus the definition of violence as abnormal is surprisingly imprecise, even within a single section of the health services.

Violence appears to be becoming more common in the community in general, and also appears to be becoming more frequent in health care settings, after a period in which it appeared to be declining as a result of the introduction of effective medication.

While the use of aggression in a controlled way is culturally acceptable as already discussed, problems begin when patients ignore the conventional taboos that normally limit aggressive behaviour. Coffey (1976) reviewed the literature on violence in psychiatric, mental handicap, and general hospitals. Violence may arise from the consequences of a poor environment for patient care, characterized perhaps by overcrowding and poor leadership. Other violence arises from the disease process itself, such as uncontrolled epilepsy or toxic states. The review looks at violence in general hospitals and in accident and emergency departments, noting, for example, that patients and their motives are frequently

unknown to the staff of casualty departments. It highlights
the need to study the occurrence of violence in the community and in the hospital more carefully before rushing into
ill-considered ways of controlling it.

The concept of psychologically abnormal behaviour thus
extends beyond the field of what is commonly accepted as
psychological oddity. The definition of psychological abnormality cannot readily aspire to objectivity in the natural
scientific sense, and to claim otherwise conceals the many
cultural biasses and methodological difficulties inherent in
such a definition. Another aspect of scientific objectivity
is maintaining a division between observer and observed.
This objectivity cannot always be maintained when attempting
to define abnormality in relationships, since a relationship
involves more than one person. Understanding your own contribution to a relationship is a necessary preliminary to
understanding the relationship itself.

References

Bishop, V. (1981)
This is the age of the strain. Nursing Mirror, August,
18-19.

Chapman, C. (1977)
Image of the nurse. International Nursing Review, 24,
166-167 and 170.

Coffey, M. (1976)
The violent patient. Journal of Advanced Nursing, 1,
341-350.

Kinsey, A.C., Pomeroy, W.B. and Martin, C.E. (1948)
Sexual Behavior in the Human Male. Philadelphia: W.B.
Saunders.

**Kinsey, A.C., Pomeroy, W.B., Martin, C.E. and Gebhard,
P.H.** (1953)
Sexual Behavior in the Human Female. Philadelphia: W.B.
Saunders.

Macilwaine, H. (1981)
How nurses and neurotic patients view each other in
general hospital psychiatric units. Nursing Times, July,
1158-1160.

Moses, E. and Roth, A. (1979)
Nurse power: what do statistics reveal about the na-
tion's nurses. American Journal of Nursing, 79, 1745-
1756.

Ruiz, M.C.J. (1981)
Open-closed mindedness, intolerance of ambiguity and
nursing faculty attitudes toward culturally different
patients. Nursing Research, 30, 177-181.

Wilson-Barnett, J. (1980)
Prevention and alleviation of stress. Nursing, 10, 432-
436.

5

Knowledge of self
D. Bannister

What is self?

Definition is a social undertaking. As a community we negotiate the meaning of words. This makes 'self' a peculiarly difficult term to define, since much of the meaning we attach to it derives from essentially private experiences of a kind which are difficult to communicate about and agree upon. Nevertheless, we can try to abstract from our private experience of self qualities which can constitute a working definition. Such an attempt was made by Bannister and Fransella (1980) in the following terms.

Each of us entertains a notion of our own separateness from others and relies on the essential privacy of our own consciousness
Consider differences between the way in which you communicate with yourself and the way in which you communicate with others. To communicate with others involves externalizing (and thereby blurring) your experience into forms of speech, arm waving, gift giving, sulking, writing and so on. Yet communicating with yourself is so easy that it seems not to merit the word communication: it is more like instant recognition. Additionally, communicating with specific others involves the risk of being overheard, spied upon or having your messages intercepted and this contrasts with our internal communications which are secret and safeguarded. Most importantly, we experience our internal communications as the origin and starting point of things. We believe that it is out of them that we construct communications with others. We know this when we tell a lie because we are aware of the difference between our experienced internal communication and the special distortions given it before transmission.

We entertain a notion of the integrity and completeness of our own experience in that we believe all parts of it to be relatable because we are, in some vital sense, the experience itself
We extend the notion of me into the notion of my world. We think of events as more or less relevant to us. We distinguish between what concerns and what does not concern us. In this way we can use the phrase 'my situation' to indicate the boundaries of our important experience and the ways in

which the various parts of it relate to make up a personal
world.

**We entertain the notion of our own continuity over time; we
possess our biography and we live in relation to it**
We live along a time line. We believe that we are essentially the 'same' person now that we were five minutes ago
or five years ago. We accept that our circumstances may have
changed in this or that respect, but we have a feeling of
continuity, we possess a 'life'. We extend this to imagine a
continuing future life. We can see our history in a variety
of ways, but how we see it, the way in which we interpret
it, is a central part of our character.

**We entertain a notion of ourselves as causes; we have
purposes, we intend, we accept a partial responsibility for
the consequences of our actions**
Just as we believe that we possess our life, so we think of
ourselves as making 'choices' and as being identified by our
choices. Even those psychologists who (in their professional
writing) describe humankind as wholly determined, and persons as entirely the products of their environments, talk
personally in terms of their own intentions and purposive
acts and are prepared to accept responsibility, when
challenged, for the choices they have made.

**We work towards a notion of other persons by analogy with
ourselves; we assume a comparability of subjective
experience**
If we accept for the moment the personal construct theory
argument (Kelly, 1955, 1969) and think not simply of 'self'
but of the bipolar construct of self versus others, then
this draws our attention to the way in which we can only
define self by distinguishing it from and comparing it to
others. Yet this distinction between self and others also
implies that others can be seen in the same terms, as 'persons' or as 'selves'. Our working assumption is that the
rest of humankind has experiences which are somehow comparable with, although not the same as, our own and thereby
we reasonably assume that they experience themselves as
'selves'.

We reflect, we are conscious, we are aware of self

Everything that has been said so far is by way of reflecting, standing back and viewing self. We both experience and
reflect upon our experience, summarize it, comment on it and
analyse it. This capacity to reflect is both the source of
our commentary on self and a central part of the experience
of being a 'self'. Psychologists sometimes, rather quaintly,
talk of 'consciousness' as a problem. They see consciousness
as a mystery which might best be dealt with by ignoring it
and regarding people as mechanisms without awareness. This
seems curious when we reflect that, were it not for this
problematical consciousness, there would be no psychology to

have problems to argue about. Psychology itself is a direct expression of consciousness. Mead (1925) elaborated this point in terms of the difference between 'I' and 'me', referring to the 'I' who acts and the 'me' who reflects upon the action and can go on to reflect upon the 'me' reflecting on the action.

Do we or do we not know ourselves?

The question 'do you know yourself?' seems to call forth a categorical 'yes' by way of answer. We know, in complete and sometimes painful detail, what has happened to us, what we have to contend with and what our thoughts and feelings are. We can reasonably claim to sit inside ourselves and know what is going on.

Yet we all have kinds of experience which cast doubt on the idea that we completely know ourselves. A basic test (in science and personal life) of whether you understand someone is your ability to predict accurately what they will do in a given situation. Yet most of us come across situations where we fail to predict our own behaviour; we find ourselves surprised by it and see ourselves behaving in a way we would not have expected to behave if we were the sort of person we thought we were.

We also sense that not all aspects of ourselves are equally accessible to us. There is nothing very mysterious in the notion of a hidden storehouse. We can confirm it very simply by reference to what we can readily draw from it. If I ask you to think about what kind of clothes you wore when you were around 14 years old you can probably bring some kind of image to mind. That raises the obvious question: where was that knowledge of yourself a minute ago, before I asked you the question? We are accustomed to having a vast knowledge of ourselves which is not consciously in front of us all the time. It is stored. It is not a great step to add to that picture the possibility that some parts of the 'store' of your past may not be so easily brought to the surface. We can then go one stage further and argue that although parts of your past are not easily brought to the surface they may nevertheless influence the present ways in which you feel and behave.

The best known picture of this kind of process is the Freudian portrait of the unconscious. Freud portrayed the self as divided. He saw it as made up of an id, the source of our primitive sexual and aggressive drives; a super-ego, our learned morality, our inhibitions; and an ego, our conscious self, struggling to maintain some kind of balance between the driving force of the id and the controlling force of the super-ego. Freud argued that the id is entirely unconscious and a great deal of the super-ego is also unconscious, and that only very special strategies such as those used in psychoanalytic therapy can give access to the contents of these unconscious areas of self. We do not have to accept Freud's particular thesis in order to accept the idea of different levels of awareness, but it may well be that the enormous popularity of Freudian theory is due to the fact that it depicts what most of us feel is a 'probable' state of affairs; namely, that we have much more going on in us than we can readily be aware of or name.

Indeed, if we examine our everyday experience then we may well conclude that we are continually becoming aware of aspects of ourselves previously hidden from us.

A great deal of psychotherapy, education and personal and interpersonal soul-searching is dedicated to bringing to the surface hitherto unrecognized consistencies in our lives.

How do we know ourselves?

There is evidence that getting to know ourselves is a developmental process: it is something we learn in the same way that we learn to walk, talk and relate to others. In one study (Bannister and Agnew, 1977), groups of children were tape-recorded answering a variety of questions about their school, home, favourite games and so forth. These tape-recordings were transcribed and re-recorded in different voices so as to exclude circumstantial clues (names, occupations of parents and so forth) as to the identity of the children. Four months after the original recording the same children were asked to identify their own statements, to point out which statements were definitely not theirs and to give reasons for their choice. The children's ability to recognize their own statements increased steadily with age, and the strategies they used to pick out their own answers changed and became more complex. Thus, at the age of five, children relied heavily on their (often inaccurate) memory or used simple clues such as whether they themselves undertook the kinds of activity mentioned in the statement; 'That boy says he plays football and I play football so I must have said that'. By the age of nine, they were using more psychologically complex methods to identify which statements they had made and which statements they had not made. For example, one boy picked out the statement 'I want to be a soldier when I grow up' as definitely not his because 'I don't think I could ever kill a human being so I wouldn't say I wanted to be a soldier'. This is clearly a psychological inference of a fairly elaborate kind.

Underlying our notions about ourselves and other people are personal psychological theories which roughly parallel those put forward in formal psychology. A common kind of theory is what would be called in formal psychology a 'trait theory'. Trait theories hinge on the argument that there are, in each of us, enduring characteristics which differentiate us from others, who have more or less of these characteristics. The notion that we or someone else is 'bad-tempered' is closely akin to the notion in formal psychology that some people are constitutionally 'introverted' or 'authoritarian' and so forth. The problem with trait descriptions is that they are not explanatory. They are a kind of tautology which says that a person behaves in a bad-tempered way because he is a bad-tempered kind of person. Such approaches tend to distract our attention from what is going on between us and other people by firmly lodging 'causes' in either us or the other person. If I say that I am angry with you because I am 'a bad-tempered person' that relieves me of the need to understand what is going on specifically between you and me that is making me angry.

Environmental and learning theories in psychology have their equivalents in our everyday arguments about our own nature. The fundamental assertion of stimulus-response psychology, that a person can be seen as reacting to his environment in terms of previously learnt patterns of response, is mirrored in our own talk when we offer as grounds for our actions that it is all 'due to the way I was brought up' or 'there was nothing else I could do in the circumstances'. Those theories and approaches in formal psychology which treat the person as a mechanism echo the kinds of explanation which we offer for our own behaviour when we are most eager to excuse it, to deny our responsibility for it and to argue that we cannot be expected to change.

Any theory or attempt to explain how we come to be what we are and how we change involves us in the question of what kind of evidence we use. Kelly (1955) argued that we derive our picture of ourselves through the picture which we have of other people's picture of us. He was arguing here that the central evidence we use in understanding ourselves is other people's reactions to us, both what they say of us and the implications of their behaviour towards us. He was not saying that we simply take other people's views of us as gospel. Obviously this would be impossible because people have very varying and often very disparate reactions to us. He argued that we filter others' views of us through our view of them. If someone you consider excessively rash and impulsive says that you are a conventional mouse, you might be inclined to dismiss their estimate on the grounds that they see everyone who is not perpetually swinging from the chandelier as being a conventional mouse. However, if someone you consider very docile and timid says that you are a conventional mouse, then this has quite different implications. You do not come to understand yourself simply by contemplating your own navel or even by analysing your own history. You build up a continuous and changing picture of yourself out of your interaction with other people.

Do we change ourselves? That we change in small ways seems obvious enough. Looking at ourselves or others we readily notice changes in preferred style of dress, taste in films or food, changes in interests and hobbies, the gaining of new skills and the rusting of old and so forth.

Whether we change in large ways as well as small involves us in the question of how we define 'large' and 'small' change. Kelly (1955) hypothesized that each of us has a 'theory' about ourselves, about other people, and about the nature of the world, a theory which he referred to as our personal construct system. Constructs are our ways of discriminating our world. For many of them we have overt labels such as nice-nasty, ugly-beautiful, cheap-expensive, north-south, trustworthy-untrustworthy and so forth. He also distinguished between superordinate and subordinate constructs. Superordinate constructs are those which govern large areas of our life and which refer to matters of central concern to us, while subordinate constructs govern the minor detail of our lives.

If we take constructs about 'change in dress' at a subordinate level then we refer simply to our tendency to switch from sober to bright colours, from wide lapels to narrow lapels and so forth. If we look at such changes superordinately then we can make more far-reaching distinctions. For example, we might see ourselves as having made many subordinate changes in dress while not changing superordinately because we have always 'followed fashion'. Thus at this level of abstraction there is no change because the multitude of our minor changes are always governed and controlled by our refusal to make a major change: that is, to dress independently of fashion.

Psychologists differ greatly in their view of how much change takes place in people and how it takes place. Trait psychologists tend to set up the notion of fixed personality characteristics which remain with people all their lives, which are measurable and which will predict their behaviour to a fair degree in any given situation. The evidence for this view has been much attacked (e.g. Mischel, 1968). Direct examination of personal experience suggests that Kelly (1955) may have been right in referring to 'man as a form of motion and not a static object that is occasionally kicked into movement'.

Psychological measurement, to date, suggests that people change their character, if only slowly, and have complex natures so that behaviour is not easily predictable from one situation to another. Psychologists have also tended to argue that where change takes place it is often unconscious and unchosen by the person. The issue of whether we choose change or whether change is something that happens to us is clearly complex. One way of viewing it might be to argue that we can and do choose to change ourselves, but that often we are less aware of the direction which chosen change may eventually take.

A person in a semi-skilled job may decide to go to night-school classes or undertake other forms of training in order to qualify themselves for what they regard as more challenging kinds of work. They might be successful in gaining qualifications and entering a new field. Up to this point they can reasonably claim to have chosen their direction of personal change and to have carried through that change in terms of their original proposal. However, the long-term effect may be that they acquire new kinds of responsibility, contacts with different kinds of people, new values and a life style which, in total, will involve personal changes not clearly envisaged at the time they went to their first evening class.

On the issue of how we go about changing ourselves, Radley (1974) speculated that change, particularly self-chosen change, may have three stages to it. Initially, if we are going to change, we must be able to envisage some goal; we must have a kind of picture of what we will be like when we have changed. He argued that if we have only a vague picture or no picture at all then we cannot change; we need to be able to 'see' the changed us in the distance. He went on to argue that when we have the picture then we can enact the role of a person like that. That is to say, we do not at heart believe that we are such a person but we can behave as if we were such a person, rather like an actor playing a role on stage or someone trying out a new style. (This may relate to the old adage that adolescence is the time when we 'try out' personalities to see which is a good fit.) He argued that if we enact in a committed and vigorous way for long enough then, at some mysterious point, we become what we are enacting and it is much more true to say that we are that person than that we are our former selves. This is very much a psychological explanation, in that it is about what is psychologically true, rather than what is formally and officially true. Thus the student who qualifies and becomes a teacher may officially, in terms of pay packet and title, be 'a teacher'. Yet, in Radley's terms, the person may still psychologically be 'a student' who is enacting the role of teacher, who is putting on a teaching style and carrying out the duties of a teacher but who still, in his heart of hearts, sees himself as a student. Later, there may come a point at which he becomes, in the psychological sense, a teacher.

However, we are also aware that there is much that is problematic and threatening about change. The set expectations of others about us may have an imprisoning effect and restrict our capacity to change. People have a picture of us and may attempt to enforce that picture. They may resist change in us because it seems to them unnatural, and it would make us less predictable. Phrases such as 'you are acting out of character', or 'that is not the true you', or 'those are not really your ideas' all reflect the difficulty people find and the resistance they manifest to change in us. Often the pressure of others' expectations is so great that we can only achieve change by keeping it secret until the change has gone so far that we can confront the dismay of others.

This is not to argue that we are simply moulded and brainwashed by our society and our family so that we are merely puppets dancing to tunes played by others. We are clearly influenced by others and everything, the language we speak, the clothes we wear, our values, ideas and feelings, is derived from and elaborated in terms of our relationships with other people and our society. But the more conscious we become of how this happens, the more likely we are to become critical of and the less likely automatically to accept what we are taught (formally and informally), and the more we may independently explore what we wish to make of ourselves as persons.

Equally, when we attempt to change we may find the process personally threatening. We may lose sight of the fact that change is inevitably a form of evolution: that is to say, we change from something to something and thereby there is continuity as well as change. If we lose faith in our own continuity we may be overwhelmed by a fear of some kind of catastrophic break, a fear of becoming something unpredictable to ourselves, of falling into chaos. Whether or not we are entirely happy with ourselves, at least we are something we are familiar with, and quite often we stay as we are because we would sooner suffer the devil we know than the unknown devil of a changed us. Fransella (1972) explored the way in which stutterers who seem to be on the verge of being cured of their stutter often suddenly relapse. She argued that stutterers know full well how to live as 'stutterers'; they understand how people react and relate to them as 'stutterers'. Nearing cure they are overwhelmed with the fear of the unknown, the strangeness of being 'a fluent speaker'.

onitoring of self

One of the marked features of our culture is that it does not demand (or even suggest) that we formally monitor our lives or that we record our personal history in the way in which a society records its history. True, a few keep diaries, and practices such as re-reading old letters from other people give us glimpses into our past attitudes and feelings. For the most part, our understanding of our past is based on our often erratic memory of it. Moreover, our memory is likely to be erratic, not just because we forget past incidents and ideas but because we may actively 're-write' our history so as to emphasize our consistency and make our past compatible with our present.

Psychologists have tended to ignore the importance of personal history. The vast majority of psychological tests designed to assess the person cut in at a given point in time; they are essentially cross-sectional and pay little heed to the evolution of the person. It would be a very unusual psychology course that used biography or autobiography as material for its students to ponder. There are exceptions to this here-and-now preoccupation. In child psychology great emphasis is laid on the notion of 'development' and a great deal of the research and argument in child psychology is about how children acquire skills over a period, how they are gradually influenced by social customs and how life within the family, over a period of years, affects a child's self-value. Additionally, clinical psychologists involved in psychotherapy and counselling very often find themselves engaged in a joint search with their clients through the immediate and distant past in order to understand present problems and concerns. This does not necessarily argue that a person is simply the end product of their past. We need to understand and acknowledge our past, not in order to repeat it but in order either to use it or to be free of it. As Kelly (1969) put it, 'you are not the victim of your autobiography but you may become the victim of the way you interpret your autobiography'.

Obstacles to self-knowledge and self-change

To try and understand oneself is not simply an interesting pastime, it is a necessity of life. In order to plan our future and to make choices we have to be able to anticipate our behaviour in future situations. This makes self-knowledge a practical guide, not a self-indulgence. Sometimes the situations with which we are confronted are of a defined and clear kind so that we can anticipate and predict our behaviour with reasonable certainty. If someone asks you if you can undertake task X (keep a set of accounts, drive a car, translate a letter from German and so forth) then it is not difficult to assess your skills and experience and work out whether you can undertake the task or not. Often the choice or the undertaking is of a more complex and less defined nature. Can you stand up in conflict with a powerful authority figure? Can you make a success of your marriage to this or that person? Can you live by yourself when you have been used to living with a family? The stranger the country we are entering the more threatening the prospect becomes; the more we realize that some degree of self-change may be involved, the more we must rely upon our understanding of our own character and potential.

In such circumstances we are acutely aware of the dangers of change and may take refuge in a rigid and inflexible notion of what we are. Kelly (1955, 1969) referred to this tendency as 'hostility'. He defined hostility as 'the continued effort to extort validational evidence in favor of a type of social prediction which has already been recognized as a failure'. We cannot lightly abandon our theory of what we are, since the abandonment of such a theory may plunge us into chaos. Thus we see someone destroy a close relationship in order to 'prove' that they are independent or we see teachers 'proving' that their pupils are stupid in order to verify that they themselves are clever.

Closely connected to this definition of hostility is Kelly's definition of guilt as 'the awareness of dislodgement of self from one's core role structure'. Core constructs are those which govern a person's maintenance processes; they are those constructs in terms of which identity is established and the self is pictured and understood. Your core role structure is what you understand yourself to be.

It is in a situation in which you fail to anticipate your own behaviour that you experience guilt. Defined in this way guilt comes not from a violation of some social code but from a violation of your own personal picture of what you are.

There are traditional ways of exploring the issue of 'what am I like?' We can meditate upon ourselves, ask others how they see us, or review our history. Psychologists have devised numerous tests for assessing 'personality', though in so far as these are of any use they seem to be designed to give the psychologist ideas about the other person rather than to give the people ideas about themselves. Two relatively recent attempts to provide people with ways of exploring their own 'personality' are offered by McFall (in Bannister and Fransella, 1980) and Mair (1970).

McFall offers a simple elaboration on the idea of talking to oneself. His work indicated that if people associate freely into a tape-recorder and listen to their own free flow then, given that they erase it afterwards so that there is no possible audience other than themselves at that time, they may learn something of the themes, conflicts and issues that concern them; themes that are 'edited out' of most conversation and which are only fleetingly glimpsed in our thinking. Mair experimented with formalized, written conversation. Chosen partners wrote psychological descriptions of each other (and predictions of the other's description) and then compared and discussed the meaning and the evidence underlying their written impressions.

Although we have formal ways of exploring how we see and how we are seen by others (the encounter group), and informal ways (the party), it can be argued that there is something of a taboo in our society on direct expression of our views of each other. It may be that we fear to criticize lest we be criticized, or it may be that we are embarrassed by the whole idea of the kind of confrontation involved in telling each other about impressions which are being created. Certainly if you contemplate how much you know about the way you are seen by others, you may be struck by the limitations of your knowledge, even on quite simple issues. How clear are you as to how your voice tone is experienced by other people? How often do you try and convey to someone your feelings and thoughts about them in such an oblique and roundabout way that there is a fair chance that they will not grasp the import of what you are saying?

Psychologists are only very slowly seeing it as any part of their task to offer ways to people in which they may explore themselves and explore the effect they have on others.

Role and person

Social psychologists have made much use of the concept of 'role'. Just as an actor plays a particular role in a drama it can be argued that each of us has a number of roles in our family, in work groups, in our society. We have consistent ways of speaking, dressing and behaving which reflect our response to the expectations of the group around us. Thus within a family or small social group we may have inherited and developed the role of 'clown' or 'hardheaded practical person' or 'sympathizer'. Jobs often carry implicit role specifications with them so that we perceive different psychological requirements in the role of teacher from the role of student or the role of manager from the role of worker. We are surprised by the randy parson, the sensitive soldier, the shy showbusiness person. Society also prescribes very broad and pervasive roles for us as men or women, young or old, working-class or middle-class and so forth. It is not that every word of our scripts is pre-written for us, but the broad boundaries and characteristics of behaviour appropriate to each role are fairly well understood. These social roles can and do conflict with personal inclinations and one way of defining maturity would be to look on it as the process whereby we give increasing expression to what we personally are, even where this conflicts with standard social expectations.

Kelly chose to define role in a more strictly personal sense in his sociality corollary which reads: 'to the extent that one person construes the construction processes of another he may play a role in a social process involving the other person'. He is here emphasizing the degree to which, when we relate to another person, we relate in terms of our picture of the other person's picture of us. Role then becomes not a life style worked out by our culture and waiting for us to step into, but the on-going process whereby we try to imagine and understand how other people see the world and continuously to relate our own conception to theirs.

The paradox of self-knowing

We reasonably assume that our knowledge of something does not alter the 'thing' itself. If I come to know that Guatemala produces zinc or that the angle of incidence of a light ray equals its angle of reflection, then this new knowledge of mine does not, of itself, affect Guatemala or light. However, it alters me in that I have become 'knowing' and not 'ignorant' of these things. More pointedly, if I come to know something of myself then I am changed, to a greater or lesser degree, by that knowledge. Any realization by a person of the motives and attitudes underlying their behaviour has the potential to alter that behaviour.

Put another way, a person is the sum of their understanding of their world and themselves. Changes in what we know of ourselves and the way in which we come to know it are changes in the kind of person we are.

This paradox of self-knowledge presents a perpetual problem to psychologists. An experimental psychologist may condition a person to blink their eye when a buzzer is pressed, simply by pairing the buzzer sound with a puff of air to the person's eyelid until the blink becomes a response to the sound of the buzzer on its own. But if the person becomes aware of the nature of the conditioning process and resents being its 'victim' then conditioning may cease, or at least take much longer. Knowledge of what is going on within that person and between the person and the psychologist has altered the person and invalidated the psychologist's predictions. Experimental psychologists seek to evade the consequences of this state of affairs by striving to keep the subject in ignorance of the nature of the experimental process or by using what they assume to be naturally ignorant subjects: for example, rats. But relying on a precariously maintained ignorance in the experimental subject creates only a mythical certainty in science. Psychotherapists, on the other hand, generally work on the basis that the more the person (subject, patient, client) comes to know of themselves, the nearer they will come to solving, at least in part, their personal problems.

This self-changing property of self-knowledge may be a pitfall for a simple-minded science of psychology. It may also be the very basis of living, for us as persons.

References

Bannister, D. and Agnew, J. (1977)
The Child's Construing of Self. In A.W. Landfield (ed.),
Nebraska Symposium on Motivation 1976. Nebraska:
University of Nebraska Press.

Bannister, D. and Fransella, F. (1980)
Inquiring Man (2nd edn). Harmondsworth: Penguin.

Fransella, F. (1972)
Personal Change and Reconstruction. London: Academic
Press.

Kelly, G.A. (1955)
The Psychology of Personal Constructs, Volumes I and II.
New York: Norton.

Kelly, G.A. (1969)
Clinical Psychology and Personality: The selected
papers of George Kelly (ed. B.A. Maher). New York:
Wiley.

Mair, J.M.M. (1970)
Experimenting with individuals. British Journal of
Medical Psychology, 43, 245-256.

Mead, G.H. (1925)
The genesis of the self and social control.
International Journal of Ethics, 35, 251-273.

Mischel, W. (1968)
Personality and Assessment. New York: Wiley.

Radley, A.R. (1974)
The effect of role enactment on construct alternatives.
British Journal of Medical Psychology, 47, 313-320.

6

Psychopathology
D. A. Shapiro

'Psychopathology', literally defined, is the study of disease of the mind. Our society entrusts most of the care of individuals whose behaviour and experience are problematic or distressing to medical specialists (psychiatrists). Being medically trained, psychiatrists see their work as requiring diagnosis and treatment of 'patients'. Psychologists, on the other hand, have sought alternative means of understanding abnormal behaviour, and the aim of this chapter is to outline the progress that has been made in this direction.

The varieties of psychopathology

A good way to appreciate the great variety of problems we are concerned with is to examine the system of classification used by psychiatrists, summarized in table 1. Readers requiring more detailed descriptions of these should consult a psychiatric textbook. In the NEUROSES, the personality and perception of reality are fundamentally intact, although emotional disturbances of one kind or another, usually involving anxiety or its presumed effects, can make life very difficult for the individual. The PSYCHOSES, on the other hand, are characterized by gross impairments in perception, memory, thinking and language functions, and the individual is fundamentally disorganized, rather than merely emotionally disturbed. However, there is no clear-cut brain disease, and so the disorder cannot be explained in purely biomedical terms. The layman's conception of 'madness' is based on the symptoms of schizophrenia, including delusions (unshakeable, false beliefs), hallucinations (such as hearing 'voices') and thought disorder (manifested in 'garbled' speech). The third category of table 1, personality disorders, comprises deeply ingrained, motivational and social maladjustments. Table 1 also includes organic syndromes, which are behaviour disorders associated with identified brain disease. Not included in the table are the important group of psychosomatic illnesses. These are characterized by physical symptoms whose origins are in part psychological (emotional). They include asthma, high blood pressure, gastric and duodenal ulcers. More generally, psychological stress is increasingly implicated in many physical illnesses.

Table 1

Major category	Neuroses (milder disturbances)				
Illus-trative syndromes	Anxiety state	Obsessive-compulsive disorders	Phobias	Conversion reactions	Neurotic depression
Charac-teristic symptoms	Palpitation, tires easily, breathless-ness, ner-vousness anxiety	Intrusive thoughts, urges to acts or rituals	Irrational fears of specific objects or situations	Physical symptoms, lacking organic cause	Hopelessness dejection

Major category	Psychoses (severe Non-organic disturbances		Personality disorders (antisocial disturbances)	Organic syndromes		
Illus-trative syndromes	Affective disorders	Schizo-phrenia	Psycho-pathic persona-lity	Alcoholism and drug dependence	Epilepsy	Severe mental handicap
Charac-teristic symptoms	Distur-bances of mood, energy and activity patterns	Reality distor-tion, social withdrawal, disorga-nization of thought, perception and emotion	Lack of conscience	Physical or psycho-logical dependence	Increased suscepti-bility to convulsions	Extremely low intelli-gence, social impairments

The medical model of psychopathology

Before describing psychological approaches to behaviour disorder, it is necessary to examine critically the predominant medical approach. This makes three major assumptions, which are considered in turn.

The diagnostic system
The first assumption of the medical model is that the various kinds of abnormal behaviour can be classified, by diagnosis, into syndromes, or constellations of symptoms regularly occurring together. This diagnostic system has already been summarized in table 1. It has a number of disadvantages. First, some disorders appear to cut across

the boundaries of the system. Thus an individual whose
severe anxiety is associated with fears of delusional
intensity may defy classification as 'neurotic' or 'psychotic'. Second, scientific studies of the ability of psychiatrists to agree on the diagnosis of individuals have
suggested that the process is rather unreliable, with
agreement ranging from about 50 per cent to 80 per cent
depending upon the circumstances (Beck, Ward, Mendelson,
Mock and Erlbaugh, 1962). Third, research also suggests that
the diagnosis given to an individual may bear little relationship to the symptoms the individual has (Zigler and
Philips, 1961). Fourth, the diagnosis of psychiatric disorder is much more subjective and reflective of cultural
attitudes than is the diagnosis of physical illness; one
culture's schizophrenic might be another's shaman; similar
acts of violence might be deemed heroic in battle but
psychopathic in peacetime. Careful comparisons of American
and British psychiatrists have shown that the two groups use
different diagnostic criteria and hence classify patients
differently.

Despite these limitations, the psychiatric classification persists. This is largely because no better descriptive system has been developed, whilst improvements have
been obtained in the usefulness of the system by refining it
in the light of earlier criticisms. For example, agreement
between psychiatrists has been improved by standardization
of the questions asked in diagnostic interviews and the use
of standard decision-rules for assigning diagnoses to
constellations of symptoms. But it is still necessary to
bear in mind that the diagnostic system is not infallible
and the 'labels' it gives individuals should not be
uncritically accepted.

Physiological basis of psychopathology

The second assumption of the medical model is that the
symptoms reflect an underlying disease process, physiological in nature like those involved in all illnesses,
causing the symptoms. Three kinds of evidence are offered
in support of this. First, the influence of hereditary
factors has been assessed by examining the rates of disorder
among the relatives of sufferers. To the extent that a
disorder is heritable, its origins are considered biological
in nature. For example, comparison between the dizygotic
(non-identical) and monozygotic (identical) twins of
sufferers suggests that there is some hereditary involvement
in schizophrenia, anxiety-related disorders, depression and
antisocial disorders, with the evidence strongest in the
case of schizophrenia (Gottesman and Shields, 1973). Studies
of children adopted at birth also suggest that the offspring
of schizophrenic parents are more liable to suffer from
schizophrenia than other adopted children, despite having no
contact with the biological parent. On the other hand, the
evidence also shows that hereditary factors alone cannot
fully account for schizophrenia or any other psychological

disorder. Even amongst the identical twins of schizophrenics, many do not develop the disorder. Both hereditary
and environmental influences are important.

The second line of evidence for a 'disease' basis of
psychopathology concerns the biochemistry of the brain. This
is a vastly complex subject, and one whose present methods
of investigation are almost certainly too crude to give
other than an approximate picture of what is going on. Over
the years, a succession of biochemical factors have been
suggested as causes for different forms of psychopathology.
Unfortunately, the evidence is not conclusive, as biochemical factors found in sufferers may be consequences
rather than causes. Hospital diets, activity patterns or
characteristic emotional responses may influence the brain
biochemistry of disordered individuals.

Despite these problems, there are some promising lines
of biochemical research. For example, it has been suggested
that schizophrenia may be caused by excess activity of dopamine, one of the neurotransmitters (substances with which
neurons stimulate one another: see Snyder, Banerjee, Yamamura and Greenberg, 1974). This suggestion is supported by
the similarity in molecular structure between dopamine and
the phenothiazine drugs which are used to alleviate schizophrenia, suggesting that these drugs block the reception of
dopamine by taking its place at receptors which normally
receive it. These drugs also cause side effects resembling
the symptoms of Parkinson's disease, which is associated
with dopamine deficiency. Although this and other evidence
support the dopamine theory of schizophrenia, some research
has failed to support it, and so the theory has yet to be
universally accepted. In sum, biochemical evidence is sug-
gestive, and consistent with presumed physiological origins
of psychopathology, but it is not conclusive, nor can such
evidence make a psychological explanation redundant. It is
best seen as an important part of our understanding of
psychopathology, whose causal significance varies from one
disorder to another.

The third line of evidence for the physiological basis
of psychopathology concerns disorders with clear organic
causes. Disease or damage to the brain can result in severe
disturbance of behaviour. A classic example of this is
'general paresis of the insane', whose widespread physical
and mental impairments were discovered in the last century
to be due to the syphilis spirochete. This discovery encouraged medical scientists to seek clear-cut organic causes
for other psychological abnormalities. A large number of
organic brain syndromes have been established, in which
widespread cognitive and emotional deficits are associated
with damage to the brain by disease, infection, or injury.
Epilepsy, in which the individual is unusually susceptible
to seizures or convulsions, is associated with abnormal
patterns of brain activity measured by the electro-
encephalogram (EEG) even between seizures. Many individuals
with severe mental handicap (cf. Clarke and Clarke, 1974),

who attain very low scores on tests of general intelligence and show minimal adaptation to social requirements and expectations, suffer from clear-cut organic pathology, often accompanied by severe physical abnormalities.

On the other hand, all of these disorders are affected by the person's individuality, experience and environment. For example, similar brain injuries result in very different symptoms in different individuals. Those suffering from epileptic seizures can make use of their past experience to avoid circumstances (including diet and environmental stimuli) which tend to trigger their convulsions. Most mentally handicapped people do not have clearly identifiable organic illnesses. Even amongst those who do, the environment can make a big difference to the person's ability to learn the skills of everyday living. Psychologists have found that special training can help mentally handicapped people who might otherwise appear incapable of learning.

Medical treatment of psychopathology

The third assumption of the medical model concerns how psychopathology should be managed. Physical treatments are offered in hospitals and clinics to persons designated 'patients'. It is beyond our present scope to describe the extensive evidence supporting the effectiveness of drugs and electro-convulsive therapy (ECT), the major physical treatments currently employed. However, there are several reasons why psychologists are often inclined to question the support this evidence gives to the medical model. First, individuals differ in their responsiveness to physical treatments, and nobody really understands why some individuals are not helped. Second, the fact that abnormal behaviour can be controlled by physical means does not prove that its origins are physical. Third, the physical treatments often lack a convincing scientific rationale to explain their effects.

The medical model: conclusions

In sum, the medical model gains some support from the evidence, but is sufficiently defective and incomplete to warrant the development of alternative and complementary approaches. Although the diagnostic system is of some value, it must be used with caution. Although hereditary influences, biochemical abnormalities and organic pathology have a part to play in our understanding of psychopathology, they cannot explain its origins without reference to environmental and psychological factors. The apparent efficacy of physical treatment does not establish the physical origins of what they treat. The remainder of this chapter is concerned with five alternative approaches developed by psychologists and social scientists, and assesses their contribution with respect to some of the most important kinds of psychopathology. The evidence presented is, of necessity, very selective, and a full appreciation of these approaches can only follow more extensive study. It should also be borne in mind that the present emphasis on origins of disorder entails a relative neglect of research on treatment.

The statistical model

The statistical model identifies individuals whose behaviour or reported experience is sufficiently unusual to warrant attention on that basis alone. Abnormal individuals are those who greatly differ from the average with respect to some attribute (such as intelligence or amount of subjective anxiety experienced). For example, according to Eysenck (1970), people who score highly on dimensions known as 'neuroticism' (very readily roused to emotion) and 'introversion' (quick in learning conditioned responses and associations) are likely to show what the psychiatrist calls 'anxiety neurosis'. Although this approach is commendably objective, it is not very helpful alone. Not all unusual behaviour is regarded as pathological. Exceptionally gifted people are an obvious case in point. Some statistically abnormal behaviours are obviously more relevant to psychopathology than are others, and we need more than a statistical theory to tell us which to consider, and why. But the model is of value for its suggestion that 'normal' and 'abnormal' behaviour may differ only in degree, in contrast to the medical model's implication of a sharp division between them.

The psychodynamic model

The psychodynamic model is very difficult to summarize, based as it is on theories developed early in the century by Freud, and revised and elaborated by him and subsequent workers within a broad tradition (Ellenberger, 1970). Like the medical model, it seeks an underlying cause for psychopathology, but this is a psychological cause, namely, unconscious conflicts arising from childhood experiences. Freudians have developed a general theory of personality from their study of psychopathology. Freud viewed the personality as comprising the conscious ego, the unconscious id (source of primitive impulses) and partly conscious, partly unconscious super-ego (conscience). The ego is held to protect itself from threat by several defence mechanisms. These are a commonplace feature of everyone's adjustment, but are used in an exaggerated or excessively rigid manner by neurotic individuals, and are overstretched to the point of collapse in the case of psychotic individuals.

For example, neurotic anxiety is learnt by a child punished for being impulsive, whereupon the conflict between wanting something and fearing the consequences of that desire is driven from consciousness (this is an example of the defence mechanism known as repression). According to this theory, pervasive anxiety is due to fear of the person's ever-present id impulses, and phobic objects, such as insects or animals, are seen as symbolic representations of objects of the repressed id impulses. Dynamic theory views depression as a reaction to loss in individuals who are excessively dependent upon other people for the maintenance of self-esteem. The loss may be actual (as in bereavement) or symbolic (as in the misinterpretation of a rejection as a total loss of love). The depressed person expresses a child-like need for approval and affection to restore self-esteem. In psychotic disorders such as schizophrenia, the collapse of the defence mechanisms leads to the predominance of primitive 'primary process' thinking.

Despite its considerable impact upon the ways in which we understand human motivation and psychopathology, psychodynamic theory has remained controversial. Most of the evidence in its favour comes from clinical case material, as recounted by practising psychoanalysts, whose work is based on the belief that unconscious conflicts must be brought to the surface for the patient to recover from the symptoms they have engendered. Whilst this method often yields compelling material which is difficult to explain in other terms (Malan, 1979), it is open to criticism as insufficiently objective to yield scientific evidence. It is all too easy for the psychoanalyst unwittingly to influence material produced by the patient, and the essential distinction between observations and the investigator's interpretations of them is difficult to sustain in the psychoanalytic consulting-room. The abstract and complex formulations of psychodynamic theory are difficult to prove or disprove by the clear-cut scientific methods favoured by psychologists, and the patients studied, whether in Freud's Vienna or present-day London or New York, are somewhat unrepresentative.

There is some scientific evidence which is broadly consistent with psychodynamic theory; for example, the defects in thinking found in schizophrenia are compatible with the dynamic concept of ego impairment, and loss events of the kind implicated by dynamic theory are associated with the onset of depression. Although psychologists hostile to dynamic theory can explain these findings in other terms, there is little doubt that the theory has been fruitful, contributing to psychology such essential concepts as unconscious conflict and defence mechanism.

The learning model

The learning model views psychopathology as arising from faulty learning in early life, and conceptualizes this process in terms of principles of learning drawn from laboratory studies of animals and humans. The most basic principles are those of Pavlovian or 'classical' conditioning (in which two stimuli are presented together until the response to one stimulus is also evoked by the other), and 'operant' conditioning (whereby behaviour with favourable consequences becomes more frequent). According to proponents of the learning model, the symptoms of psychopathology are nothing more than faulty habits acquired through these two types of learning. The 'underlying pathology' posited by the medical and psychodynamic models is dismissed as unfounded myth.

For example, it is suggested that phobias are acquired by a two-stage learning process; first, fear is aroused in response to a previously neutral stimulus when this stimulus occurs in conjunction with an unpleasant stimulus; then the person learns to avoid the situation evoking the fear, because behaviour taking the person away from the situation is rewarded by a reduction in fear. Another learning theory is that schizophrenic patients receive more attention and other rewards from other people, such as hospital staff, when they behave in 'crazy' ways, thereby increasing the frequency of this behaviour. Again, depressed people are seen as failing to exercise sufficient skill and effort to 'earn' rewards from situations and from other people; a vicious circle develops and activity reduces still further in the absence of such rewards.

In general, the learning model provides a powerful set of principles governing the acquisition of problem behaviour. But it has severe limitations. For example, the fact that fears and phobias can be established by processes of conditioning in the laboratory does not prove that this is how they come about naturally. The theory cannot readily explain how people acquire behaviours which lead to such distress (it is hardly 'rewarding' to suffer the agonies of depression or anxiety, and learning theorists acknowledge their difficulty over this fact by referring to it as the 'neurotic paradox'). Recently, learning theorists have examined the important process of imitative learning or modelling, whereby the behaviour of observers is influenced by another's actions and their consequences. Fear and aggression can be aroused in this way, with obvious implications for the transmission of psychopathology from one person (such as a parent) to another. But human thinking is considered by many psychologists too complex to be understood in terms of these relatively simple learning theories. Hence the development of the cognitive approach, to which we now turn.

The cognitive model

The cognitive model focusses upon thinking processes and their possible dysfunctions. 'Neurotic' problems are seen as due to relatively minor errors in reasoning processes, whilst 'psychotic' disorders are held to reflect profound disturbances in cognitive function and organization.

For example, it is well known that depressed people hold negative attitudes towards themselves, their experiences and their future. According to cognitive theory, these attitudes give rise to the feelings of depression (Beck, 1967). Although an episode of depression may be triggered by external events, it is the person's perception of the event which makes it set off depressed feelings. Experiments in which negative beliefs about the self are induced in non-depressed subjects have shown that a depressed mood does indeed follow. But whether similar processes account for the more severe and lasting depressive feelings of clinical patients is another matter, although the promising results of 'cognitive therapy', in which the attitudes of depressed patients are modified directly, may be taken as indirect evidence for the theory.

Cognitive theory also embraces people's beliefs about the causation of events (known as attributions). For example, it has been suggested that the attributions one makes concerning unpleasant experiences will determine the impact of those experiences upon one's subsequent beliefs about oneself; thus, if a woman is rejected by a man, this is much more damaging to her self-esteem if she believes that the main cause of the event is her own inadequacy, than if she attributes the event to the man's own passing mood. An attributional approach suggests that failure experiences are most damaging if individuals attribute them to wide-ranging and enduring factors within themselves. Consistent with this, depressed people have been found to attribute bad outcomes to wide-ranging and enduring factors within themselves, whilst they attribute good outcomes to changeable factors outside their control.

Psychologists have devoted considerable efforts to precise descriptions of the cognitive deficits of schizophrenic patients through controlled laboratory experiments. For example, schizophrenics have difficulty performing tasks requiring selective attention to relevant information and the exclusion from attention of irrelevant information. Schizophrenics are highly distractable. This may help to explain how irrelevant features of a situation acquire disproportionate importance and become interpreted as part of their delusional systems of false beliefs, or how speech is disorganized by the shifting of attention to irrelevant thoughts and mental images which other people manage to ignore.

The cognitive approach is of great interest because it combines the systematic and objective methods of experimental psychology with a thoroughgoing interest in an important aspect of human mentality. It is a very active 'growth area' of current research, and shows considerable promise. It is perhaps too soon to evaluate many of its specific theories, however, and it does carry the risk of neglecting other aspects of human behaviour.

The socio-cultural model

The final model to be considered attributes psychopathology to social and cultural factors. It focusses upon malfunctioning of the social or cultural group rather than of an individual within that group.

In terms of the socio-cultural model schizophrenia, for example, has been considered both in relation to the quality of family life and to larger socio-economic forces. Within the family, behaviour labelled schizophrenic is seen as a response to self-contradictory emotional demands ('double binds') from other family members, notably parents, to which no sane response is possible. Although graphic accounts have been offered of such patterns in the family life of schizo-phrenic patients, there is no evidence that these are peculiar to such families. If anything, the research evidence suggests that abnormalities of communication within the families of schizophrenics arise in response to the behaviour of the patient, rather than causing the disorder. Looking beyond the family, the higher incidence of schizo-phrenia amongst the lowest socio-economic class, especially in inner city areas, is attributed to the multiple depriva-tions suffered by this group. Episodes of schizophrenia are triggered by stressful life events, some of which are more common, or less offset by social and material supports, amongst lower-class people. On the other hand, cause and effect could be the other way round, with persons developing schizophrenia 'drifting' into poverty-ridden areas of the city. Indeed, schizophrenic patients tend to achieve a lower socio-economic status than did their parents.

The socio-cultural approach is of undoubted value as a critical challenge to orthodox views, and has generated useful research into social and cultural factors in psycho-pathology. Its proponents have also made valuable contri-butions by bringing a greater humanistic respect for the personal predicament of troubled individuals, and to the development of 'therapeutic communities' and family therapy as alternatives to individually-centred treatments. However, many of its propositions concerning cause-effect relation-ships have not stood the test of empirical research.

The psychology of illness

It is well known that certain physical illnesses are related to psychological factors. These 'psychosomatic disorders' include ulcerative colitis, bronchial asthma and hyper-tension. It is not so widely appreciated, however, that psychological factors may be involved in any physical ill-ness. This is because the physiological changes associated with stress (for instance, the release of the 'stress hormones' such as adrenalin) can suppress immune responses and so increase the individual's susceptibility to many diseases, ranging from the common cold to cancer (Rogers, Dubey and Reich, 1979). Many aspects of a person's life have been implicated in ill-health, presumably because of their effects on such physiological mechanisms. These include physical stresses such as noise, highly demanding and/or repetitive jobs (whether physical or mental), catastrophic life events (such as accidents, illness or bereavement) and major emotional difficulties (such as marital discord).

However, for physical illness as for psychopathology, the cause-effect relationship is not simple. Some indivi-duals are more constitutionally stress-prone than others, it appears. Some people live in congenial and supportive surroundings, enabling them to withstand pressures which might otherwise lead to illness. Most of the events impli-cated in psychological distress and ill-health are in part the results of the individual's own state and behaviour. For example, marital conflict may reflect prior strains felt by the individuals involved. Furthermore, the impact of a stressful event or circumstance depends on the individual's appraisal of it. For example, noise is less distressing if we know we can silence it should it become unbearable. Thus consideration of psychological factors in ill-health demonstrates clearly the interaction between features of individuals and of their surroundings. For physical illness as for psychopathology, we must realize that there are many interacting causes rather than imagine that any one factor is alone responsible for the problem at issue.

Conclusions

Each of the approaches surveyed has contributed to our understanding of psychopathology. The evidence presented for each can only illustrate the massive amounts of research which have been carried out. Nonetheless, several clear themes emerge which have profound implications for our present and future knowledge of psychopathology.

First, the system of classification is inadequate, and research shows that different people within the same broad diagnostic group (such as schizophrenia) behave very differently; it therefore follows that different causes may be found for the difficulties experienced by these sub-groups of people.

Second, the different approaches could profitably be integrated rather more than they have been in the past. For example, elements of the medical, statistical, sociocultural and cognitive approaches have been combined in recent work on schizophrenia, in which the vulnerability of an individual to the disorder is seen as reflecting both heredity and environment; this vulnerability determines whether or not a person experiences schizophrenia when faced with stresses which are too much to cope with (Zubin and Spring, 1977). The fact that psychopathology generally has multiple causes lends particular urgency to the need to construct broad theories incorporating the facts which were hitherto regarded as supporting one or another of the competing approaches.

Third, the different approaches have more in common than is often acknowledged. In relation to schizophrenia, for example, the breakdown of ego functioning described by psychodynamic theory resembles the inability to process information identified by cognitive theory.

Fourth, the limitations of existing models have encouraged the growth of alternative approaches. For example, the 'transactional' approach emphasizes the importance of the individual's active part in bringing about apparently external stressful events and pressures (Cox, 1978). This approach views the individual as neither a passive victim of circumstances, nor as irrevocably programmed from birth to respond in a particular way. Person and environment are seen as in continuous interaction, so that one-way cause-effect analysis is inappropriate. For example, harassed executives and mothers of small children bring some of the stress they suffer upon themselves as they respond sharply to colleagues or children and thus contribute to a climate of irritation or conflict. Research using this approach has only recently begun, but it holds considerable hope for the future.

Finally, what can this psychological study of psychopathology offer the professional? There are as yet no certain answers to such simple questions as 'What causes schizophrenia?' or 'Why does Mrs Jones stay indoors all the time?' If and when such answers become available, they will not be simple. They will involve many interacting factors. Meanwhile, the psychological approach teaches us a healthy respect for the complexity of the human predicament, and is a valuable corrective to any tendency to offer simplistic or unsympathetic explanations of human distress. Furthermore, professionals will often find it illuminating to apply some of the approaches outlined here to help understand distressed individuals they encounter in their daily work.

References

Beck, A.T. (1967)
Depression: Clinical, experimental and theoretical aspects. New York: Harper & Row.

Beck, A.T., Ward, C.H., Mendleson, M., Mock, J.E. and Erlbaugh, J. (1962)
Reliability of psychiatric diagnosis II: a study of consistency of clinical judgments and ratings. American Journal of Psychiatry, 119, 351-357.

Clarke, A.M. and Clarke, A.D.B. (1974)
Mental Deficiency: The changing outlook (3rd edn). London: Methuen.

Cox, T. (1978)
Stress. London: Macmillan.

Ellenberger, H.F. (1970)
The Discovery of the Unconscious. London: Allen Lane/ Penguin.

Eysenck, H.J. (1970)
The Structure of Human Personality. London: Methuen.

Gottesman, I.I. and Shields, J. (1973)
Genetic theorising and schizophrenia. British Journal of Psychiatry, 122, 15-30.

Malan, D.H. (1979)
Individual Psychotherapy and the Science of Psychodynamics. London: Tavistock.

Rogers, M.P., Dubey, D. and Reich, P. (1979)
The influence of the psyche and the brain on immunity and disease susceptibility: a critical review. Psychosomatic Medicine, 41, 147-164.

Snyder, S.H., Banerjee, S.P., Yamamura, H.I. and Greenberg, D. (1974)
Drugs, neurotransmitters and schizophrenia. Science, 184, 1243-1253.

Zigler, E. and Philips, L. (1961)
Psychiatric diagnosis and symptomalogy. Journal of Abnormal and Social Psychology, 63, 69-75.

Zubin, J. and Spring, B. (1977)
Vulnerability – a new view of schizophrenia. Journal of
Abnormal Psychology, 86, 103-126.

softspotITTER

Understanding yourself and other people: Part II Questions

1. Describe some of the ways in which your understanding of yourself has increased.
2. Discuss the problem of defining self.
3. How do parents influence their children's idea of self?
4. People are born with a fixed character which they cannot alter. Is this true?
5. Examine ways in which a person's idea of self is affected by the nature of their work.
6. To what extent is our picture of ourselves influenced by our physical state and appearance?
7. From your knowledge of psychology, explain why patients and their nurses may each have different perceptions of the same situation.
8. How can chronic disability affect ideas of self?
9. How would you respond if a patient of the opposite sex told you that he or she had fallen in love with you?
10. How would you respond if you realized that you had developed an unreasonable dislike of a particular patient?
11. Some wards and departments meet regularly for staff to discuss how their personal differences affect their work. Is this a good idea?
12. Do defence mechanisms have a positive value in helping us to adjust to everyday circumstances?
13. Deafness tends to evoke less sympathy than blindness. Why?
14. Why do people contribute more generously to charities for animal welfare than to charities for the mentally ill and handicapped?
15. Is masturbation normal?
16. Is the concept of disease useful in understanding psychological disturbance?
17. How useful is it to think of depression as arising from negative attitudes towards self?
18. Prejudice, like aggression, is simply inevitable. Is this true?
19. Is there any evidence to support the view that violence creates violence?
20. How might an understanding of learning theory help in the understanding of neurotic disorders?
21. Violence in the family is increasing. How does it develop in an individual family?

22. Discuss the contribution of psychological and social factors to the establishment of a chronic gambling problem.
23. How does a knowledge of psychological concepts help in understanding confused patients?
24. To what extent are genetic factors relevant in the causation of mental handicap?
25. What effect does social class have on the incidence and long-term course of schizophrenia?
26. What would lead you to suspect that a patient in your ward is developing an anxiety state?
27. What are the main problems in understanding people with a chronic schizophrenic disorder?
28. What types of disturbed behaviour do you find most difficult to tolerate from those around you in your home life?
29. What types of disturbed behaviour do you find most difficult to tolerate from the patients in your care in a medical or surgical ward?
30. What are the possible consequences for the nurse of being continually in contact with strange and unusual behaviour?

Part three
Assessment

7

Assessing people and patients
John Hall

Assessing people and patients

Nursing assessment

The recent development of the 'nursing process' has introduced nurses to the concept of assessment as a major aspect of the nurse's work. In nursing process terms, assessment of the patient is the first step to be carried out before the nursing intervention is planned, before the plan is implemented, and before an evaluation is carried out. In practice, these four steps can be so inter-related that they are all part of any one nursing activity.

Assessment is not some procedure that is distinct from the everyday concerns of the clinical nurse. An assessment is taking place every time a nurse takes a temperature, records the volume of urine that has drained into a collecting bag, or notices that a patient is now eating more food after an operation. An assessment is being recorded when a nurse makes an entry in a Kardex or in case-notes about the progress of a patient.

In this part of the book, assessment refers to the formation of impressions, and the making of judgements about others. Psychological assessment does not refer only to the use of standardized tests, but also to the use of a wide range of structured and semi-structured techniques. To some nurses, the term assessment may already have a special meaning, being used to refer to the evaluation of a trainee or student nurse by a supervisor or more senior nurse. For most nurses, the process of assessment will involve them in obtaining information about patients as a preliminary step to planning treatment to be carried out by them or by someone else. Sometimes it is not the patient but the relatives of the patient who have to be assessed, as when determining whether an elderly lady can safely be returned to the care of her equally elderly husband. Some nurses will be interested in assessing other nurses, or would-be nurses, because of their involvement in staff recruitment and personnel work, or because of their educational and training responsibilities. Although people are usually the focus of assessment, the environment of the patient may be equally deserving of a careful appraisal and assessment, as when a house needs to be inspected to see whether handrails should be fitted, or steps replaced by a ramp, for the benefit of a physically handicapped child.

The total amount of information potentially assessable in most nursing and community settings is vast. A skilled nurse has to become a skilled assessor of those aspects of the patients' behaviour and functioning which are of relevance to their care. Yet, for any one patient, only a proportion of the information available will be assessed by even the most skilled nurse. A compromise usually has to be made between collecting a lot of information about a patient rather crudely, and collecting less information more carefully. There is usually an inverse relationship between bandwidth (the amount and complexity of information processed) and fidelity (the precision with which information is transmitted). Hence it can sometimes be helpful to consider assessment as a two- or multi-stage process, beginning an assessment from a broad bandwidth approach, and then carrying out a much more limited and narrow high-fidelity assessment of the behaviour or function of special interest.

Skill in the clinical assessment of patients can be highly specific. The experienced nurse on a post-operative surgical ward may identify signs of recovery in the colour and texture of a wound which would be missed by an equally, but differently, skilled nurse from the renal dialysis unit. For most skilled assessment decisions, an amount of clinical experience is helpful: but the experience must be recent, as the type of knowledge used in this sort of skill is dependent on ready recall of other similar patients, and on knowledge of the effect of particular medical and surgical treatments, which can sometimes change quickly over only one or two years.

This part of the book discusses a number of concepts, such as validity, which are central to an understanding of the psychology of assessment. It also discusses some of the assumptions underlying particular assessment techniques, most of which are intended for the assessment of patients, but some of which are relevant to personnel and educational uses. The section describes particular techniques, so that the relevance of them to the overall care of the patient can be appreciated.

Integrity in assessment

Haward (1964) commented upon some of the difficulties he had encountered in working with nurses in three clinical research studies. The first study was a trial of suppositories in large general hospitals: the ward sisters were asked to report on the effect of the suppository immediately after the action was complete. When the six-week trial was over, it was noticed that the entries on the forms from one hospital contained large gaps in the entries on the forms. When this was pointed out to the sister, she generously offered to complete the forms from memory if they were returned to her! In another of the studies the respiration rate of patients before and after treatment was recorded in a study of the effects upon respiratory stress of artificial pneumo-thorax and pneumo-peritoneum. In a ward of tuberculous patients, irrespective of age, constitution, and

whether or not they were inflated with two litres of air,
each patient showed a respiration of 20/minute! The conclusion drawn from these studies was that all nurses participating in a research study, even if only having an assessment role, should understand the need for integrity in
providing research data, and should be trained in the use
of the particular procedures.

The nurse as assessor

Nurses probably do not see themselves as assessors, as distinct from the rest of the functions they carry out while
involved in nursing. Equally, patients probably do not
construe nurses as constantly assessing them. Yet it is
implicit in a hospital setting that a patient in a ward is
subject to a high degree of nursing observation and assessment, including observation of personal acts, such as defe-
cation, which are normally intensely private. Indeed, the
very design of a ward may be intended to permit maximum
possible observation.

There is increasing evidence that many assessment procedures are highly reactive: that is, the behaviour of
patients is determined in part by their expectation of the
person assessing them, and the reactions of the assessor to
their behaviour. This means that the way in which the nurse
observes and assesses the patients may affect the result of
the assessment. Interview methods of assessment are particularly reactive, so that the attitude taken by the nurse
to the patient, and the way in which questions are phrased,
will determine the quantity and quality of information
yielded by the interview. For most of the assessment methods
described in this section, the way in which they are used by
the nurse is as important as the particular method chosen.
By viewing themselves as assessors, nurses then place upon
themselves the responsibility of collecting and recording
information as systematically and sensitively as possible.

Self-assessment

There is no reason why patients should not be encouraged to
assess themselves: this places some responsibility upon them
for their own case, and also permits self-checking at intervals, without needing to rely on the help of professional
staff. While self-assessment for breast cancer by women is
widely published, there has been little concern about testicular cancer in men. Murray and Wilcox (1978) described a
simple self-examination procedure for the testicles; the
article also refers to teaching materials which are available, including a film, illustrating the importance of
teaching correct procedures whenever self-assessment is
encouraged.

Observation and assessment in clinical nursing

By far the most important form of patient assessment used
by nurses is direct observation, either of the behaviour or
state of the patient, or of the readings of various measuring devices. The four senses of sight, touch, hearing and

smell, are used constantly in nursing care. Nurses will see the colour of the urine, and note the smoky or red colour indicating the presence of blood. They will use their fingers and thumb to take the patient's radial pulse beat and, by taking the pulse on both sides simultaneously, might detect a slight delay on one side indicative of some abnormality. They will listen through stethoscopes for the sudden change in sound that signals the diastolic blood pressure when using a sphygmomanometer. They will catch a whiff of faeces and know that someone on the ward has been incontinent.

A number of phrases are used to describe a patient's level of consciousness, such as 'semi-comatose', 'stuporous' and 'lethargic'. The meaning of these terms is not always clear, but level of consciousness is an important function in the monitoring of many patients. Jones (1979) outlined how the Glasgow Coma Scale is used in the University of Texas Medical Branch. The scale consists of three parts, eye-opening assessment, verbal response, and best motor response. Each section of the scale can be scored on a numerical scale which ranges from a total of 14, for a normal person, to three, which is compatible with, but not necessarily indicative of, brain death. Reliability studies have shown that different staff can use the scale with little variability between observers. The scale is an example of the way in which a clinical assessment can be graded to facilitate repeated assessment.

The importance of awareness in clinical assessment

The routine act of taking a temperature illustrates some important aspects of clinical assessment. Although the notional 'normal' body (skin) temperature is 98.4 degrees Fahrenheit, or 36.9 degrees Centigrade, there are known limits to the normal range of temperature. Yet since normality is defined statistically, there will be some healthy individuals who have a stable body temperature outside the 'normal' range. A number of factors affect the temperature recorded by a thermometer, such as the site where the temperature is taken (the mouth, skin or rectum), the level of activity of the patient immediately before taking the temperature, and individual differences between nurses in the way in which they interpret readings when the mercury surface lies on the borderline between two gradations. Thus, even when taking temperatures, the interpretation of a reading depends on a good knowledge of 'normality' and its range, and on a knowledge of the effect of minor variations in procedure.

Sims-Williams (1976) reviewed the ways in which the clinical glass thermometer is used, drawing attention to the way in which the procedure 'stands in danger of becoming ... a ritual'. She discussed the factors affecting normal temperature variation, and choice of the appropriate site. She points out, for example, that a careful nursing assessment is needed before even embarking on a temperature recording:

'it cannot be blindly assumed that an adult patient is fit for oral temperature recording'. The available evidence suggests that even with an accepted clinical procedure such as this, nurses need to give more time in order to make recordings accurate. On the other hand, the main value of taking temperatures may be in promoting nurse-patient contact, and could be replaced by 'informed talking' for an equivalent period of time.

Relying on direct observation implies that the patient is available and in sight of the nurse carrying out the observation. In psychiatric hospitals it is not unusual for there to be a patient who leaves the ward very early in the day, and who can only be observed by the ward staff for a very small proportion of the day. This may mean that someone other than a nurse, even a hospital gardener or porter, may be the best source of information on the everyday pattern of behaviour of some patients.

Apart from direct observation, the second most important form of nursing assessment involves talking to the patient. Some conversations with patients may be wholly casual – asking the name of favourite football teams – but can still be used in retrospect to assess some aspects of the patient's functioning. Other information may need to be gained by talking to the patient in a more focussed way. 'Interview' may sound too formal as a description of most conversations with patients intended to yield information about them, but it is helpful to regard such conversations as interviews. We are all familiar with the various types of interviews conducted in everyday life, such as enquiring at a DIY shop about the availability of a particular brand of paint, or going as parents to see the teacher at school about our children. There are common features to all interviews, no matter who is interviewing whom, and clinical interviewing techniques can be improved by considering the findings of research conducted on interview techniques in general.

Whatever the degree of formality or informality of an interview or chat with a patient, the questions have to start somewhere. The order in which information is collected may be determined by the order in which items are written down on a standard hospital form. Yet the order in which such items are written may not be the order in which they should be asked. Some information may need to be collected very early on in a nurse's contact with a patient, such as information about current medication when a patient attends a casualty department. Other information can often wait: patients can be distressed or irritated by having to recount painful, embarrassing, or simply lengthy and detailed material, immediately on admission.

Suggested means of interdisciplinary assessment
The progress of patients in rehabilitation has traditionally been depicted mainly in terms of activities of daily living. However, this approach is rather narrow, and it may be

better to assess progress on a wider basis, using a range of behavioural indicators. Fenwick (1979) described the development of an interdisciplinary assessment tool, which covered five areas of information, to describe readiness for discharge:

* assessment of the patient's medical state of readiness;
* assessment of the patient's functional readiness;
* assessment of the patient's and family's psychosocial readiness;
* assessment of the patient's readiness in communication skills;
* assessment of the patient's and family's expressed readiness for future living patterns.

The assessment sheets would normally be completed prior to the monthly team meeting, so that each member could contribute appropriate information to the decision of the team.

Ways of gathering information

Interviews may start from exploring the presenting problem of the patient in front of you; but very often some written material, such as a referral letter or old case-notes, is available to help structure an assessment interview. Records can be very good at giving certain categories of factual information about family history, medical history, etc., but they tend to be less good at giving a clear picture of the day-to-day level of functioning of the patient. Some form of rating scale or check-list can be very helpful in providing information relating to activities of the daily life of the patient, which can then be reassessed several years later, using the same scale.

There are many ways in which different assessment procedures can be combined to form an assessment schedule for a research project. If a series of assessments are to be carried out, it is worth while considering carefully the sequence in which the assessing nurse or the patient has to complete them. For example, if patients complete a structured forced-choice questionnaire on their attitudes to hospital they are forced to think in an organized way about the subject. This might make it difficult for them then to answer a second open-ended interview on the same subject without being affected by the questionnaire. In such circumstances, it might be better to use the less structured method before the more highly structured approach.

For some assessment procedures, such as taking the temperature, pulse, and respiration rate of a patient, standard recording forms are available. Careful layout of a record form is an integral part of a well-thought-out assessment system. It ensures that the required information is entered and that crucial information is unlikely to be omitted. It is important that, whenever possible, a record is made of an assessment as soon as practicable after it has been carried out, consistent with the needs of patient care.

Delay in recording the information leads to the possibility of error.

Many qualified nurses are involved in the assessment of people to see if they are fitted for particular posts. This is normally done through selection interviews and is supplemented by information supplied by the candidates and referees. A considerable amount of work has been done to establish whether student nurses can usefully be selected on the basis of psychological test results, and a number of personality and ability tests have been tried for this purpose. A good example of this type of assessment procedure is the educational test of the General Nursing Council for England and Wales. This particular test is of considerable importance since it acts as a selection instrument for those candidates for training who do not possess either the minimum educational qualifications set by the Council, or the higher educational standards which may be set by individual hospitals.

Selection of staff

Good selection of new nurses leads to satisfaction for both employer and employee, and reduces the costs of high staff turnover. Kaiser (1978) set out her views on how to interview applicants for jobs as ten separate steps. Some of these steps were: before the interview, review the written material on the application form to generate questions for the interview (step 1); describe the job accurately to applicants, including both positive and negative aspects of the job (step 5); evaluate the results of your interviews by carrying out a follow-up of people employed, and asking questions about the interviews of the people employed (step 10). Included in the article are a number of tips for applicants, such as 'Watch your body language ... calmness and self-control are considered desirable traits.'

Appraisal of staff

Another type of staff assessment is known as staff appraisal, a procedure for monitoring the performance of staff. This involves the completion of a check-list (often standardized) by the immediate superior of each member of staff, and very often also involves feedback interviews, when staff members are told how well they have been functioning.

Of equal concern to nurse tutors is the appraisal of trainee nurses, either in the course of training, or as the final stage of qualification. Since nursing is a registered profession, and since minimum standards of competence need to be established to protect the public, the final appraisal of assessment of student nurses is, in effect, a licence to practise. There have been major changes in the way in which the competence of nurses, as well as other health care professionals, has been finally assessed in recent years. In virtually all cases this has involved a shift away from reliance on traditional essay-type questions. A comprehensive approach to educational evaluation should include an assessment and evaluation not only of the students, but also of the training course and the teachers.

The performance of nurses in written examinations often bears little relationship to their clinical proficiency in the ward. Boreham (1977) described the development of a case history test, which simulates the situations that student nurses encounter on the ward, and requires them to apply, in a practical way, the principles of nursing care they have learnt. The major steps in developing the test were: the initial choice of a case history, selecting the appropriate parts of the history to include in the test, the decision to distribute questions about the history throughout the test rather than all at the end, and careful drafting of the questions. The test was well received by both nurse teachers: 'I like to relate issues to a patient: the case history test enables this to be done'; and by students: 'It's more real - it mixes up the systems.'

The effect of environment

All the examples of assessment so far considered have been of people. But people live in environments; for patients these environments include out-patient departments, health centres and sites of accidents, as well as their own homes. The behaviour of people can be markedly affected by the setting in which they are observed. The child who is a tantrum-throwing brat at home may genuinely behave like an angel in a paediatric ward, because the constraints are different. Mentally handicapped adults may apparently be unable to feed themselves in their own ward simply because appropriate implements have never been placed before them under conditions where they have time to feed themselves without disturbance from other patients. The constraints upon a patient may not be physical, but may be organizational: the use that a psychiatric patient can make of local shops may depend on local hospital regulations regarding the total amount of money patients are allowed to hold at any one time.

An awareness of the effect of this type of physical and organizational variation has led to the development of a number of measures (e.g. measures of ward atmosphere and of ward restrictiveness) which can be valuable supplements to patient-centred assessments. Whenever some event (such as visits to the patient by a particular friend) or some environmental factor (such as the level of noise) appears to consistently affect a patient, there may be a case for developing a simple, but systematic, assessment procedure. This can be used in order to examine the strength of relationship between the external event and the alleged change in the patient.

References

Boreham, N.C. (1977)
The use of case histories to assess nurses' ability to solve clinical problems. Journal of Advanced Nursing, 2, 57-66.

Fenwick, A.M. (1979)
An interdisciplinary tool for assessing patients' readiness for discharge in the rehabilitation setting. Journal of Advanced Nursing, 4, 9-21.

Haward, L.R. (1964)
The nurse as a research associate. International Journal of Nursing Studies, 1, 211-217.

Jones, C. (1979)
Glasgow Coma Scale. American Journal of Nursing, 79, 1551-1553.

Kaiser, P. (1978)
Ten steps to interviewing job applicants. American Journal of Nursing, 78, 627-629.

Murray, B. and Wilcox, L. (1978)
Testicular self examination. American Journal of Nursing, 78, 2074-2075.

Sims-Williams, A.J. (1976)
Temperature taking with glass thermometers: a review. Journal of Advanced Nursing, 1, 481-493.

8

Interviewing
Russell P. Wicks

If there is one universally applied technique to be found
in behavioural research it is 'interviewing'. If there is
one technique basic to all professional practice it is the
interaction between people that is called 'interviewing'. It
is the nature of this interaction between people which is
the concern of this chapter. It is to be hoped that what
is said can be applied not simply to 'the interview' in
'an interview situation' but to all purposive contacts
between individuals; the critical feature, it is claimed,
being the purposive nature of the encounter. The participants bring hopes, fears, expectations, misconceptions and
many other cognitions to the situation, most times in the
hope that their wishes will be met, fears reduced and so on.
Customarily this view is found in the characterization of an
interview as a 'conversation with a purpose'. So it is, but
all those participating in an interview have their purposes
and not simply, for example, the interviewer. In the complex
transactions of getting and giving information we observe
effort aimed at achieving purposes. Thus the psychologist
testing a client by means of, say, the Wechsler Adult
Intelligence Scale is conducting an interview as defined.
The purpose from one point of view is to help the client in
some way, from the other to be helped. In the exchange of
information each has purposes and expectations that they
hope will be met. Each may be optimizing their strategies
towards fulfilling these purposes. Roles will be assumed
constraining and shaping behaviour. If participants in
interviews can become more skilful and aware of the processes involved there is some hope of raising levels of
satisfaction. It is, therefore, the aim of this chapter to
examine such interview processes with this goal in mind. For
this purpose a simple model of an interview is described
(see figure 1) and for illustrative purposes reference made
to three particular interview situations; occupational
counselling, job interviews and research interviewing.

Initiation

The view that it is the purposive nature of the interview that is crucial leads us to consider the motives of
the participants. An individual approaching a counselling
situation may be motivated by a complex of needs, and

Figure 1

Model of an interview

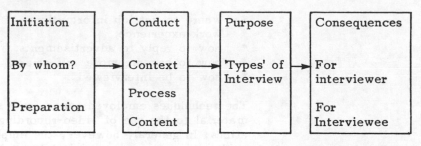

voluntary or compulsory attendance may be crucial in structuring these needs. Whether these needs are shared and whether they can be fulfilled is another matter. It may well be the case that some frequently voiced criticisms of interviews arise, in part, from a failure to make explicit the needs and expectations of the parties involved. Nowhere is this more important than in those situations with a high level of emotional involvement. Two people may look back on an interview as a total failure because each had different expectations which unfortunately were not fulfilled. We all, interviewers and interviewees, bring hopes and fears to the task. Just as Orne (1962) draws our attention to the 'demand characteristics' of the experimental situation as a result of which subjects perform as they believe they are expected so to do, so participants in interviews will seek a role that they perceive as being appropriate. Not always, unfortunately, do they choose correctly.

In analysing an interview it follows, therefore, that attention to preliminaries and preparation is vital. Many writers on interviewing stress the physical preparations needed, literally setting the scene. Here, 'cognitive' scene setting is judged to be more important; for example, in employment interviewing paying attention to providing information about the organization, or providing an adequate job description. Considering the contribution of application forms and references, together with other 'scene setting' activities, will go a long way towards minimizing the cognitive gap that may occur. Furthermore, such preparations are in fact part of the information exchange that lies at the heart of an interview. In general, preparation from the interviewer's point of view means careful planning of all aspects of the situation. Briefing oneself, rehearsing the interview, anticipating needs; all contribute to an efficiently managed, worth-while encounter.

Recently, increasing attention has been given to preparation on the part of the interviewee, especially for those about to be interviewed for a job. For example, a great deal of work stemming from careers work with young people has resulted in programmes aimed at developing 'life skills'. There is clear evidence that all can profit from paying attention to the activities and skills involved in job seeking. The material included in such programmes varies widely but may cover:

*   where to get job information;
*   work experience;
*   how to reply to advertisements;
*   how to become more self-aware;
*   how to be interviewed.

The techniques employed range from self-instructional material to the use of video-recording of role-play situations. In general, however, the emphasis is on providing guidelines, improving social skills, self-presentation and making people more aware of the processes of social interaction.

Conduct

Context

What effect on the behaviour of the participants in an interview might the following environments have: a police station; a doctor's surgery; a street corner; a psychology laboratory? Clearly the effect can be dramatic. We have the clearest evidence here for the importance of the frame of reference, role expectations and construal of the situation upon behaviour in an interview. Indeed, the subtlety of the rules of the 'games' played out in different contexts is such that we spend our lives refining and editing our private rule books. Within each context there may be a range of indicators signalling to us how to behave, how to address people, what to say and what not to say, an obvious example being dress, particularly a uniform which may be anything from a pin-stripe suit to a white coat. What is the experience of people who customarily wear a 'uniform' when they discard it? What might people say to a priest in mufti that they would not say if he donned his clerical garb? Thus our perception of the interview context is an essential part of the scene setting previously discussed. Most interviewers, being aware of this, go to some trouble to ensure that the physical setting signals what they wish it to: they dress in a particular style, arrange the seats appropriately, adjust the lighting, ensure that interruptions do or do not occur. They try to ensure that the interview is conducted in a 'good mannered' way.

A further aspect is that participants bring substantial resources to the task: their background knowledge, and skills expectations. Whilst these resources may bring benefits to an interview, they sometimes create problems. Such difficulties have been extensively investigated by Rosenthal and his co-workers (e.g. Rosenthal and Rosnow, 1969) in studies of the characteristics of 'volunteers' in research and studies of the expectations of subjects in experiments, as well as the experimenters. Avoiding bias and error arising from these factors is a major concern of investigators; thus one should be aware that volunteers for survey research tend to be better educated; if male, they score higher on IQ tests; and they are better adjusted than non-volunteers. Such factors should be taken into account in evaluating data. Similarly, the survey interviewer asked to find a sample of five people, even though certain characteristics of the sample are specified, may unwittingly choose those they feel it would be 'nice' to interview.

Process

A great deal of what we know about interpersonal communication has been learnt by systematic study of interviews, especially the face-to-face two-person encounter. What is offered here, however, is a general communication model which may be used to analyse an interview (see figure 2). The utility of this model as a tool for examining interpersonal behaviour rests upon the conceptualization of communication as a system; the model is dynamic because it has independent parts with provision for feedback.

Figure 2

A communication model

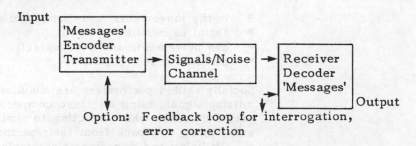

Such a model could stand for many communication systems: radio or television transmission; a nervous system; or, in this case, an interview. A useful procedure arising from the 'system' model is that we can examine its integrity. In other words, we can see what happens when one part of the system is distorted or eliminated.

In this model, 'message' is taken to stand for that which we wish to transmit. Embedded in this is the difficult problem of meaning, and an obvious use of the model is to compare inputs and outputs according to some criterion of meaningfulness. Such a comparison is the basis of an often hilarious game in which the distortion occurring when a 'message' is passed along a line of people by word of mouth is examined. Bartlett (1972) showed in his method of serial reproduction the simplifications and intrusions which occur in this process.

Within the interview, 'meaning' arises at a number of levels. First, it arises at the level of verbal content. What was the question and what is the answer? Much has been written about asking the right sort of question in an interview, whether to use direct or indirect questions, the appropriate form of words, and the dangers of certain questions such as leading or multiple forms. Skilful interviewers do not seem to be constrained by rigid rules but show flexibility, constantly probing and following up interesting leads. They tend to ask: 'Tell me', 'When was that?', 'How was that?', 'What did you do?' and perhaps the most difficult question of all, 'Why?'

Second, the question of meaning arises at the level of recording the interview material. What gets lost or distorted when an interviewer distils a reply into notes or makes a decision? Third, a consideration arising especially in the research interview is: what has happened to the original meaning when a response is coded, probably into a pre-determined category, and is lumped together with others when the study is reported?

However, the verbal content of the message is only a small part of the signal. Many researchers assert that the non-verbal component of a signal is of greater importance. Argyle (1973, 1975) in particular has drawn our attention to the role of non-verbal communication factors such as:

* bodily movements: body language: gestures;
* facial expression;
* eye movements and eye contact;
* personal space: proximity.

Socially skilled performers are simultaneously transmitting signals using all these components together with verbal material whilst reacting to similar signals constituting feedback from their partners.

Utilizing and decoding this complex of information involves us in consideration of interpersonal perception, a key area in the analysis of interviewing. How we form judgements about other people is at the heart of interview decisions: the substantial literature on this topic, for example Cook (1979), suggests that the information we use includes:

* a person's actions;
* the situation in which the person is observed;
* appearance (including facial expression, physique, speech characteristics and dress style);
* non-verbal cues mentioned previously.

The powerful influence of some cues is seen most clearly in the study of stereotypes. Picking up one piece of information and building often unwarranted assumptions upon it is the classic error in judging others. Reacting to a regional accent, to hair colour, to ethnic origin or any other isolated item is all too common. Such a reaction, especially to irrelevant information, is usually dubbed the 'halo effect'. Since the judge or interviewer is striving for cognitive consistency, information is often interpreted in such a way that it fits this single judgement. Thus favourable material or even attributions will be ascribed to a liked person. Contrariwise, undue weight may be given to negative indications in the case of dislike. Clearly, interviewers must be constantly on their guard against introducing bias of this kind. Awareness of their prejudices and the sorts of errors we make in judging others will help.

It is the process component of interviewing which has received most attention in the training of interviewers. Such training commonly takes the form of general social skills training together with exercises directed at the specialization of the interviewer; for example, obtaining clinically relevant material in the hospital setting. Just how effective training may be is not easy to assess. Largely this is so because published studies of interview training tend to use different criteria, thus making comparisons difficult. The benefits to the trainee probably come from receiving informed feedback in role-playing or group tasks about their performance together with enhanced self-awareness.

Content

The point has been made that the absence of a shared common aim or the lack of a clear plan in an interview leads to many difficulties. Specifically, criticisms in terms of interview decisions tend to the view that they may leave much to be desired. It is claimed, for example, that the research literature points overwhelmingly in this direction. Without wishing to dismiss the many studies leading to this conclusion, it must be pointed out that they cover a wide range of interview outcomes made by many interviewers at different levels of experience and training with their decisions based on imprecise criteria. The message of these studies seems to be that all concerned with interviews should be aware of the shortcomings and take steps to overcome them. Apart from errors arising from factors already mentioned in describing context and process aspects at an interview, the principal source is often the lack of a clear plan for an interview; in other words, content must be tailored to the particular aim in mind, each interview requiring careful planning with preparation related to a desired outcome. By way of illustration let us consider the content of interviews within the three professional contexts of counselling, job interviews and research interviewing.

COUNSELLING: OCCUPATIONAL GUIDANCE. What is the aim of an occupational guidance procedure? At one time the approach was modelled upon the notion of talent matching: specify the job, specify the person and attempt to match the two. On the job side of the equation, techniques of task analysis, job description and content specification were developed whilst evidence of congruent relevant behaviour was sought from the interviewee. It is no coincidence that the heyday of this approach coincided with the early boom in psychological test production. Aptitude tests, occupational interest guides, and tests of specific skills were all produced to aid the matching. Today, with the application of computer-based matching procedures, the approach is enjoying a revival. The role of the interview in this model was largely to establish the congruence of job and applicant profiles by comparison through discussion. From this approach evolved the contemporary developmental model, with an emphasis on career decision making as a process over time, starting in the early years with educational counselling, proceeding to occupational counselling and then to career development counselling, with perhaps counselling for retirement in later years. Thus there may be many interviews within this model each with a specific aim, the sum aimed at the overall development of the individual. Among the sub-goals of this process we can recognize the following:

* self-appraisal: equipping the client to achieve realistic self-assessment;
* self-perception: providing frames of reference, categories of occupationally significant behaviours;
* job perception: acquiring the skills required to assess the world of work in terms of job content, values, roles and life style;
* reality testing: matching aspirations and goals with opportunities within one's limitations;
* setting goals and objectives: specifying attainable goals and precise objectives;
* hypothesis generation: helping the client to generate occupational 'theories';
* interaction of the person and the job environment: examining the complexities of the person/work situation interaction;
* sharing information: providing the client with educational and occupational information, and providing the counsellor with perceptions of the client;
* task setting: translating immediate goals into discrete tasks, such as finding an address, seeking information, reading a pamphlet, etc.

The task of the interviewer/counsellor therefore becomes that of achieving these goals at the appropriate time and in a manner which meets the client's needs. Flexibility, wide background knowledge and the ability to relate to the client are clearly prerequisites on the part of the counsellor. Similar goals are shared by modern staff appraisal schemes and staff development procedures.

JOB INTERVIEWS. Being interviewed for a job, for promotion

or for annual assessment is probably the most commonly
experienced form of interview. It has certainly attracted a
substantial body of folk-lore, myth, jokes and hard-luck
stories. That this is so is, in itself, of considerable
psychological significance. The job interview comes in many
varieties, not least the panel interview. Here especially
the crucial importance of planning an interview is seen. The
justifiable criticism of such encounters is frequently due
first to poor interviewing skills on the part of the individual board members, and second to the lack of an agreed
role for each.

Whilst not normally included under the heading of
interviews, such behavioural observation techniques as role-
playing by candidates, group discussions, problem-solving
exercises and others raise the same problems previously
mentioned of reliable and valid judgements about other
people.

Two examples of interview plans used in job interviews
will be presented here: one is a general approach commonly
employed, namely, the biography; the second a well-known
technique called the Seven-Point Plan.

1. The biography: the majority of job interviews employ
this approach, often, however, in an undisciplined fashion,
hunting and pecking at a person's history. However, a simple
structure which can be readily shared consists of establishing landmarks within relevant areas; commonly times of
change such as leaving school. Bearing in mind the selec-
tivity of recall, in itself an important indicator within an
interview, and that the recent past may be more accessible,
one should not expect uniform coverage of a life history.
This raises the problem of breadth and depth within the
interview in relation to the relevance of the information.
Too often an interviewer will spend time on an irrelevant
area, missing the opportunity to explore a significant point
in detail.

However, a plan such as that shown in figure 3 provides
a secure frame of reference for interviewer and interviewee.
Not least, the interviewee can be assembling information
and anticipating questions; the task is not unlike talking
through a curriculum vitae. A final benefit of this approach
is that it enables the interviewer to check dates, spot gaps
in the account and draw out the inter-relationships between

Figure 3

	Education	Interests	Home	Work
The past	Dates			
Landmarks				
The present				

events. This approach is underpinned by application forms and curricula vitae, which are customarily set out in biographical order.

2. The Seven-Point Plan: probably the best known of all assessment and interview formats, the plan was originally developed by Alec Rodger within the framework of the talent matching approach to occupational guidance. It was intended to apply to both candidates and jobs, to obtain relevant information about people and, by asking the same questions of a job, to facilitate matching.

The plan was rapidly adopted for job interviewing and has undoubtedly been highly influential in so far as it provides the unskilled interviewer with a robust, easily understood framework within which to work. Over the years, a number of modifications have been suggested to the original plan. Similarly based schemes have been published, but what is essentially the original is presented here (Rodger, 1974).

1. Physical characteristics:
   Physical abilities of occupational importance.
   State of health. Vision, hearing. Appearance. Speech.
2. Attainments (and previous experience):
   Educational background, achievements. Occupational and professional training. Experience. How well has this person done? Personal achievements in any area: sports, pursuits, etc.
3. General ability:
   Especially general intelligence and cognitive skills – words, numbers, relationships.
4. Special aptitudes:
   Particularly occupationally applicable talents – scientific, mechanical, mathematical, practical, literary, artistic, social skills.
5. Interests:
   Often the core information: type of interests, how they are pursued, to what effect. Intellectual, practical, physical, social and artistic interests may be occupationally significant.
6. Personality:
   What is this person like? Especially in terms of self-perception. Social relationships, behaviour indicative of self-reliance, dependability.
7. Circumstances:
   The context of the person's life in so far as it affects his aspirations. Family circumstances, financial background, current problems.

The first six points apply particularly to the study of jobs. What physical characteristics, what attainments and so on are required for this job? It should be added that Rodger emphasized the importance of paying attention to individual likes and dislikes, to difficulties or distastes mentioned by people, and to the individual's strengths and weaknesses when applying the plan; in particular, stressing the importance of negative information in making selection decisions and the noting of danger signs.

Finally, in considering job interviews it should be noted that advice and preparation for interviewees is widely available in relation to the job interview. Social skills training and self-presentation courses are examples.

RESEARCH INTERVIEWS. The place of the interview in social research is central. Its contribution ranges from preliminary information gathering to a place as the principal research tool. Clearly it takes many forms but the main dimension along which it varies is that of being unstructured/structured, from free to semi-structured to structured. Here, the highly structured form typically found in market research and surveys is considered, the characteristics of the unstructured form being similar to counselling interviews. For the structured approach a unique feature is the use of an interview schedule: in effect, a carefully prepared script meticulously adhered to by the interviewer. A great deal of thought is put into preparing the schedule in order that question form and content, question order, response mode, use of response aids and other factors can be taken into account.

Customarily these factors are checked by conducting pilot studies. Another feature of research interviewing is the attention paid to teaching interviewers how to present a particular schedule, together with supervision of their work in the field. Finally, since it is often the case that large numbers of respondents are involved, it is usual to design the schedules with data analysis in mind: for example, the coding of responses by interviewers for data entry.

As an example of research interviewing the approach of the Government Social Survey is now described. The Social Survey began work dealing with wartime problems of the 1940s. It is now a Division of the Office of Population Censuses and Surveys carrying out a wide range of studies of social and economic interest for public departments. A detailed description of the practices and procedures it employs is to be found in the handbook for interviewers (Atkinson, 1971).

Steps in producing such surveys include:

* identifying research question: decide on form and content of survey, consider costs;
* draft proposals: content of schedule, sampling of respondents;
* pilot stage: explore degree of structure appropriate, such as free to highly. Coding of replies. Analyse pilot material;
* brief and train interviewers: careful training including practice on schedule. How to contact the public. Identifying the person to be interviewed (e.g. by age,

sex, role). Putting over the purpose of the survey; problem of refusals or lack of co-operation. Conducting the interview: defining the roles of interviewer and informant;

* timetable: prepare addresses, number of interviewees, target dates;
* carry out field survey: interviewers adhere to research officers' instructions on each question. Comprehend the purpose of each question: (i) factual information; (ii) expression of opinion; (iii) attitude measures.
Deploy response modes without distortion: open questions with free response, closed/forward choice questions with pre-coded or scaled responses. Interviewers practise use of response aids: prompt cards for scaled responses, self-completion scales, repertory grids, examples of products in market research.
Interviewers pay particular attention to prompting and probing. Guard against distortion in recording data: both precoded and open response items are susceptible;
* coding: check schedules and categorize response;
* computing: produce tables, analyse data;
* conclusion: write report.

Purpose

At this stage in the discussion of our model of an interview it must be clear that so many varieties exist as to demand careful consideration of each in terms of purpose. The variety of purposes has been mentioned, and also that the approach may vary from structured to unstructured according to purpose. Thus a number of recognizable forms of interview have emerged to meet particular needs. Examples include:

* non-directive counselling, client-centred therapy;
* psychotherapeutic encounters of many kinds;
* depth interviews emphasizing motivational factors;
* group interviews involving a number of respondents in a discussion group type format;
* psychological testing, especially individual tests such as WAIS (Wechsler Adult Intelligence Scale);
* problem-solving interviews such as individual role-playing for a variety of purposes.

Consequences

Accepting the purposive nature of the interview implies that outcomes are important for all concerned and that their nature depends on the situation, and not least how the situation is perceived. For the interviewer, this will involve achieving the particular aims which have been identified together with maintenance of professional competence; for example, in the research interview maintaining the validity, reliability and precision of data with errors eliminated as far as possible.

For the interviewee or respondent one might ask: what do they get out of the experience? All too often what might be called the public relations aspect of interviewing is ignored. Symptoms of this include fears on the part of correspondents regarding the confidentiality of data, or that in some way they are being threatened. Such considerations appear to bring us full circle, for if attention is paid to the initiation stage of the proceedings by way of setting the scene such alarms can be reduced. Nevertheless, the sometimes necessary use of subterfuge in research needs to be handled with great care, a minimum requirement being the provision of an adequate explanation after the event or an account of the research.

References

Argyle, M. (1973)
Social Interaction. London: Tavistock.

Argyle, M. (1975)
Bodily Communication. London: Methuen.

Atkinson, J. (1971)
A Handbook for Interviewers (2nd edn). London: HMSO.

Bartlett, F.C. (1932)
Remembering. Cambridge: Cambridge University Press.

Cook, M. (1979)
Perceiving Others. London: Methuen.

Orne, M.T. (1962)
On the social psychology of the psychological experiment. American Psychologist, 17, 776-783.

Rodger, A. (1974)
Seven Point Plan. London: NFER.

Rosenthal, R. and Rosnow, R.L. (1969)
The volunteer subject. In R. Rosenthal and R.L. Rosnow (eds), Artifact in Behavioral Research. New York: Academic Press.

9
Personality and individual assessment
P. Kline

In this chapter we examine individual differences among human beings, how such differences are measured, and the psychological implications of such differences for understanding personality and behaviour. First of all we discuss psychological tests and testing techniques, for it is by the application of these measures that individual differences have been discovered.

Characteristics of good psychological tests and how these may be achieved

Efficient testing devices must be (i) reliable, (ii) valid and (iii) discriminating.

Reliability

Reliability has two meanings: first, self-consistency. Tests must be self-consistent; each item should measure the same variable. An instrument, for example, which measured in part pressure as well as temperature would not give a reliable measurement of either of these. The second meaning is consistency over time: that is, test-retest reliability. If a test is administered a second time to a person then, unless a real change has taken place, the score on the two occasions should be the same. Reliability is measured by the correlation coefficient, an index of agreement running from +1 (perfect agreement) to -1 (perfect disagreement). A correlation of 0 shows random agreement. Good tests should have a reliability coefficient of at least 0.7 which represents 49 per cent agreement (square the coefficient).

1. FACTORS INFLUENCING RELIABILITY

* Test length: it can be shown that reliability increases with the length of a test. The typical university essay exam has only four items (four essays) and is thus not highly reliable. To increase reliability, most psychological tests have a large number of items. Twenty items are about the minimum necessary for reliability.
* Objective scoring: scores should be objective: that is, there should be no personal judgement required of the scorer. Where judgement is required, as in essays, differences arise, often large, between different markers and with the same markers if they rescore the

test. A good test has items that are objectively scored.

If a test is reliable then it can be valid. Notice the 'can'. It is possible to devise a highly reliable test that measures virtually nothing. A test for measuring the length of people's noses would be easy to devise and would be highly reliable, but it is unlikely to be a valid test of intelligence or personality. On the other hand, an unreliable, inconsistent test which gives different scores on different occasions cannot possibly be valid.

Validity

A test is said to be valid if it measures what it claims to measure. This may sound obvious but many tests are quite invalid. For example, essay-type tests of scientific subjects are highly unlikely to be valid since essay writing demands verbal ability, and ability in physics is somewhat different from this. The term validity is used in psychological testing (psychometrics) in several ways.

1. FACE VALIDITY: this refers to the appearance of a test which is said to be face valid if it looks as if it measures what it claims to measure. This is important in testing adults who may balk at doing tests which look absurd. They may simply refuse to co-operate or even treat the test as a bit of a joke. Children, however, are used to overlooking such niceties. Face validity is not usually related to true validity.

2. CONCURRENT VALIDITY: this refers to studies of the validity of a test made on one occasion. For example, the concurrent validity of a new test of intelligence would be assessed by its correlation with well-established intelligence tests; does the new test give a similar score to the score on an existing test? Concurrent validity studies are beset by problems of criteria: what tests or other measurement should be used in establishing the concurrent validity of a test? If other similar tests are used, and the correlation is very high, the question arises as to what value the new test has since it is measuring the same variable as the old.

3. PREDICTIVE VALIDITY: this refers to the capacity of a test to correlate with some future criterion measure. This can be the most powerful evidence for the validity of a test. Some examples will clarify this point. A good test of anxiety should be able to predict future attendance at the psychiatric clinic, and a good test of intelligence given at 11 years of age should correlate with future academic performance in GCE examinations and subsequently. Thus the test predicts events external to itself.

4. CONSTRUCT VALIDITY: the construct validity of a test

is defined by taking a large set of results obtained with the test and seeing how well they fit in with our notion of the psychological nature of the variable which the test claims to measure. Thus it embraces concurrent and predictive validity. In effect, we set up a series of hypotheses concerning the test results and put these to the test. For example, if our test was a valid measure of intelligence we might expect:

*   high-level professional groups would score more highly than lower-level professionals;
*   children rated highly intelligent by teachers would score more highly than others;
*   scores would correlate positively with level of education;
*   scores would correlate highly with scores in public examinations;
*   scores would correlate highly with scores on other intelligence tests;
*   scores would not correlate with scores on tests not claiming to measure intelligence.

If all these hypotheses were supported then the construct validity of our test would be demonstrated. It is deserving of note that it is always useful to show (as in the final point above) what tests do not measure, a technique used by Socrates in his examination of the meaning of words.

Unlike reliability, for which there can be clear unequivocal evidence, the validity of a test is to some extent subjective. Nevertheless, most well-known tests, especially of ability, have now accumulated so much evidence relating to validity that there is no dispute about them. It is more difficult to demonstrate the validity of personality tests but, as we see later, it can be done. Many psychological tests have little support for their validity and a large number are clearly invalid.

Discriminatory power

Good psychological tests should be discriminating: that is, they should produce a wide distribution of scores. For example, if we test 10 children and all score 15 we have made no discriminations at all. If four score 13, three score 12 and three score 14 then we have made only three discriminations. If, on the other hand, each child scores a different score, then the distribution of scores is wide. The scatter of scores in a distribution is known as the variance and the standard deviation is the usual measurement. A good test has a large standard deviation.

With reliable, valid and discriminating tests it is possible to investigate the nature of individual differences in human beings. In fact, this has been going on since the turn of the century when Binet began the assessment of the educability of Parisian children.

ypes of tests and
ategories of individual
fferences

Individual differences among human beings fall into relatively independent categories for which different types of
tests have been developed.

Intelligence and ability tests

The most important ability as studied by psychometrists is
general intelligence, the ability to educe correlates; a
general reasoning ability which underlies much problem-
solving ability. Modern studies of this general reasoning
factor (e.g. Cattell, 1971) tend to reveal two aspects: (i)
fluid ability which is close to inherited reasoning ability;
and (ii) crystallized ability, which is fluid ability as it
is evinced in a culture. The old-fashioned 11+ intelligence
tests were largely concerned with crystallized ability. More
will be said later about intelligence.

Other typical abilities are: verbal ability, V; numerical ability, N; and spatial ability, K. Performance on
various tasks will depend upon our status on these variables. For example, a writer and an engineer may both score
much the same on general intelligence, but on verbal ability
the writer should be higher, whereas on numerical and spatial ability the engineer should be superior. Intelligence
can be thought of as a general factor, while verbal and
numerical ability are group factors. Intelligence plays its
part in almost all skills, while verbal ability is involved
only in certain groups. Some factors are more narrow than
this; auditory pitch discrimination would be an example.

Aptitude tests

Aptitude tests comprise a group of tests related to tests of
ability. Aptitude tests tend to be of two different kinds.
One type may be identical with the group tests discussed
above. Thus it would be difficult to distinguish between
verbal ability and verbal aptitude. However, computer
aptitude tests are clearly different; they should test the
collection of traits (perhaps more than just abilities)
necessary for this particular job. In some instances, such
as clerical aptitude, the necessary skills are quite disparate and unrelated to each other. Generally, aptitude
tests measure the separate abilities demonstrated to be
important for a particular job or class of jobs.

Personality tests

Personality tests can be divided into tests of temperament,
mood and dynamics. Temperament tests measure how we do
what we do. Temperamental traits, such as dominance and
anxiety, are usually thought of as enduring and stable.
Dynamic traits are concerned with motives; why we do what we
do. These attempt to measure drives such as sexuality or
pugnacity. Moods refer to those fluctuating states that we
all experience in our lives: anger, fatigue or fear.

Temperament tests

The most used type of temperament test is the personality

questionnaire. These consist of lists of items concerned with the subject's behaviour. Typical items are: do you enjoy watching boxing? Do you hesitate before spending a large sum of money? Items come in various formats. Those above would usually require subjects to respond 'Yes' or 'No'; or 'Yes', 'Uncertain' or 'No'. Sometimes items are of the forced choice variety; for example, 'Do you prefer: (i) watching boxing; (ii) going to a musical; or (iii) sitting quietly at home reading?'

The disadvantages of questionnaires are considerable, yet in spite of them many valid and highly useful personality questionnaires have been constructed. These disadvantages are outlined below.

* They are easy to fake: that is, subjects may not tell the truth for one reason or another. This makes them difficult to use in selection, although for vocational guidance or psychiatric help, where subjects have no reason to fake, this is not too serious.
* They require a degree of self-knowledge and some subjects, while attempting to be honest, may respond quite unrealistically.
* They are subject to response sets. An important set is social desirability, the tendency to endorse the socially desirable response. People like to present themselves in the best possible light. For example, to the item 'Do you have a good sense of humour?', the response 'Yes' would be given by about 95 per cent of subjects. The other serious response set is that of acquiescence; the tendency to put 'Yes' or 'Agree' to an answer, regardless of content. Balanced scales, with some responses keyed 'No', obviate this to some extent.

OBJECTIVE TESTS: these, defined by Cattell (cf. Cattell and Kline, 1977) as tests of which the purpose is hidden from the subject and which can be objectively scored (see the section on reliability), have been developed to overcome the disadvantages of questionnaires. Ironically, because their purpose is hidden from subjects, considerable research is necessary to establish their validity and as yet most are still in an experimental form. These tests will probably take over from questionnaires when the necessary research has been done. The following examples indicate their nature.

* Balloon blowing: subjects are required to inflate a balloon as much as they can. Measures taken are the size of the balloon, time taken in blowing it up, whether they burst it, and delay in beginning the task. This test may be related to timidity and inhibition.
* The slow-line drawing test: subjects are required to draw a line as slowly as possible. The measure is the length of line over a fixed time.

In fact more than 800 such tests have been listed and more can easily be developed, depending upon the ingenuity of the researcher. The technique is to administer a large battery of such tests and to determine experimentally by so-called validity studies what each of them measures.

PROJECTIVE TESTS: these essentially consist of ambiguous stimuli to which the subjects have to respond. These are some of the oldest personality tests and one, the Rorschach test (the inkblot test), has achieved a fame beyond psychology. The rationale of projective tests is intuitively brilliant: if a stimulus is so vague that it warrants no particular description, then any description of it must depend on what is projected on to it by the subject. Projective testers believe that projective tests measure the inner needs and fantasies of their subjects.

A serious problem with projective tests lies in their unreliability. Responses have to be interpreted by scorers and often considerable training, experience and expertise is necessary. Inter-marker reliability is low. Generally, too, it is difficult to demonstrate test validity. However, the present writer has experimented with entirely objective forms of scoring these tests and some evidence has now accrued that this is a useful procedure.

PROJECTIVE TEST STIMULI: although any ambiguous stimulus could be used as a test, the choice of stimulus is generally determined by the particular theory of personality which the test constructor follows. For example, a psychoanalytically-orientated psychologist would select stimuli relevant to that theory, such as vague figures who could be mother and son (the Oedipus complex) or figures with knives or scissors (the castration complex). The TAT (Thematic Apperception Test) developed by Murray uses pictures which, it is hoped, tap the inner needs held by Murray to be paramount in human behaviour.

Mood and motivation tests
Mood and motivation tests are essentially similar to temperament tests, but relatively little work has been done with these and their validity is not so widely attested as that of temperament tests.

Mood tests generally use items that concentrate, as might be expected, on present feelings rather than on usual ones. With these, high test-retest reliability is not to be expected. However, fluctuations in scores should not be random but should be related to external conditions. Thus experiments can be conducted in which the tests, if they are valid, can be retaken. If the experimental manipulations are good and the tests valid, the relevant scores should change in response to these changes in mood.

The results of motivation tests should be similarly fluctuating, according to whether drives are satisfied or frustrated. In one study the scores of a single subject over a 28-day period were related to a diary recording all that happened to her and everything she felt or thought (Kline and Grindley, 1974). In fact, the relation of scores to diary events was close. For example, the fear drive rose each weekend when the subject went touring in a dangerous car. The career drive was flat except on the day when the subject was interviewed for a course in teacher-training, and so on.

Motivation tests can be of the questionnaire variety, although objective and projective tests are more frequently used. For moods, questionnaire tests are more usually employed though they suffer, of course, from the same response sets as bedevil questionnaire measures of temperamental traits.

Interest tests
The tests of motivation described above are very general: that is, they measure variables thought to account for a wide variety of human behaviour. Vocational and industrial psychologists, however, have long felt the need for more specific measures of motivation, assessing the variables which seemed of immediate relevance to them: for instance, interests. We all know of motoring enthusiasts who seem to have an all-embracing interest in cars, which seems to account for much of their behaviour and conversation.

A number of interest tests have been developed which attempt to assess the major interests such as outdoor, mechanical, or interest in people. In some tests, the scoring of items is in terms of occupational groups. The performance of particular occupational groups on the tests is known and if, for example, foresters score high on a particular item then this item contributes to the 'interest in forestry' score. In other tests, the scoring involves little more than subjects having to rank jobs. In other words, interest tests of this type are like formalized interviews.

Generally, the correlations of interest test scores with success in a job relevant to those interests are modest and little better than the correlation obtained between job success and the subject's response to the question of whether the job would be enjoyable or not.

Attitude tests
Social psychologists have attempted to measure attitudes for many years now. Usually, the attitudes tested apply to important aspects of an individual's life: for example, attitudes to war, or to coloured people (in white populations) or to religion. Obviously, if efficient measures of such attitudes are possible then progress can be made in understanding how such attitudes arise or are maintained; important knowledge, it is thought, in a complex multi-racial society. There are three kinds of attitude test, differing in their mode of construction.

1. THE THURSTONE SCALES: in these tests items are given to the judges to rank 1-11 (favourable-unfavourable) in respect of an attitude. Items on which there is good agreement among the judges are then retained. The subject then taking the test is given the highest judged rank score of the items with which he agrees. The reason for this is clear if we consider a few examples. (1) 'War is totally evil' would probably be ranked high as unfavourable to war. (2) 'Wars sometimes have to be fought if there is no alternative': this is clearly against war, but not strongly. (3) 'Wars are not always wrong': this is yet further down the scale, while the item (4) 'Wars are good: they select the finest nations' is favourable. Thus a subject who agreed with (1) would not agree with (2), (3) or (4). Similarly, a subject agreeing with (3) would not agree with (4). These tests are difficult to construct because much depends on obtaining a good cross-section of judges. A more simple alternative is the Likert scale.

2. LIKERT SCALES: in the Likert scales statements relevant to the attitude being measured are presented to the subject who has to state on a five-point scale the extent of his agreement. Thus a 'Hitler' would score 100 on a 20-item attitude to war scale. A 'Ghandi' would score zero, one presumes. To make the scale less obvious, items are so written that to agree with items represents both poles of the attitude.

3. THE GUTTMAN SCALE: this is a scale constructed so that if the items are ranked for positive attitude, then any subject who endorses item 10 will also endorse items 1-9 below it. While this tends to happen by nature of its construction with the Thurstone scale, such perfect ordering of items can usually only be achieved by leaving huge gaps between the items (in terms of attitude) which means few items and rather coarse measurement.

Such, then are the main types of psychological tests with which individual differences are measured in psychology. Needless to say, these are not the only kinds of test. In the remainder of this chapter we briefly describe some intelligence tests, discuss some of the substantive findings that have emerged from these tests and examine their application in practical psychology.

Intelligence tests

Intelligence has been most widely studied of all test variables and, since it is a topic of considerable importance in applied psychology and education, let us examine in detail some intelligence tests to help us to understand the nature of intelligence as conceptualized by psychologists.

Individual intelligence tests

Some intelligence tests are given to subjects individually. This enables the tester to measure not only the intelligence

117

of the subject but also to see whether a child panics at difficulties or goes on and on obsessionally even when it is obvious that no solution will result. Similarly, it can be seen whether an individual is easily distracted, and all this is valuable in attempting to understand any educational difficulties which may arise.

The WISC

The Wechsler Intelligence Scale, WISC (Wechsler, 1938), consists of the following sub-tests which fall into two groups: verbal tests and non-verbal tests. A total IQ score is obtainable, as are a verbal IQ and a performance IQ. Large differences between these two sub-scores are of some psychological interest and call for further study. Some of our examples are taken from Kline (1976).

1. THE VERBAL TESTS

*   Vocabulary: a straightforward vocabulary test. Vocabulary is highly related to intelligence although social class differences in reading habits do, obviously, affect this particular sub-test. Nevertheless, if forced to make a selection of intelligent children or adults as quickly as possible, the vocabulary sub-test would be about the best measure obtainable.
*   Information: a test of general knowledge.
*   Arithmetic: an ordinary arithmetic test.

These three tests are heavily affected by school learning and social class. They therefore reflect what Cattell called crystallized intelligence, or the result of cultural influences upon innate ability.

*   Comprehension: this is an interesting test because it presents problems which are dependent upon how much the child is capable of making sensible decisions on its own initiative. One example (which is not in the test) might be a question like 'What would you do if you saw a burglar in the house next door?' Two points would be scored by a response such as 'Phone the police - dial 999'; one point by the response 'Run and tell Mummy', and no points by 'Shoot him with my bow and arrow' or 'Push his car over'. At the higher level this sub-test requires abstract analytical reasoning on such questions as 'Why is there a Hippocratic oath?'
*   Similarities: a common form of intelligence test item, simple to write and easy to vary the level of difficulty. For example, 'What is similar about peaches and prunes?' The correct response requires that the essential similarity (fruit) is recognized.
*   Digit span (forward and reverse): digits are read out and the subjects repeat them immediately. Seven or eight digits is the usual span for bright adults.

In the majority of cases most psychologists give five of the six tests, the last two of which in part measure fluid ability.

2. THE NON-VERBAL TESTS: these are generally quite novel to most subjects, so they are more a measure of fluid (inherited) ability than are the verbal tests. Large disparities between the verbal and performance score are often found in middle-class children whose upbringing is highly verbal. The performance sub-tests are as follows.

* Block design: patterns are presented to the child in a booklet and he must then make them up by arranging building blocks such that their top surfaces represent the pattern. This test can be made of varying difficulty. It is also one which indicates well how a child tackles a strange problem.
* Picture arrangement: here series of strip cartoons tell stories. Each series is presented in jumbled order and the child must put them in their correct sequence: a neat way of testing a child's ability to work out the relationships involved.
* Object assembly: this is a timed jigsaw-like task of arranging broken patterns.
* Mazes: the child is required to trace the way through pencil and paper mazes.
* Coding: here the key to a simple cipher system is given. The child then completes as many examples as possible (presented in random order) in a fixed time.
* Picture completion: pictures with a missing element, often only a small detail, are shown to the subject who is required to spot this.

This, then, is the Wechsler Intelligence Scale, one of the standard individual intelligence tests. The verbal and performance IQ scores are highly reliable, as is the total score: all around 0.9 or beyond.

The WISC is an individual test. It is obviously not suitable for group administration. Let us now look at some item types used in group intelligence tests (rather than examine any one test in detail) since these are widely used in applied psychology.

roup intelligence tests

Items can be verbal or non-verbal, testing largely fluid or crystallized ability.

1. ANALOGIES

Easy: a is to c as g is to ...
            sparrow is to bird as mouse is to ...

Difficult: Samson Agonistes is to Comus as the
            Bacchae are to ...

With analogy items all kinds of relationships may be tested, as in the examples where we find sequence, classification, double classification (by author and type of play, for example), and opposites. Analogy is thus a useful form for encapsulating a wide variety of relationships. We can use shapes for this type of item, as distinct from verbal forms.

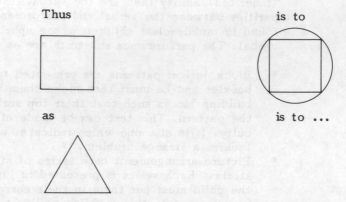

Thus   is to

as   is to ...

Here we would supply possible answers in multiple choice form, for example:

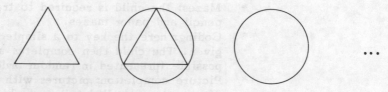

2. ODD-MEN-OUT

Odd-men-out items also allow us to test wide varieties of relationships in many materials. Some examples are given below.

* carrot, turnip, swede, beetroot, cabbage
* valley, coomb, hillock, gorge, chasm
* early, greasy, messy, swiftly, furry

For these three examples some knowledge is required of vegetables, geography and grammar, but this alone is not enough.

3. SIMILARITIES

These are essentially the same item form (where the common relationship must be worked out), but are more difficult to write for a group test, because the multiple choice answer will give the game away.
Non-verbal odd-men-out items are simple to produce; see the following examples.

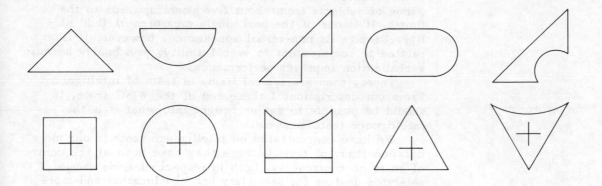

4. SEQUENCES AND MATRICES

Numbers, of course, offer easy ways of creating complex
relationships without needing any special knowledge of
mathematics and hence sequences are a useful item form. For
example, 20, 40, 60, 80 ... is entirely unequivocal. Sequences allow also for the development of highly complex or
multiple relationships.

A matrix involving several sequences might be of the
following form:

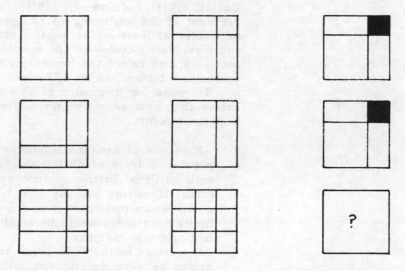

followed by a multiple choice

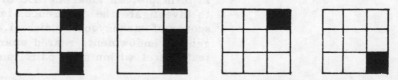

Raven's Matrices is an example of a test composed entirely of such sets of non-verbal items. Many forms have been produced and it is capable of extending the intelligence of subjects from about five years upwards to the limits. It is one of the best single measures of fluid ability. Despite its non-verbal appearance, however, it is related to some extent to verbal ability, presumably because verbalization improves performance.

These, then are typical items in tests of intelligence. From our description of these and of the WISC scale, it should be possible to get an insight into what it is that intelligence tests measure.

We have concentrated on intelligence tests in our more detailed study of tests because they have been at the centre of so much controversy, both in respect of their use as selection devices for secondary school education and more recently in respect of the heritability of success in these tests. It is to this latter topic, which is of great social importance and intellectual interest, that we now turn, a further reason for ensuring that the nature of such tests is fully appreciated.

The heritability of intelligence test scores

This is so large and complex a subject that inevitably our summary must be somewhat assertive and dogmatic. To make it even more difficult, well-known writers reviewing the same evidence come to opposite conclusions. For example, Cattell (1971) and Eysenck (1971) conclude that about 80 per cent of the variance in intelligence test scores is heritable, at least in the west. Kamin (1974), reviewing the same evidence, comes to the conclusion that there are no sound data to reject the hypothesis that differences in test scores are determined by different life experiences.

To make our discussion of this matter comprehensible rather than comprehensive let us first establish a number of important points.

* All results of heritability studies refer only to the population from which the sample was drawn. Thus results in Great Britain are not applicable in other cultures. If culture has any effect, then in a country with a diverse cultural background (such as India) the heritability index would be smaller than in a more homogeneous culture.
* All workers in the field argue that there is an interaction between genetic and environmental determinants of intelligence test scores. Where there is disagreement is in the matter of how large is the influence of each factor.
* In principle, an ideal method of studying the topic is to investigate the differences in intelligence test scores of monozygotic twins (i.e. twins with the same genetic endowment) reared apart. All differences in test scores within such pairs must be environmentally

determined (ignoring differential effects of placental deprivations, etc., in such pairs which would exaggerate any differences).

Critics of this approach argue that it is vitiated by the fact that twins are, by definition, a different population from singleton children. Furthermore, there is a tendency for identical twins to be placed in foster homes similar to each other, thus making their scores similar.

* Burt carried out the most extensive twin studies. His data, however, must be ignored. It appears, alas, that he doctored the figures.
* However, other twin studies show the same results, namely that in America and Great Britain there is a substantial hereditary component in the determination of test scores, the critical finding being that identical twins reared apart show less differences in intelligence test scores than do non-identical twins reared together.
* Kamin's (1974) arguments attempting to refute these results are statistically weak, as has been fully exposed by Fulker (1975).
* More sophisticated methods of statistical analyses known as biometric genetic methods, which have been demon- strated as powerful in animal work, have been employed in the study of human intelligence test scores. These can assess the kind of gene action and the mating system in the population by analysing within and between family differences and their interactions. The results of these methods are difficult to impugn and it appears from such studies that: (i) around 70 per cent of the variance in IQ score is heritable in Great Britain and the USA; (ii) there is a polygenic dominance for IQ and that assorta- tive mating is an important influence.
* Such biometric methods can be applied to any variable to reveal its heritability. The major personality vari- ables such as extraversion, neuroticism and psychoti- cism, are also similarly highly genetically determined.

The factorial description of personality

Factor analysis is a statistical technique for simplifying correlations: this is extremely useful in the study of personality by questionnaires, of which there are very large numbers. Factor analysis reveals dimensions which can mathematically account for the observed correlations. For example, almost all tests of ability are highly correlated together. Factor analysis reveals that this is largely due to the operation of two related factors: fluid and crystallised ability.

Personality questionnaires have been subjected, over the years, to factor analyses in the hope of discovering what are the basic temperamental dimensions. The main research- ers in this area have been Cattell (working in Illinois), Eysenck (in London), both students of Burt, and Guilford (in

California). Although superficially each has produced what looks like a separate set of factors, recent research in this field has enabled some sort of consensus to be arrived at (see Cattell and Kline, 1977, and Kline, 1979, for a full discussion of this work). In effect, the study of individual differences has led to the establishment of the main dimensions of personality. These dimensions are therefore those that demand study. They are outlined below.

Extraversion

The high-scoring extravert is sociable, cheerful, talkative and does not like to be alone. He enjoys excitement, takes risks and is generally impulsive: an outgoing optimist, active and lively. The introvert is the opposite of this: cold, retiring and aloof. This dimension has been related by Eysenck to the arousability of the central nervous system. Scores on tests of this factor have a large genetic component.

Neuroticism (or anxiety)

The highly anxious subject is one who worries a lot, is moody and often depressed. He is highly emotional and takes a long time to calm down. He tends to sleep poorly and to suffer from psychosomatic disorders. This variable is claimed to be related to the lability of the autonomic nervous system. These variables are both measured by the Cattell 16PF test and Eysenck's EPQ. If we know an individual's status on these two factors, then already we know a good deal about his temperament.

Psychoticism

This variable has not been as extensively studied as extraversion and anxiety and only recently (1975) has it appeared in a published questionnaire: the EPQ. Nevertheless, the nature of psychoticism is clear. The high scorer on this dimension is solitary, uncaring of people, troublesome, lacking in human feeling and empathy, thick skinned and insensitive. He is cruel, inhumane, hostile and aggressive, reckless to danger, and aggressive even to his own family. Naturally enough, most normals score low on P but many criminals score high. This factor has been related by Eysenck to masculinity, and to be related to levels of male sex hormones.

It is to be noted that these three factors have not only been clearly identified from the factor analysis of questionnaires: there is also a considerable mass of experimental data supporting their identification and nature.

These are the three second-order factors claimed by Eysenck to be the most important in accounting for temperamental differences. (Second-order factors are factors arising from the correlations among first-order factors; i.e. the factors accounting for the original correlations.) The first-order or primary factors are more problematic than the second-orders but, as the work of Cattell has shown, can be of considerable power in applied psychometrics.

In brief, the factorial analysis of personality has revealed three basic dimensions, each tied to the basic physiology of Man and hence largely heritable.

The study of individual differences, described in this chapter, has implicit within it a model of Man which might be called the psychometric model. Explanation of this model, which is remarkably simple, will make the application of results obvious.

The implicit psychometric model
This model states that any given piece of behaviour is related to that individual's status on the main factors in the sphere of ability, temperament, motivation and mood. This model does not ignore past experience because this itself affects status on these variables. The psychometric model is therefore a variant of a trait model of behaviour. Thus, for example, performance on GCE examinations depends upon intelligence, verbal and numerical ability, extra-version, anxiety, psychoticism, mood at the time of taking the exam and the various motivation variables discussed above (to take the main variables). Obviously, for different behaviours (e.g. exam passing and serving well behind a bar) different weights for each of the factors is required.

How important each factor is - that is, what its weight is - has to be determined empirically. In fact, the statistical technique of multiple correlation or regression does this precisely. Thus, the argument runs, we put all the test variables into a multiple correlation with the criterion and these are then weighted to achieve the highest possible correlation. These weights (beta weights) indicate the relative importance of the variable for the behaviour in question. Cattell and Butcher (1968) have done exactly this with academic success both in America and Great Britain and found multiple correlations around 0.7.

Thus in educational guidance and selection we find the beta weights of the variables and select and guide children accordingly. If X, Y and Z have the highest weights for academic success, then we select and encourage children high on these variables. In industrial psychology, we can choose and guide people to various jobs according to their scores on the highest weighted variables. In clinical psychology, too, we can find the tests most related to psychiatric breakdown or diagnose into clinical groups. Then we know who in the population is at risk and can avoid putting them into stressful condititions.

References

Cattell, R.B. (1971)
Abilities: Their structure, growth and action. New York: Houghton-Mifflin.
Cattell, R.B. and Butcher, H.J. (1968)
The Prediction of Achievement and Creativity. New York: Bobbs Merrill.

Cattell, R.B. and Kline, P. (1977)
The Scientific Analysis of Personality and Motivation.
London: Academic Press.
Eysenck, H.J. (1971)
Race, Intelligence and Education. London: Temple-
Smith.
Fulker, D. (1975)
The science and politics of IQ. American Journal of
Psychology, 88, 505-537.
Kamin, L.J. (1974)
The science and politics of IQ. Harmondsworth: Penguin.
Kline, P. (1976)
Psychological Testing. London: Malaby Press.
Kline, P. (1979)
Psychometrics and Psychology. London: Academic Press.
Kline, P. and Grindley, J. (1974)
A 28-day case study with the MAT. Journal of
Multivariate Clinical Experimental Psychology, 1, 13-32.
Wechsler, D. (1938)
The Wechsler Intelligence Scale for Children. New York:
Psychological Corporation.

10

Other approaches to assessment
John Hall

Other approaches to assessment

Tests are only one form of standardized psychological assessment, but to many people they are probably the most familiar type of psychological assessment procedure. During the Second World War many servicemen took some sort of test when they entered the armed forces; many middle-aged and young British adults took the '11+' examination when they were at school; many nurses have taken some sort of test as part of the selection process to enter a training school.

Some tests are thus particularly associated with psychologists. Indeed the most common stereotype people have of psychologists is probably of their carrying out tests. Many tests are restricted in availability: they can only be acquired by a psychologist or by someone specially trained in their use.

Yet tests are only one way of giving a degree of structure and objectivity to the assessment of people. Several psychologists have tried to classify the various ways in which people can be assessed. Hundleby (1973) suggested eight 'domains' of measurement:

* self-description methods, using interview or questionnaire data;
* ratings or judgement by others;
* life history information, about past events in the individual's life;
* morphology, or body build;
* expressive movement, or habitual styles of everyday behaviour;
* simulated real-life situations, or 'analogue' methods, which may be quite long and complex;
* physiological variables;
* motor-perceptual and performance measures, or performance tests.

This scheme illustrates the wide range of methods that can potentially be used. Some of the domains outlined above are of limited value to nurses interested in assessment; for example, there is now little interest in assessment of morphology, or body build, though psychologists such as Sheldon and Kretschmer carried out extensive investigations into the relationship between body-build and personality.

What sort of assessment is best?

Faced with the range of available methods, how can the best method be chosen? The answer to this question depends on the purpose of the assessment; what decision has to be taken as a result of the assessment? Most decisions in clinical practice can be considered under one of three categories.

In what group does this person fit?

This type of decision is involved in making a diagnosis. The assessment should give information that helps to separate the people under investigation into a set of groups or categories, and hence the assessment seeks to differentiate clearly between the members of these groups.

How good is this person at a particular task?

This type of decision is relevant in deciding whether patients are able to be discharged, or are capable of carrying out some procedure which has implications for their health, such as stoma care. The assessment here is intended to place an individual at some point on a dimension or continuum, along which cut-off points may be inserted to select those people suitable for some treatment or procedure.

Has this person changed?

Most medical treatments are assessed clinically, without the need for special assessment techniques. When a treatment is complex, such as the rehabilitation of people with spinal injuries, it may be helpful to use some assessment procedure to indicate the degree or rate of improvement in the functioning of the limbs. The requirement here is that change in the individual person's behaviour is reflected in changes in the assessment scores.

In clinical practice, the information relevant to these decisions cannot always be obtained from psychological tests. It may, however, be obtained by directly observing the behaviour of the patient in the ward, or in the physiotherapy gymnasium. It may not be obtainable from the doctor, but only from those staff, or indeed family members, who are in regular day-to-day contact with the patient. The information may not even be externally observable, but can be obtained only by using devices which tell us about patterns of activity within the body.

This chapter outlines a number of assessment methods which are widely used by psychologists as well as by other professional staff and which are relevant to the work of nurses. These methods do not require any special professional background for use, although some training is usually required if the methods are to be used to maximum benefit. They clearly offer a valuable form of assessment when no other alternative is readily available as, for example, on a ward in a mental handicap hospital. An attractive feature of many of the methods is that they are flexible, and can be adapted to the needs of the individual researcher or user.

Assessment methods have a number of characteristics which separate them from tests. Intelligence and ability tests commonly assess the person's 'best' performance, whilst other methods usually assess 'typical' performance of the individual. A number of tests involve a highly structured assessment setting, whereas other assessment techniques are carried out in a normal or 'neutral' setting. Most personality and ability tests rely on the person saying or doing something in response to particular questions, and hence the person is aware of being assessed: for other types of assessment, the person may not even be aware of the assessment and thus does not behave any differently from usual.

Despite these differences, the requirements of reliability and validity that apply to tests apply to other modes of assessment. Reliability has been described in the previous chapter as self-consistency. With the types of assessment considered here a major cause of poor consistency is lack of agreement between observers or raters on what they have seen. Hence the degree of agreement between observers, known as inter-observer reliability, is usually the most important type of reliability to check. But even the same observers can vary in their reliability because of tiredness, boredom, or distraction by other tasks; so it can be useful to look at intra-observer reliability as well.

Validity is assessed in the same way as for tests. One way of categorizing validation methods is to distinguish between concurrent validity and predictive validity (see chapter 9).There can be major difficulties in finding suitable independent ways of looking at the person's behaviour to enable concurrent validity to be examined. For example, schizophrenia is difficult to diagnose reliably over the whole range of schizophrenic patients, and any measure of schizophrenia cannot be more valid than the reliability of the diagnosis itself. The validity of an assessment technique can only be established within a particular context: a technique which might be highly valid for one type of decision might not be valid for another which superficially appears similar; for example, a rating scale which proved to be useful in selecting those residents of an old peoples' home who could manage in a warden-supervised hostel might not be useful in selecting patients from a chronic psychiatric ward who were to manage in a group home. Views on the best way to think about validity are changing, and a lot of attention is now being paid to the views of Cronbach, Glesser, Nanda and Rajaratnam (1973). They have introduced the alternative concept of 'generalizability', and this promises a clearer way of looking at the meaning of assessment data.

Types of assessment method

Four main categories of assessment are examined here, covering the first, second, fifth and seventh domains in Hundleby's scheme outlined above.

1. BEHAVIOURAL ASSESSMENT METHODS. These rely on

direct observation and immediate recording of the person's behaviour. They rely on objective categorization of behaviour, with as little interpretation or opinion being required from the observer as possible.

2. CHECK-LISTS AND QUESTIONNAIRES. Some of these were described in the previous chapter with reference to the assessment of personality. Questionnaires have been developed to assess a wide range of categories of behaviour. The term check-list is often used interchangeably with questionnaire or inventory, but the former may be used more specifically to record simply the presence or absence of a symptom or problem, whereas questionnaires characteristically refer to the quality of behaviour.

3. RATING SCALES. These are standardized methods of obtaining opinions or judgements from an observer about a person's behaviour. They may rely on the observer's recollection of several days, or even weeks, of observation, and they may demand a certain degree of interpretation from the observer.

4. PSYCHOPHYSIOLOGICAL TECHNIQUES. These usually involve the recording at the skin surface of physiological events which are mainly controlled by the autonomic nervous system. These techniques are used in the treatment known as biofeedback.

Behavioural assessment methods

In the simplest form of behavioural assessment the specific aspects of the person's behaviour under investigation are counted as discrete or separate events, or timed, noting the duration or frequency of each event. For satisfactory observations a simple counting device (such as a stop-watch) may be needed. Data are entered as soon as possible on a suitable record form or sheet, and very often the figures can subsequently be produced in graph form.

It is usually necessary to develop a coding system when the behaviour to be assessed is complex. In a setting where the behaviour of physically handicapped people in a workshop is to be studied, the following sort of code might be developed.

1. BODY POSTURE

* Standing
* Sitting
* Walking

2. POSITION OF HEAD

* Directed to work
* Directed to other person
* Directed to own body/clothes

* Other

3. POSITION OF HANDS

* In contact with work tools or materials
* In contact with work surfaces
* Holding food or cigarette
* In pockets
* Other

This code would then be used by an observer, and at specified points in time the person's behaviour would be coded separately under each of the three categories of behaviour 1, 2 and 3. There are obvious limits to the number of different categories of behaviour, and to the number of options within each category, which any one observer can use efficiently.

Usually observers are interested in recording the actual behaviours of a person. If the severity of epilepsy was being assessed in a child, then an accurate count of the number of fits would be one appropriate measure of severity. However, it can sometimes be useful to record the consequences, or results, of the behaviour, rather than merely the behaviour itself. This can be appropriate where there is some objective permanent record of a person's behaviour. Thus counting the number of cigarette burns on the clothes of a long-term patient would be one measure of the degree of deterioration in smoking habits. In a well-known study Ayllon (1963) modified the towel-hoarding habits of one patient, and the index of change that was chosen was the number of towels the patient had in her room at any one time.

It is often necesssary to obtain a measure of behaviour that is representative of a person's overall behaviour. It is not usually possible to observe people continuously and so some attempt has to be made to ensure that a representative sample of observations is obtained, perhaps covering all the day and the various places where the person goes. This process of obtaining a set of scores by observing the person systematically through a set period is known as time-sampling. It is normally done by ensuring that observations are made exactly every 30 minutes, or every hour, or other convenient interval of time. Event-sampling is used when the behaviour studied is relatively infrequent and perhaps rather lengthy, so that time-sampling would not allow sufficient observations. In this procedure, the event is sampled so that every event is noted, but only every fifth event (or perhaps every tenth) would be fully coded.

If a group of people (say, ten patients) have to be assessed it is possible to work out a group time-sampling schedule, so that every hour each patient is observed at 30-second intervals. Thus in 4½ minutes all the patients are observed, and no further observation is made until the next hour. Provided that the coding system is relatively simple, and that adequate time is given for observers to record their observations, this type of procedure can be relatively efficient for monitoring the behaviour of quite large numbers of people.

Check-lists and questionnaires

Personality questionnaires typically comprise a large number of items, sometimes several hundred, and the results may be interpreted in terms of relatively complex factorial structures. Simpler types of questionnaire have been developed to assess marital interaction, work interests, etc. The importance of questionnaires and check-lists is that typically they require no skilled professional time to administer; that is, they can be self-administered by the person.

The standard questionnaires that are available have a wide range of purposes. They may be used to identify targets for treatment; to identify potential rewards or reinforcers for use in a behavioural programme; or to assess covert or internal processes or thoughts which do not normally result in outward action or words. Because they are so uncomplicated to use, it is necessary to guard against bombarding people with questionnaires and asking them so many questions that they feel overwhelmed.

As with all assessment procedures, they should be chosen with care; they must be relevant to the people taking them and they must appear to be relevant. Some standard questionnaires relating to depression, for example, should be introduced carefully even when used for research studies only: the questions may lead to introspection in some subjects, while some questionnaires may irritate subjects so that they either refuse to complete the questionnaire, or give false or facetious answers.

Zung (1965) has developed a 20-item self-assessment scale of depression. This questionnaire is widely used and has been carefully standardized with groups of patients of known diagnosis and severity, and is useful both to assess the degree of depression and to monitor changes in level of depression. Other published questionnaires relate to more specific types of problem. A number of questionnaires on particular phobias have been developed, such as fear of snakes, fear of heights, and even fear of mathematics! Denny and Sullivan (1976), for example, produced a 60-item questionnaire describing various aspects of spider phobia, which is perhaps not a crippling sort of phobia but one which is certainly relatively common.

Check-lists are useful as initial screening devices in that they usually record the simple presence or absence of a particular symptom or problem. They allow a large number of items to be rapidly checked without the need to consider carefully the degree of abnormality or deviation.

A check-list could be needed, for example, to monitor the problems presented by a child who was having difficulty in getting to school on time. The early morning routine of getting up, going to the lavatory, washing, dressing, having

breakfast, cleaning teeth, and perhaps meeting deadlines for
catching buses or trains is a major problem for many residents in institutions, not to mention parents of young
children! A period of time in a residential setting or hostel may make such problems worse, since this long and complex chain of behaviour comes under the external control of
the institutional regime, rather than under the child's
internal control. A check-list of the chain of activities
involved in this routine would thus be both a useful and
initial assessment tool, and also could be used to check
progress. Here is such a check-list.

Figure 1

Check-list for early morning routine

Name of resident ....

Date check-list completed ....

Completed by ....

SKILLS:

☐ Wakes up when alarm/bell is rung

☐ Gets out of bed (feet outside bed) within
ten minutes of alarm

☐ Washes unprompted before breakfast

☐ Toilets unprompted before breakfast

☐ Selects appropriate clothes unaided

☐ Dresses unaided

☐ Eats breakfast unaided

☐ Tidies utensils unaided

PROBLEMS:

☐ Argues with other children

☐ Engages in irrelevant behaviour

☐ Eats in a messy way

Rating scales

Rating scales may consist of a single item or of a series of
many items. For each item the rater is required to make a
judgement about the person's behaviour in terms of a set of
available responses. This judgement is usually expressed
in terms of the quality, intensity, or frequency of the

behaviour in question. Examples of single-item rating scales are shown in figure 2.

Figure 2

A. Was the patient aggressive? ... Twice or more during the week
... Once in the week
... No aggression seen

B. Dressing ability
1. Patient dressed self without help
2. Patient needed some help to get dressed
3. Considerable help needed to get dresssed
4. Fails to co-operate in getting dressed

C. Speech

-3	-2	-1	0	+1	+2	+3
mute	very little speech	less than average	aver-age	more than aver-age	mark-edly talk-ative	talks with very few pauses

---

Some rating scales are designed to be filled in soon after the behaviour has happened, while others (particularly those using nurses as raters) may require the rater to think back over several days when making the rating. This means that the rater must be able to remember what the person has done over the stated period, and also of course that the rater has actually observed the person over a reasonable proportion of that period. Senior ward staff may have a number of administrative and other commitments which reduce the possibility of their observing patients at all times of the day, so that nursing assistants or aides may be the staff best equipped to act as raters.

A wide range of standard rating scales is available to assess the behaviour of various groups of patients (the elderly, the mentally ill, the physically handicapped) at a range of activities (activities of daily living, work tasks, social competence) and in a range of settings (home, hostel, day-centre, ward). For example, Pattie and Gilleard (1979) have developed a special system of assessment for older people, known as the Clifton Assessment Procedure for the Elderly (CAPE). This consists of two parts, one being a short test of the patient's ability, the other of which is a standard rating scale of general behaviour. CAPE has been evaluated with various diagnostic groups of older people in hospital and hostels, so that it can be used widely as a standard assessment of the elderly. By contrast, the Adaptive Behaviour Scale developed by Nihira, Foster, Shellhaas and Leland (1974) is designed for use with the mentally handicapped. It is characterized by extremely detailed items, which are suited to the careful step-by-step planning of training programmes often necessary for this group of clients.

Psychophysiological techniques

Although we may 'know' what happiness or fear means for ourselves, it is sometimes hard to know exactly what other people mean when they use the same words. Although there is a sense in which we can never know the inner feelings of other people, we can examine the physiological changes that often accompany such reactions as fear or sexual arousal. We may be interested in the relationship between emotion and physiology for its own sake, or we may wish to use this relationship as an index of treatment response, or indeed as a method of treatment in itself.

There are a number of different functions which can be assessed using physiological techniques. Measurement of electrical activity in the muscles (EMG) is one of the most frequently used techniques. This type of activity can be measured by surface electrodes, or by needle electrodes implanted in the muscle fibres. Muscular relaxation training is widely used as a component of the treatment for psychological disorders, such as phobias, and EMG measures can be used to evaluate the effectiveness of this type of training.

Measures of cardio-vascular activity are also important in psychophysiological assessment. The characteristics of heart-beat can be recorded by an electro-cardiograph (ECG), which will reveal the wave form, and such irregularities as cardiac arrhythmia. Heart-rate is one of the most error-free psychophysiological measures. Blood pressures can be measured in a number of ways. The occlusion cuff is used commonly in clinical medicine but is subject to some difficulties, such as the difficulty in interpreting the Korotkoff sounds. Ultra-sound techniques can be used, and direct cannulation, but these require fairly sophisticated equipment. Other ways of assessing cardio-vascular activity rely on measures of blood flow. Temperature measures at body sites such as the face or the fingers provide an indirect measure of blood flow. Photoplethysmography can also be used: this relies upon the fact that blood absorbs light of certain wavelengths so that putting an ear-lobe, for example, between a light source and a photo-sensitive cell permits the blood-flow through the lobe to be measured.

Other techniques include the measurement of electrical resistance between electrodes placed on the skin (usually of the palm or fingers). This simple procedure leads to a number of possible measures, skin resistance and skin conductance being the most commonly used. Levels of sexual arousal in men can be assessed by penile plethysmography, which indicates changes in volume of the penis. Other techniques have been developed to measure respiration, gastro-intestinal activity, and changes in size of the pupil of the eye.

All of these psychophysiological measures require appropriate instruments, which are now usually electronic, to detect and amplify the electrical signal, and feed it into some appropriate display or recording device. The signal detector, or transducer, picks up the signal: in most cases it is important that the transducer is held as firmly as possible against the skin surface (and in some cases electrode jelly and specialized adhesives are necessary). The display and recording device can be modified to give the most suitable sort of output, which may be a variable tone or noise, or a light which varies in intensity, or some permanent record on a moving-paper record, like that used for EEGs. All of these instruments are becoming progressively lighter, smaller, and relatively cheaper. They offer opportunities for direct recording of psychophysiological functioning with a fully mobile patient that were unthinkable even a few years ago. None the less, these instruments need careful calibration and the measures they yield can be influenced by such factors as humidity and slight variation in electrode placement. Devices which are operated from the mains electricity supply must be used with extreme care, and following the procedures set out in the instruction manual.

Flexibility in assessment

An attractive feature of many of the methods outlined in this chapter is that they can be adapted to the needs of the individual patient or particular project, unlike standard tests. Precisely because of this flexibility, there is a risk that they will be used incorrectly or thoughtlessly, or under conditions which will not yield reliable data. Virtually anyone can put together some questions on general physical health and call it a 'Health Questionnaire'. But there are a number of criteria which should be met by any assessment technique.

Does the technique cover the appropriate topics?
The content of a rating scale or questionnaire should adequately sample the range of events within the stated coverage of the scale. Content can be chosen on the basis of several different criteria.

* How often does it happen?
* Is it clearly associated with treatment outcome?
* Do staff think it is important?

Hall (1977) carried out a survey of nurses to find out what content should be included in ratings of chronic patients, and his report discusses this topic in more detail.

Is the technique likely to be understood by those who have to use it?
Scales and questionnaires as well as behavioural assessment

methods should be designed to be as simple as possible to
fill in. This can be achieved by careful layout of the form
and, for example, setting out all the items so that they
require a similar sort of response. Less confusion will
result if all the questions need a tick, or if all need one
answer circled, than if the first ten need circling, the
next three need underlining, the next six need the wrong
answers crossed out, and so on. The words used in the instructions and on the form should be at such a vocabulary
level that they can be understood by the users of the form.
'Chooses the right clothes' is better than 'Selects appropriate garments'!

Are the instructions clear?

The steps that a rater or observer has to make should be
clearly described; for example, it is usually important that
the data, and possibly even the time, is recorded on the
form. Is the direction of the period of observation clearly
stated and, if a time-keeping device is needed, has the observer got one that works? It is often helpful to provide a
space for any additional comments to be noted by the observer.

Is there any check of reliability?

The procedure should be carried out as intended. Perhaps the
observers can be videotaped to make sure they are doing it
properly. At least every now and then an additional observer
should carry out a repeat or duplicate assessment, and compare the results. By laying out the results as a simple
series of paired scores, it is often possible to see if
reliability is poor. The example below (figure 3) shows the
scores obtained by raters A and B on a four-item rating
scale with five patients.

gure 3

| | | Patients | | | | | | | | |
| | | P | | Q | | R | | S | | T | |
		A	B	A	B	A	B	A	B	A	B
ms 1		1	0	2	2	0	2	1	1	1	0
2		1	1	2	2	1	0	2	2	2	1
3		2	1	1	1	1	0	2	1	2	0
4		1	1	2	2	2	1	1	1	2	2
tals		5	3	7	6	4	3	6	5	7	3

A simple check like this makes several points clear, without
any need to calculate reliability formally. Rater A is consistently scoring higher than rater B. Some patients are
scored more reliably than others: there is disagreement on

all four items for patient R, but on only one item for patient Q. Some items are scored more reliably than others: there is only one disagreement for item 4, but four for item 3. This sort of simple check can be used to correct at least the most obvious sources of unreliability.

Planning and recording an assessment schedule

Very often one particular assessment technique may stand out as the most appropriate one to use for a particular purpose. Again, practical constraints on the amount of time that can be given to assessments usually mean that only one method can be used. However, when several different methods are used in the same project it may be found that one is more sensitive to change than another; but it is not always possible to predict which one it will be. If the exact nature of a problem is unclear, or if the response to a treatment is difficult to predict, it is good practice to choose two or three different types of assessment rather than two or three varieties of the same type of assessment. Rather than use three questionnaires on social functioning to assess the outcome of a social skills training programme, it would be better to use a time-sampling measure of interaction, plus a self-report questionnaire of social functioning, plus a rating of social competence by someone else.

Assessment can take a lot of time, and the value of the assessment has to be evaluated at least in part in terms of how long it takes. If a large number of people have to be assessed it is possible to work out how many can be reasonably be assessed each week, and so allow enough time for all the people to be assessed at that rate. If new patients are being assessed in a hospital it is often possible to work out from local or national statistics the probable rate of referral or incidence of that category of patient so it is then possible to calculate how long it will take to gather a sample of, say, 50 patients. Some patients may refuse to co-operate in a study, others may be too ill to co-operate, and others may return incomplete or spoilt questionnaires; a short pilot run of an assessment schedule can indicate how many respondents are likely to be lost in these ways.

Increasing attention is being paid to organizing nursing and clinical notes so that they more reasily lead to formulation of a treatment plan. One way of so organizing notes is called a Problem Orientated Record (Weed, 1969). This form of record keeping consists of four logical stages:

data base - problem list - plans - follow-up

This approach means that in stating the problems presented by a patient it is also necessary to give the supporting evidence or data for its existence. Formal assessment data would need to be incorporated in this evidence. This should be included in the notes in such a way that they are permanent and readily intelligible to the staff who are going to have to interpret that data.

Conclusions

There is a wide range of psychological assessment methods other than tests, questionnaires and interviews. Depending on the question that has to be answered, and on the decision that then has to be made, these other methods can be very useful. They are particularly useful because many of them do not require a particular professional background to be used properly. They may also be useful because they enable observers, such as ward staff, with a close and detailed knowledge of the person's everyday behaviour to contribute assessment data in a structured and standardized way.

References

Ayllon, T. (1963)
Intensive treatment of psychotic behaviour by stimulus satiation and social reinforcement. Behaviour Research and Therapy, 1, 53-61.

Cronbach, L.J., Glesser, G.C., Nanda, H. and Rajaratnam, N. (1973)
The Dependability of Behavioral Measurement: Theory of generalizability for scores and profiles. New York: Wiley.

Denny, D.R. and Sullivan, B.J. (1976)
Desensitization and modeling of spider fear using two different types of scene. Journal of Consulting and Clinical Psychology, 44, 573-579.

Hall, J.N. (1977)
The content of ward rating scales for long-stay patients. British Journal of Psychiatry, 130, 287-293.

Hundleby, J. (1973)
The measurement of personality by objective tests. In P. Kline (ed.), New approaches in psychological measurement. Chichester: Wiley.

Nihira, K., Foster, R., Shellhaas, M. and Leland, H. (1974)
AAMD Adaptive Behavior Scale. Washington, DC: American Association of Mental Deficiency.

Pattie, A.H. and Gilleard, C.J. (1979)
Clifton Assessment Procedures for the Elderly (CAPE). Sevenoaks: Hodder & Stoughton Educational.

Weed, L.L. (1969)
Medical Record, Medical Education and Patient Care. Cleveland, Ohio: Press of Case Western Reserve University.

Zung, W.W.K. (1965)
A self-rating depression scale. Archives of General Psychiatry, 12, 63-70.

Assessment: Part III questions

1. What is meant by the validity of an assessment procedure?
2. Why should psychological tests be reliable?
3. Why are observations by nurses so important?
4. Why is immediate recording of information important?
5. Give a brief description of the main types of psychological test.
6. What are the advantages and disadvantages of the interview as a method of assessment?
7. Compare projective and questionnaire approaches to 'testing' personality.
8. Are IQ tests simply a measure of performance on the test, or do they measure intelligence?
9. What are the reasons for the wide use of psychological tests?
10. What are the major limitations of tests?
11. Why is the establishment of norms so important in interpreting test results?
12. Give a simple account of the relevance of factor analysis to the study of personality.
13. What aspects of the context, or setting, of an interview most affect its conduct?
14. What special precautions need to be taken when using interviews in research studies?
15. Which types of non-verbal behaviour are important in interviews?
16. Describe the main methods of sampling behaviour when using direct observation.
17. What is the effect of using (i) patients, or (ii) relatives as assessors instead of staff?
18. Outline the main steps that should be taken to train ward staff in the use of a standard published rating scale.
19. Discuss some of the factors which are relevant in designing a record chart to be placed on the wall of the ward office and filled in daily by ward staff.
20. What are some of the effects of the same nurse repeatedly using the same assessment procedure with the same patients?
21. What attributes might predict the success of student nurses in training?

22. Using psychological methods, how could you assess whether a nurse has mastered a specific nursing procedure?
23. What aspects of the physical environment of a ward could justify assessment?
24. Why is the period of time immediately after admission to hospital a poor one for collecting information from a patient?
25. Which aspects of long-term residents of psychiatric hospitals could convey to the general public the fact that they are not 'normal'?
26. A 10-year-old boy knows that his parents are keeping a systematic diary of his self-mutilation: how will this knowledge possibly affect the data obtained?
27. An 18-year-old is assessed by personality tests as being highly introverted and hysterical. What observations of the patient's behaviour would confirm that view?
28. An agricultural worker has fallen from the roof of a barn on to the frame of a farm machine, fracturing a rib and with suspected internal injury. What observations would be carried out, and why?
29. A special unit for developmentally handicapped children wants to develop self-help skills programme, concentrating on dressing. What would be the detailed items to include on an assessment chart?
30. A 70-year-old lady is admitted to your ward. How could her nursing needs be assessed?

Part four

The Early Years

11

Early life
John Hall

New-born children are almost completely helpless. Maybe to
their parents they have sorts of potential, and to relatives
they may resemble all sorts of distant relations. But to the
detached observer, babies are capable of only a limited
range of actions, and we cannot really say what infants are
feeling, or what their individual needs are.

No new-born infant could survive without all sorts of
care and attention: indeed, human babies are unusual in the
animal world in the length of time they take to reach maturity and in the degree of protection they require in their
early life. The child at the point of birth has already
survived nine months of inter-uterine life, protected physically from the outer world, and should be able to look forward to a further 15 or 20 years of social and emotional
protection before entering into adulthood.

Each new-born baby is an individual. From the moment
of fertilization, the aspects of the child's development
which are genetically determined are fixed. Equally from
that moment the genetic endowment interacts with the environment, first of the womb and then of the outside world,
to produce a unique person. Nurses who care for the newly
born, and health visitors in contact with young children,
know that they differ markedly in temperament from the
earliest hours of their life. Not only do they differ in
their behaviour, but they differ in their response to their
environment so that, for example, some young children adapt
to a reduction in sleep by apparently needing less, while
other children react by becoming lethargic or irritable.

Most children are brought up in families. The psychology
of the family is discussed fully in the next part of the
book, but the effect of the family upon the young child
cannot be overestimated. Parents care physically for the
young child, and it is upon their vigilance and discernment
that the physical health of the child depends. For example,
the decision whether to carry out a tonsillectomy upon a
child depends more on the persistence and attitudes of the
parents, allied to opinions of the family doctor, than upon
the clinical condition of the child. If a child becomes
demanding and manipulative, the probability of the parents
seeking help is related more to whether they see the behaviour as a problem than to any external assessment of the
child's shouting and screaming.

From a nursing point of view, children pose particular problems. They often cannot decribe clearly what is wrong with themselves; they may be very upset at having to come to the clinic or into hospital; and their state can quickly vary from one extreme to another, embarrassing mothers by their quiet play when the doctor arrives hot-foot after an anguished call.

Slack (1979) was concerned about the piecemeal nature of health service provision for children. There are maternity units for mothers and children; paediatric units for sick children; child health clinics for preventative services. She wrote of the difficulties that this dispersed provision poses for comprehensive health and nursing services to children and their families. Her article includes a diagram showing the range of health, social service, and educational agencies that are available to children. It illustrates the need to plan around the needs of child and family. Her article concludes by commenting on 'the number of young able nurses and health visitors who have a remarkably clear idea of what is meant by integrated services', and the need for co-ordinated management of nursing services to children.

This part of the book looks at the early years of the child and adolescence. However, the period before birth, the pregnancy, is of special interest to midwives and the special problems of sick children are of concern to many other nurses, not only those on paediatric wards.

Pregnancy: starting a family

Pregnancy is a nine-month prelude to major changes in the lives of parents. It is a period of important physical and social change for the expectant mother, and a time of preparation for the rest of the family.

While having a baby is undoubtedly a female event, it may not, paradoxically, be perceived as feminine. To many women 'feminine' means being young and attractive, while being 'motherly' may mean feeling less attractive in a romantic sense. Thus impending motherhood may mean that a woman sees herself as becoming less physically attractive to her mate.

Even at this stage the unborn child can become an interloper between mother and father. The father may become aware of the mother's increasing preoccupation with the foetus within her, and fear yet more neglect following the birth, especially if he has not yet become secure in his role as husband. Apart from the mother's view of her own body, the husband's view of his wife's body is important in ensuring the continuation of sexual relations during pregnancy. There is some evidence that sexual attitudes and performances before pregnancy are related to the ease of labour, and this provides additional evidence that the happiness of the mother in pregnancy is related to the quality of the marital relationship beforehand. There is no reason why sexual contact should be diminished, though the usual position adopted by the couple may be uncomfortable, and alternative positions may be helpful.

There are a number of stereotypes of pregnancy which carry with them associated attitudes and expectations, and these can affect not only the mother-to-be, but other family members.

Pregnancy as an illness

Pregnancy is not an 'illness', but the people who look after pregnant women are clearly doctors and nurses, and the overwhelming majority of babies in Britain are born in hospital and not at home. Thus some women may see their pregnancies as confirming their wish for medical attention and support, and lead them to seek a similar type of attention from others. Nonetheless, pregnancy is essentially a natural process, in the course of which many women feel exceptionally well physically and emotionally.

Pregnancy as a duty

There may be strong implicit and explicit pressures upon a couple to start a family, not necessarily for their own satisfaction but to supply a grandchild, nephew or niece to other family members. A childless couple may come to feel guilty about not having children. Couples who, for right reasons for them, delay starting a family may be endlessly prodded on the matter. In some countries they give medals to mothers of large families!

Pregnancy as a crisis

A crisis may be benign in its effects, not necessarily pathological. With the growth of employment for women pregnancy is, for an increasing proportion of women, an escape or a break from a work routine and a transfer to a different life style. For others it may have serious career or economic consequences and other implications for an anticipated style of family life when an 'accidental' pregnancy occurs later in life to a mother with children already in their teens.

As with all stereotypes, attitudes to pregnancy are modified by exposure to reality. Most mothers have at least a second child, so that their attitudes to subsequent pregnancies are modified by their own personal experience. This means that events which occurred in the first pregnancy, such as a very long time in labour, may condition expectations in later pregnancies even though the events are unlikely to be repeated.

An important first step in pregnancy is confirmation that the woman is in fact pregnant. A woman who has several children may 'know' she is pregnant, but others may delay medical confirmation for some weeks. Confirmation of pregnancy may immediately lead to other medical checks, such as an amniocentesis to check for certain abnormalities in the foetus. These may in turn lead to an abortion being considered. In association with a termination, or subsequent to it, a sterilization may be performed. It has been thought that elective sterilization itself carries a risk of emotional disturbance, but this does not appear to be the case. Other pregnancies are stopped by a miscarriage. If a miscarriage occurs later on in the pregnancy, then there may be a sense of bereavement and loss, possibly accompanied by a traumatic memory of the loss itself, at which the father or other family members may have been present.

If there is an appreciable age gap between existing children and the child-to-be, one function of the pregnancy is allowing the older children to prepare for the new baby, so they can learn what is happening in the pregnancy, and also so that incipient problems of sibling rivalry can be minimized. New babies need a lot of care, and older children can quite correctly detect the reduction in parental attention after the birth. Some older children, on the other hand, can be exploited by the mother in that they are asked to bear an unreasonable burden in preparing for and caring for the younger child.

Pregnancy is a time of major physical and hormonal change for the mother, so it is not surprising that a proportion of mothers-to-be experience emotional disturbance. Changes in levels of hormones, especially progesterone and oestrogen, are associated with pregnancy. Since many women have experienced mood changes associated with hormonal contraceptives they may expect that hormonal changes will affect them in pregnancy, but the role of these hormones in emotional changes in pregnancy is not clear. In the course of pregnancy there are several possible foci for anxiety, including risk of handicap to the child, or a preoccupation with the degree of cleanliness necessary in caring for young children.

The birth

Birth is hard work for the mother and the baby. It is also associated with 'pain' for many mothers. Natural childbirth approaches, with their varying techniques, have the effect of directly producing muscular relaxation, and also promote more positive expectations of the birth process itself. Most of the techniques are a mixture of relaxation and focussed-attention techniques, which do lead to better tolerance of birth pain. Some of the techniques have wider objectives, so that the Le Boyer method emphasizes the continuation of close contact between child and mother immediately after birth, with the aim of improving mother-child bonding. Some psychodynamic writers have attributed considerable significance to the birth process in determining later personality deveopment, but the evidence for this view is uncertain.

For generations fathers have been carefully excluded from the build-up to birth. In some countries this has led to a separate 'birth' routine for the father, when the father experiences abdominal pain simulating childbirth. Fathers are now able to be present, not simply as passive observers, but as key members of the birth team. There are a number of tasks which the father can perform which are a direct support and help to the mother, reducing the possibility of loneliness for the mother during labour, and also incidentally reducing the father's own anxieties!

There is little information on the effects that sharing in the childbirth process has on fathers. Early interaction between mothers and infants appears to lead to more 'attachment behaviour' on the part of such mothers, but most information on attachment between fathers and new-born children has either been retrospective, or obtained from the mothers. Bowen and Miller (1980) studied 48 fathers and their children to examine the relationship between attendance at parenthood classes, presence at delivery, state of the child and the related pattern of father-infant attachment. The subjects were divided into three groups depending on whether they attended classes and were present at delivery (21 fathers), present at delivery but non-attenders at the classes (eight fathers), or whether they neither attended classes nor were present at the birth (17 fathers). For each father the way in which he behaved towards his new child was observed, using a time-sampling method of observation, between 12 and 72 hours after delivery. It was found that presence at delivery was an important variable, leading to stronger attachment behaviour of fathers to their children, but attendance at classes did not make any difference to this aspect at least of the father's behaviour. This study only looked at one aspect of father-child interaction; and it suggests a need to examine the more complex pattern of interaction between mother, father and infant taken as a group.

The sick child

The early months of childhood can be physically very tiring for parents, and they may need both support and clear, positive advice on how to cope with their baby. While breast feeding, for example, is 'an art as ancient as the human race', there are changes in fashion among both mothers and professional staff about the relative merits of breast feeding and artificial feeding. Maclean (1977) carried out a study to examine opinions on infant feeding, hypothesizing that advice given to mothers is often variable and contradictory and that it causes confusion and frustration. The study was a questionnaire survey of midwives and health visitors, and 88 questionnaires were returned on the subject of breast feeding, and 99 on artificial feeding. The report of the study examined some selected topics in detail. For example, there was a wide range of responses to an item asking how often preparation of the feed should be demonstrated. Slightly more than a quarter of the respondents thought once was enough, an equal proportion thought twice was adequate, whilst others thought four times were needed, and yet others thought that no demonstrations were necessary! The greatest variation occurred in the age at which it was considered that mixed feeding should be introduced: replies ranged from two weeks to twelve months.

The study recommended that attitudes of both staff and parents needed to be examined further and that the British Government report 'Present Day Practice in Infant Feeding' should be more widely read by nursing staff. Plentiful literature may well be available, but even the most able parent may be uncertain whether or not to ask for medical help for some childhood symptom. Most symptoms are usually identified by parents, but they may not see the significance of developmental retardation, and may have difficulty in accepting that a child who just appears slow is in fact seriously handicapped.

An important concept in all health care is 'normalization'. It stresses the need to make as many aspects of the patient's environment and routine as similar as possible to 'normal' outside life. This concept can be used by parents of chronically ill children to alleviate the feelings of being different which many of them have. Krulik (1980) followed up the mothers of 20 such children, who were aged from six to ten years. Most mothers were aware that their child felt different from their brothers and sisters, and other children of the same age, and the study identified the tactics adopted by the mother to modify these feelings.

Irrespective of the individual tactics adopted, for example, to comply with requirements for postural drainage, there were five general principles underlying all the tactics. The principles related to: preparation of the child for change; participation by the child in decision making; sharing the illness-management experience in the whole family and with the immediate neighbours and friends; and adoption of positive control by parents to counteract feelings of uncertainty.

If a child has a congenital mental or physical handicap, then present thinking encourages maintaining the child at home as far as possible. This has become possible for many children because of advances in paediatric surgery, and the improved design of aids and equipment for the disabled. None the less, the developing child needs contact with peers as well as parents, to play and to develop social skills. The policy in Britain and other countries has been to integrate educational facilities for the handicapped with normal children, to give wider opportunities to the handicapped and to reduce stigmatization of the handicapped by the others. There is evidence that aggression and self-mutilation in children is often related to boredom.

Some profoundly mentally handicapped children pose enormous nursing problems because of the extent of their handicap, or because of associated behaviour problems. While the number of children in British hospitals for the mentally handicapped has dropped considerably in recent years, there are many children attending special schools or at home who present similar difficulties, where community psychiatric nurses are often involved. Berry, Dearden, Perkins and Swarbrick (1978) described how they developed a behavioural programme in a 24-bedded ward for children whose developmental

ages ranged between six months and three years. The ward
staff, consisting of teachers, psychologist, and doctors as
well as other medical staff, agreed their respective roles
in the ward team. Following a short course on behavioural
methods, the team put the methods into practice by first of
all building up length of eye contact with some of the
children. Other programmes were later introduced, such as
a toileting programme for two children, an eating skills
programme for most of the children, and a 'play-week' to
build up the occupational skills of children. A review of
the programmes indicated several changes which could bring
further benefit, such as weekly meetings to discuss and
monitor objectives for individual children. The article
gives examples of the charts used in the programmes, which
can equally be used in home-based programmes for children
with this type of handicap.

Of course, most children are not permanently handicapped
but the majority of children suffer from infections of the
gastro-intestinal and respiratory tract, cuts and bruises,
concussion, and other minor illnesses. These are usually
treated by the family doctor, but may lead to the child
having to come to hospital, as do conditions requiring
surgical intervention.

Considerable improvement has taken place in the care of
children in hospital over the past 30 years or so. Preliminary visits to the ward can be arranged before the formal
admission. Many hospitals now provide facilities for a
parent to stay in hospital with their child, enabling the
mother to carry out some routine tasks, giving her a sense
of usefulness and the child a sense of familiarity. Unrestricted visiting is now common on children's wards. Even
during a short stay in hospital it is important that children have continual opportunities to play and to learn. This
means that play materials appropriate to the age and interests of the child must be available and used - despite the
mess - and play therapists can be used to structure and
guide play. Part-time teaching is available to children only
spending a few weeks in hospital, but full-time teaching is
provided for children staying in hospital for any length of
time.

Nurses who want to specialize in work with children who
are physically ill can, in Britain, take a separate training
for that purpose. Nurses who want to specialize in the care
of psychiatrically disturbed children cannot, however, take
a specialized basic training but must specialize later. A
similar state of affairs exists in many parts of the United
States, so that Koehler (1981) decided to introduce a child
psychiatric option for senior nursing students in the American school of nursing where she worked. She has described
both the philosophy of the course, and the range of clinical
experience the students obtain. Half the clinical experience
is gained in child psychiatric in-patient units. The other
half is gained in a community-based diagnostic/learning centre. The centre provides a number of services, such as a

'self-discovery' sensori-motor therapy programme for pre-school children with developmental disabilities. The students' experience in the centre stresses the significance of the school in the life of the child, and provides exposure to special education teachers and teaching techniques that can enhance the students' skills with other children in both hospital and community.

Some children admitted to hospital will require surgery. Children for elective surgery may be on a waiting list for some time and, like adults, have fantasies and fears about operations. Careful explanation is needed both of the procedure which will be followed, and the consequences of the operation. With very young children local anaesthesia is rarely used because of the problems in gaining co-operation. General anaesthesia may be achieved either by injection or by inhalation, but in the latter case it may be necessary to allow prior experience of the apparatus, or to use a specially modified cuddly toy which allows the gas to escape next to the child's mouth and nose.

Non-accidental injury is a term used to describe injuries inflicted on a child by an adult, often one of the parents. When non-accidental injury has occurred, the care of child and family is aimed at prevention, and often involves a number of staff and agencies. It is particularly important in such cases that there should be the fullest communication between all staff concerned, as tragic consequences can follow any delay in communication. Nurses may have some difficulty in relating to parents suspected of causing non-accidental injury to their children.

'Baby-battering' and other child abuse, is a pattern of behaviour which is strongly condemned by the public, but which can be difficult to detect because of the way in which parents conceal the extent to which their child has been injured. The use of 'At-risk' registers helps to monitor abuse, once it has been established as being likely in a particular family. It would be useful, however, to develop a model of potential child-abusers to be identified early on.

Millor (1981) evaluated three models of child abuse, which she termed the psychiatric (focussing primarily on parental psychopathology), the sociological (focussing on levels of violence in the immediate community), and the social-psychological (focussing on the interaction between parents and children). The last of these three models was chosen to to be the basis of a theoretical framework for nurses to conduct research in this topic. Ten assumptions are presented about parent-child transactions in abusive or neglectful families; for example, assumption seven states that the presence of an audience influences role enactment. This is related to the observation that when one parent physically harms a child, the other parent, if observing the incident, thereby passively tolerates such behaviour, and then subsequently the presence of that parent conveys a role expectation to the abusing parent. The article concludes by giving five examples of testable propositions arising from the model.

Older children, once they have recovered from the acute phase of their illness, may enjoy the atmosphere of the ward, and may regret leaving the ward. Nonetheless, while they are in hospital they are isolated from aspects of life outside, and when they return home they may go back to a different type of life because of their condition or the treatment they have received. Children - and indeed adults - thus need help and support when they are going home, just as they did when they came into hospital.

References

Berry, R., Dearden, R., Perkins, E. and Swarbrick, A. (1978)
Behavioural principles: a multi-disciplinary approach to the management of severely mentally handicapped children. Nursing Times, 10 August, 1327-1330.

Bowen, S. and Miller, B. (1980)
Parental attachment behaviour. Nursing Research, 29, 307-311.

Koehler, M. (1981)
Child psychiatric nursing option. Nursing Outlook, 29, 174-177.

Krulik, T. (1980)
Successful 'normalizing' tactics of parents of chronically ill children. Journal of Advanced Nursing, 5, 573-578.

Maclean, G. (1977)
An appraisal of the concepts of infant feeding and their application in practice. Journal of Advanced Nursing, 2, 111-126.

Millor, G. (1981)
A theoretical framework for nursing research in child abuse and neglect. Nursing Research, 30, 78-83.

Slack, P. (1979)
Child care - influencing the future. Nursing Focus, 1, 152-154.

12

Abilities and behaviour in childhood and adolescence
B. M. Foss

Childhood

Early development

Even at birth the differences between infants are very great, and the range of abilities and behaviour which can be called normal is large at all ages.

Apart from sleeping (80 per cent of the time), the newborn seems to spend most of his time eating, excreting or crying. There are several kinds of cry which most mothers can distinguish from each other and which can be analysed using spectographs (which break up the sound into its frequency components). The birth cry appears to be unique. Then there is a basic cry, sometimes called a hunger cry, which is the common pattern. The pain cry, which may be elicited on the first day (for instance, when a blood sample is taken), is characterized by an initial yell followed by several seconds of silence during which the baby maintains expiration and which finally gives way to a gasp and loud sobbing, which in its turn reverts to a basic cry. There is also a frustration cry which is rather like a diminished version of the pain cry. Many mothers have also recognized a different kind of cry which starts at, say, the fourth week. It seems to be a sham cry in the sense that it is caused by no specific need, but seems simply to be a way of calling for attention. Presumably this kind of cry develops into the distress which older children show when separated from their mothers.

What things does the infant attend to? Can it recognize its mother's face and voice, or are these learnt gradually over a period of time? Until recently it was believed that recognition of faces and voices did not occur until the infant was several months old, but it now looks as though infants become competent in this way very much earlier, as many mothers already suspected. At least, what they can do is distinguish between different voices and faces probably as early as the third week of life, and it is likely that they can tell difference in smell between different people as early as the second week of life, and there is some evidence that even at this age infants are particularly attracted to representations of the human face. This is a topic on which there is a conflict of evidence. What is clear, though, is that most babies have a great deal of opportunity to get to know faces, in that mothers play face-to-face

games with their babies from the very first days of life;
indeed, where they are allowed to be with the baby from
birth they will tend to play these games immediately. By the
time the baby is three weeks old it gets 'turned off' if,
when face to face with an adult, the adult fails to react to
the baby's changes in facial expression.

Perception

What seems vital for later perceptual learning is some kind
of interaction between the child and the environment. In
describing what happens it is useful to think in terms of
perceptual categories. Probably from birth, infants are
able to categorize movements and discriminate them from lack
of movement and also to categorize various colours; so they
probably have a category for 'red moving objects'. If later
in life an infant reaches out to touch such objects, a red
moving object which is a flame may be encountered, and as
a result of touching it the infant's behaviour will have
an outcome which is different from that when other kinds
of objects are touched. In such a way the infant learns to
discriminate a special sub-category of red moving objects.
Movements of all kinds - eye movements, head movements, and
body movements, and all kinds of interaction with the environment - seem to be important for the development of new
perceptions, and this leads to the possibility that perceptual development will be affected by the child's interests
(in the wider sense; that is, matters of concern): the child
is more likely to attend to and interact with those aspects
of the environment which are relevant to those interests.
One can see evidence for this kind of effect in the many
cross-cultural studies that show, for instance, that Eskimos
have many categories for snow. Similarly, small boys may
have many categories for motor cars. It will be seen that
the psychological idea of a percept is not very different
from a concept. One's perception of a dog is not only affected by the sight of the dog, but also knowing what it
sounds like, or what it feels like to be patted, or to be
bitten by, and what it smells like; and if one happens to be
a dog fancier one's perception of the dog will involve very
much finer discriminations than those made by other people.
Perception, then, is affected not only by the present state
of affairs - the stimuli from the environment, and the perceiver's attention, and motivation and emotional state - but
also by the perceiver's whole previous history, and this
leads to the possibility that different kinds of people have
rather different perceptions. The members of a gang will
perceive that gang's symbols (haircut and clothing, favourite music, favourite drink, etc.) quite differently from the
way they would be perceived by a member of an opposing
gang.

Skills

It is only about halfway through the first year of life that
a child begins to show good evidence for integrating its

movements with its perception by being able to get hold of objects in an obviously intentional way. The gradual development from these early stages through walking and various kinds of play activity to complex skills involved in sports, for instance, are well documented. It may be useful to have a model of the way in which such skills are acquired, and one such model is to regard the skill as built up of a hierarchy of lower-order habits. For instance, a child learning to write must have first learnt to hold a pencil (there is an innate grasping reflex but the child will have to relinquish this method of grasping for one using finger and thumb opposition), will have had to learn to move the pencil across the paper hard enough to leave a mark but not break the paper, will have had to learn to match shapes, to move from left to right across the page, to distinguish between mirror image letters, and so on. Many of these habits can be learnt only in a fairly definite sequence because one will depend on the acquisition of previous habits. Eventually the child will have a whole hierarchy of writing and drawing habits, and at some stage these will have to be integrated with other hierarchies of talking and hearing habits if the child is to become an ordinary literate person. The establishment of these hierarchies depends obviously on having the necessary sensory and motor abilities. They also depend on practice (one cannot learn to drive a car just by reading a book), the knowledge of results (otherwise movements will not become perfected) and on having the motivation to continue learning. One of the characteristics of these skill hierarchies is that the lower-order habits become automatic, and the skilled person does not have to think about them at all but can concentrate on the 'higher' aspects of what is being done. Such a model helps to throw light on some of the reasons why children may fail to develop skills necessary for everyday life. For instance, some sensory or motor abilities may be deficient, an essential lower-order habit may be missing, there may have been difficulty in integrating one or more hierarchies, or there may have been inadequate motivation.

Solving problems

Investigation of problem-solving has been one of the main ways in which psychologists have studied thinking. A main impetus in the study of the development of this kind of ability has been the work of the Swiss psychologist Jean Piaget. He based an elaborate theory on the way in which children develop concepts of number, space, relationships, etc., and claimed that the thinking of a child develops through a series of definite stages, rather as in the development of a skill hierarchy. His results and his theory have been called into question, and although many psychologists do not agree with his theoretical formulation, many of his empirical results have been replicated in a variety of cultures. There has, though, been a tendency to show that some of the problems which Piaget posed can be solved by children at a slightly earlier age given a different method of presenting the problem, and it turns out that sometimes the child fails to solve a problem for reasons other than those given by Piaget. For instance, the child's short-term memory may be inadequate for the storage of information necessary to solve the problem. One of the most interesting class of problems used by Piaget is concerned with what he called conservation. For instance, in testing a child's ability to show conservation of volume, the child is faced with two identical beakers filled with equal amounts of, say, lemonade. If the child agrees that there is an equal amount in each beaker the lemonade from one is then poured into a tall thin glass. The child who has not acquired the concept of conservation will choose the lemonade in the tall thin glass in preference because it will appear greater in quantity. According to Piaget, it is only in middle childhood that children acquire conservation concepts, and it is only when they are, say, 11 or 12 that full logical thinking is possible.

One major concern of psychologists has been to determine how important language is in the development of a child's thinking abilities. Perhaps it is because educationists themselves are rather verbal people that many believe language to be the most important single thing. However, there is some contrary evidence. For instance, deaf mutes who have very little vocabulary or syntax may nevertheless be rather competent in dealing with a whole range of problems varying from those found in ordinary intelligence tests to complicated problems in logic. Of all the tests which have been tried, it happens to be that conservation problems are those which seem most affected by lack of adequate language. In dealing with questions of this kind it is important to realize that there are several kinds of thinking and of intelligence. For instance, when a very broad range of intelligence tests are analysed by a technique such as a factor analysis (which is essentially a way of classifying tests), it usually turns out that there are two broad groups of tests: those involving language and those which do not, but may depend more, for instance, on being able to manipulate space and pattern. There are also large individual differences between people in this matter. Some seem to use language very much more in ordinary thinking, and there is some evidence across cultures that on the whole girls are better at language skills and boys are better at spatial skills. There is one kind of problem whose solution seems to depend on developmental stages and which may hold the key to some of the changes which occur with age. If young children are given a series of objects varying in colour, size and shape, and asked to sort them, they may do so by their colour or their shape or their size, but having sorted by one method they will be unable to see that there is a second or third method of sorting them, and it is only when they are considerably older that they can see from the start that there is an ambiguity about how sorting should be done.

Play

Play in animals and humans is usually easy to recognize
but not so easy to define. Most play does have the property
of appearing to be 'not for real', but there are difficult
borderline cases. For instance, when children are playing
together with toys there may be frequent episodes where
there is competition for toys or for territory, and this may
involve aggression which certainly appears real. Play at
first tends to be solitary even when other children are
there. There may be 'parallel play' in which children pursue
the same tasks though with no obvious co-operation. Fully co-
operative play is not seen much before children are three or
four years old. In most cultures it seems that there are sex
differences in typical play. Boys tend to play more with
boys and girls with girls, and boys show much more of what
has come to be called 'rough and tumble play'. This is the
sort of play where there is a lot of wrestling and tumbling
about and rolling over, sometimes with open-handed arm
beating, often without contact, and rapid jumping up and
down sometimes with arm slapping, and the whole thing is
often accompanied by laughter. Where there is a largish
group of children, one variant is that there is a great deal
of group running, usually in a circle and often occurring
with a lot of laughter. Chasing is another very common
variant. Another sex difference is observed when children
play with their mothers, in that girls tend to have closer
proximity to the mother than boys do, at least on the
average. When play is solitary, dolls and other playthings
and pets are sometimes made to stand for parents and for
children. Such play is often taken to reveal a child's preoccupations, and play therapy is based on the notion that
emotional preoccupations can be acted out. In older children
a lot of play becomes competitive. The dominance fighting
to establish a 'pecking order', which can be seen in all
social animals, is very evident in children. Some of it may
be symbolic and indirect, especially in girls, where dominance fighting is more likely to be verbal than physical.

Arguments about the functions of play are centuries old,
and the theories are on the whole untestable (as are most
functional theories). However, there is now a certain amount
of evidence from animals and from children regarding the
effects of deprivation of play. Harlow's experiments at
Wisconsin on the effects of various kinds of upbringing on
later behaviour in rhesus monkeys have shown that if small
monkeys are deprived of play, especially rough and tumble
play, they may become maladroit later at both sexual and
social behaviour. It is possible that play has this kind of
functional importance for humans also. A more popular theory
is that play in humans is essential for cognitive development. Many educationists believe this, and they get theoretical support from Piaget's notion that the growth of
understanding depends heavily on a child's actions with
respect to the environment. An intervention programme
has been reported in which children who appeared to be

intellectually backward as a result of malnutrition were given regular structured play sessions with toys, and as a result showed considerable development compared with children not given such a programme.

Reinforcement

This is the notion that behaviour is controlled by its consequences. In the sense in which 'reinforcement' is used by B. F. Skinner, a reinforcing state of affairs is one which, when it follows a response of an animal or human, will reinforce that response so that the probability of that response occurring in similar circumstances in the future will increase. Much of the fundamental work on reinforcement has been done on rats and pigeons but also on a very wide variety of other animals and on humans too, and it is the basis for many of the techniques used in behaviour modification. In a typical experiment a rat learns to press a lever which results in the delivery of a food pellet, and this is reinforcing to the hungry rat. Using such a simple set-up it is possible to investigate the effects of a wide variety of variables on the rate of learning. When the animal has learnt that food is no longer delivered when the lever is pressed (extinction trials) it will go on pressing for a while and then cease; but there may be spontaneous recovery. If the animal has been put on a schedule of reinforcement, in which reinforcement is not given for every response but only now and again, either regularly or irregularly and unpredictably, then the animal tends to be much more persistent in pressing the lever and will go on doing so for much longer when food is no longer delivered at all. In other words, after a schedule of reinforcement, especially if the reinforcement has been irregular, the behaviour is much more 'resistant to extinction'. A rat can also be put very much under the control of the environment, in that if a light is always on during reinforced trials but never on during unreinforced trials the animal will learn quite rapidly to press the lever only when the light is on. The light is then described as a 'discriminative stimulus'. A wide variety of things may act as reinforcers. For instance, isolated monkeys will press a lever for a view of the monkey colony or for a tape-recording of other monkeys, and these stimuli act as reinforcers. These kinds of experimental results have to be applied to humans with a good deal of caution. It is not clear how human behaviour is modified if individuals know that they are being subjected to a patterning of reinforcement; nor is it clear what the effects are of having language and being able to conceptualize the set-up.

Apart from behaviour modification techniques as used by therapists, the following are some applications which may be made. There is one kind of crying, which was mentioned earlier, whose function seems to be to get attention even though there is nothing physically wrong with the child. Such attention-getting crying may be very persistent, and attempts have been made to extinguish it by not attending to the child when he produces this kind of cry. There are several published papers indicating that this kind of procedure is effective. Getting attention, presumably benign attention, is an important reinforcer for many children. There are reports, for instance, of a child who spent most of his time in a horizontal position and crawling, and as a result obtained a lot of attention which presumably reinforced his crawling behaviour. The teachers were trained to attend to the child only when he approximated standing up and not to attend to him when he was crawling, and as a result the child learnt to produce more normal behaviour. One well-known experiment controlled the smiling of babies by reinforcing them with smiles and pleasant noises whenever they smiled. A comparison was made of babies who had been reinforced at every smile, and those who had been put on a schedule, that is, they had been reinforced only at every fourth smile. As predicted, the babies on the schedule smiled more and the smiling was more resistant to extinction. It is not known, though, how long this kind of learning persisted. One prediction of the theory would be that if a child produced a certain kind of behaviour to obtain affection, then that behaviour would be more persistent if the affection were given capriciously and, for the child, unpredictably. As Skinner himself pointed out, in everyday life most reinforcers are irregular rather than regular. This is particularly true in gambling and it is quite likely that one of the mechanisms at work in the persistent gambler is the direct result of unpredictable reinforcement. Bearing in mind the way in which an animal's behaviour can be controlled by a discriminative stimulus in the environment, one could argue that it would be much easier for a child to learn appropriate behaviour if it were made quite clear in the environment when that behaviour was appropriate and when not. To caricature the situation, if a father wore a tie whenever the child was expected to behave in a fairly orderly fashion, but not to wear a tie during playtime, then it should be much easier for the child to discriminate between those two situations. It must be very difficult for young children to know what is appropriate behaviour in a typical supermarket when everyone else is taking goods off the shelves but they themselves are not allowed to do so.

Imitation
There is some evidence that infants will imitate facial expressions when they are only a few weeks old. For instance, they will put out their tongue apparently imitatively at two or three weeks. However, it may not be true imitation since they will also put out their tongues at a pencil pointed at them at the same age. In the second half of the first year, though, a great deal of facial imitation does go on. Detailed analysis of videotape shows that in

most cases it is the mother imitating the infant and not the other way around. A lot of this imitative play seems to be a precursor of language and conversation but it is not yet known how important it is. In the second and third year and later, there is a great deal of imitation, much of it important for 'sex typing'. For instance, a three-year-old girl will spend a great deal of time imitating her mother's activities about the house. There have now been many studies of the extent to which imitation or copying occurs in middle childhood from adults or television. Boys in particular tend to copy aggressive movement, especially if the person they are imitating is a man and more especially if the man appears to be rewarded for what he is doing. It is still very unclear to what extent this sort of behaviour persists as a result of such imitation. It is still also not known in general which people children imitate most.

Freud

Many present-day theories of child development are more or less based on classical psychoanalytic theory, and many people would consider that Freud's main contribution was to focus attention on the first five years of life as being of paramount importance in determining later personality. For Freud the central concept in child development is identification, and he believed that imitation was one of the best behavioural signs that identification existed. He believed that identification with the mother figure occurred very early in life and that later, at about the time the super-ego develops, identification with the aggressor (the aggressive aspects of either mother or father figure) took place. Freud also suggested that the child passes through stages related to the way in which the libido (instinctual energy) operates. The first stage is the oral stage, in which the child's erotic life (in Freud's rather special meaning) centres on the mouth; this is followed by the anal stage, when life centres on excretion; then the phallic stage in which sexual (but of course pre-pubertal) interests centre on the genitals and the body surface as a whole. There then follows a latent period during which there is little development until the genital period is reached at adolescence. Mental illness in later life was seen as originating from traumatic experiences occurring during these periods. The situation is complicated for boys by the Oedipus situation in which the five year old sees himself as competing with his father for the love of the mother. Some of these ideas were elaborated by other psychoanalysts by devising personality typologies which were based on infantile experience. For instance, an orally-accepting type of person would be a lover of food and drink, a smoker, fond of words; the phallic type might be a lover of the body beautiful, perhaps an exhibitionist or an admirer of sculpture. Needless to say, it is extremely difficult to test the validity of such speculations.

Adolescence

In the first half of this century adolescence was treated as a period of 'storm and stress', of rebellion, of altruism, and searching for an identity. Some of these characteristics of adolescence now seem to be specific to the cultures in which the originators of the ideas lived, and this is particularly true for the notion that adolescence is a period of storm and stress. From anthropological and other studies, it is clear that in some cultures such a period does not exist. The last few decades have seen major changes occurring in the adolescent world so that many of the old generalizations no longer apply. A few decades ago the situation could be stated in fairly black and white terms: young adolescents were economically dependent; they were sexually capable but not expected to have, or were even legally forbidden from having, intercourse; and their social roles were essentially non-adult. In the course of a decade they were expected to go through a fairly clear series of transitional stages until they inevitably reached the desired position in an adult society in which their economic, sexual and social roles would all have changed utterly. At the present day sexual intercourse is often practised soon after the onset of puberty; many children, including working-class children, have considerably more spending money than their parents had at the same age; and there are now so many sub-cultures all the way from pre-adolescence to adulthood that at any age children can find themselves fully accepted within a culture, as a full member of society.

Biological factors

It is now generally accepted that the onset of puberty occurs earlier as time passes. The results of the onset of puberty on individual children seem to depend very much on what they and their peers expect those effects to be. For instance, there are large differences in the extent of menstrual pain, and those differences vary somewhat between cultures and seem to reflect the expectations within those cultures. Some studies suggest that menarche affects performance at school, whereas there are other studies giving contrary evidence. Here again much may depend on expectations. It is likely that if an individual reaches puberty long before or long after other children in the peer group, this may have considerable effect on behaviour and attitudes. It may be that ignorance of biological factors is detrimental in individual cases, but no one has yet shown what is the best way to carry out sex education, or indeed yet shown that sex education is a good thing (and it would be extremely difficult to show, since the investigator would have the problem of deciding what sex education is good for).

Social factors

Not many generations ago a person was unlikely to survive if not attached physically to a group of people. The need to belong to a group is still as great, though little is known about the psychological mechanisms involved. Avoidance of

loneliness is one powerful drive. In modern Man this need
may be satisfied by simply identifying with the group and
not necessarily belonging to it physically. A century ago a
person's choice of group was limited usually to the family,
the immediate neighbourhood, work, church, and perhaps
hobbies and sport. Now, especially in cities or where people
are mobile, groups are based more on common interests. It is
very easy these days for a person to find other people who
want to behave in the same way or have common goals. There
is a tendency for members of a group to come to look alike,
talk alike, make the same choices in food, music, beliefs,
etc.; and these tendencies are often seen in an exaggerated
form in adolescent groups, especially where the identification with the group is so complete that members see themselves as belonging to that group only and to no other. One
very noticeable thing about human groups of all kinds (and
this applies to groups at all levels of sophistication) is
that they are not only bound together by common likes but
also by common dislikes. All groups are against something.
Anything which lessens old group allegiances will also make
new groupings easier so that one would expect gangs to be
especially prevalent in new high-rise housing estates, or
with people who have just left school. One idea about adolescence, which seems not to have changed over the centuries, is that there is something called 'adolescent revolt'.
It has been observed in many cultures (though not in all)
that soon after puberty there tends to be a reaction against
the parental ways of life. The idea that there is something
primitive and possibly biological about this has been reinforced by many observations of primate societies which
show that young males tend to form breakaway groups and also
start fighting for dominance within the old group.

Dominance fighting is well accepted as an explanatory
concept applied to social animals of all kinds, and some
biologists and psychologists see it as a main source of
competitiveness in human behaviour. Besides the pressures to
belong to a group and to conform to it, there are still
these largely competitive tendencies which may take the form
of wanting to be unique, and to have a role of one's own
within the group. Very often such a role involves being best
at something. Being best may involve owning things, being
most daring, or beautiful, or cleverest. With small boys,
competitiveness may show itself in actual dominance fighting. Psychologists of various kinds have talked a lot about
the adolescent need for having an identity. It is possible
that that need may be partly and perhaps completely
satisfied once the person finds a role within a group,
especially if the role and the group are of high esteem.

Attitudes and beliefs
Sociologists and social psychologists use the concept
'reference groups'. Market researchers may want to know
how to advertise a certain kind of cosmetic product. If it
is intended to be attractive to adolescent girls, they may
well use the technique of finding out which reference group

is relevant. For instance, they may, using questionnaire techniques, ask questions of the kind designed to find out with whom adolescent girls identify when buying cosmetics. In general, one's reference group is the group of people with whom one identifies with respect to one's attitudes, beliefs and values. Developmental studies show that for young children the home provides the main reference group, but in middle childhood already there is a tendency to adopt values of heroes from stories or from television and this becomes very marked in pre-adolescence. In adolescence there may be a complete change of reference groups as has already been suggested, and if this change is very radical then it may be a source of conflict. The way in which the conflict expresses itself will, of course, vary between individuals, and any of the usual clinical manifestations are possible, such as anxiety, depression, hysterical reactions, aggression, and in some cases an attempt at a rational solution of the conflict. Attitudes towards choice of work will be affected by group pressures in just the same way as all other attitudes. The situation is affected by the fact that in many adolescent sub-cultures all the heroes and heroines are roughly of the same age as members of the sub-culture, and there is no need to look ahead to what is going to happen when one belongs to an older age group. In such cases attitudes towards work are likely to be unrealistic in terms of planning ahead.

13

Social development in early childhood
H. R. Schaffer

Introduction

Psychologists study children for two main reasons. First, they want to find out how a helpless, naïve and totally dependent baby manages in due course to become a competent, knowledgeable adult. They are interested therefore in studying the process of development. The second reason stems from the many social problems associated with childhood. Should we protect children from viewing violence on television? Are children of mothers who go out to work more likely to become delinquent? Does hospitalization in the early years produce later difficulties? How can one mitigate the effects of divorce on children? Why do some parents become baby batterers? Increasingly the psychologist is asked to examine such problems and produce answers useful to society. It is primarily to this aspect of child psychology that we pay attention here.

**The child's
socialization**

How a child develops depends very much on the people around him. From them the child learns the skills and values needed for social living, from the use of knives and forks to knowing the difference between right and wrong. Other people are always around the child, being of influence by means of example and command, and none more so at first than the members of the immediate family. On them depend the initial stages of socialization.

Disadvantaged children and their families

It is, of course, only too apparent that not every family carries out its socializing task with equal effectiveness. By way of illustration, let us look at the way in which intellectual development is shaped by the child's social environment.

At one time it was thought that intelligence is entirely determined by an individual's inborn endowment. There are few who now believe this: it seems rather that the environment in which a child is reared can have a powerful effect on development.

The issue has been much debated in relation to the poor educational achievement of 'disadvantaged' children. These are children who come from the economically and socially most deprived sectors of the community and who so often appear to be at a severe disadvantage when first starting school, because (as it has been put) 'they have learnt not to learn'. Their failure in the education system, in other words, is ascribed not so much to some genetic inferiority as to factors operating in the home, which result in an inability to make use of whatever intellectual capacities they have.

A great many schemes have been launched to counter this situation, especially in the USA. Some of the earlier efforts, designed to give children some extra training in basic cognitive skills before school entry, were clearly inadequate and produced no lasting benefits. This is partly because the schemes were too brief, partly because they came too late in the child's life, but partly also because they left untouched the home situation. Given a conflict of values about education between home and school it is highly likely that the home will always win. It is there that the child has already lived and learned for several years before ever starting school, and it is therefore significant that more recent efforts have attempted to involve the parents as well as the child or even to work solely through the parents.

There is now little doubt that parents can enhance or suppress the child's educational potential. One way in which they apparently do this is by the extent to which they foster the development of language: a function so necessary for the expression of intelligence. There are pronounced social class differences in the style of language mothers use to communicate with their children; in addition, however, it has also been shown that mothers from disadvantaged homes engage in face-to-face talking with their infants less frequently than middle-class mothers. The poorer child often lives in much noisier surroundings than the middle-class child in a quiet suburban home, but to profit from stimulation the young child must be exposed to it under the personalized conditions that only the to-and-fro reciprocity of a face-to-face situation provides. It is in this respect that many lower-class 'socially deprived children' are at a disadvantage.

Child effects on adults

Let us not now jump to the conclusion that children's development is totally a matter of what parents do to them. A child is never just a passive being that one can mould into whatever shape the adult desires. Even the youngest babies can already exert an influence on their caretakers and so help to determine how they behave towards them.

Take an obvious example: babies cry and thereby draw attention to themselves. It is a sound that can have a most compelling effect on the adult: we have all heard of the mother who can sleep through a thunderstorm, but is immediately awoken by her child's whimper in the next room. Babies, by this powerful signal, can initiate the interaction: they can thereby influence both the amount and the timing of attention which others provide.

Babies come into the world as individuals. Some are active and restless, others quiet and content; some are highly sensitive, others are emotionally robust and easy-going. The kind of care provided for one is therefore inappropriate for another, and any sensitive mother will therefore find herself compelled to adopt practices suitable for her individual child. A good example is provided by babies' differences in 'cuddliness'. Not all babies love being held and cuddled: some positively hate it and resist such contact by struggling and, unless released, by crying. It has been found that these 'non-cuddlers' tend to be more active and restless generally, and to be intolerant of all types of physical restraint (as seen when they are being dressed or tucked into bed). The mother is accordingly forced to treat her child in a manner that takes into account his 'peculiarity': when frightened or unwell these children cannot be comforted by being held close but have to be offered other forms of stimulation such as bottles, bis-cuits or soothing voices. Each mother must therefore show considerable flexibility in adjusting to the specific requirements of her child.

There is one further, and perhaps unexpected, example one can quote of the way in which parents are influenced by their children. It concerns the phenomenon of baby batter-ing, which has attracted so much attention in recent years. It is by no means a new phenomenon; historically speaking, it is probably as old as the family itself. What is new is public concern that such a thing can happen, and this in turn has given rise to the need for research into such cases. As a result of various investigations it is now widely agreed that violence results from a combination of several factors: the presence of financial, occupational and housing problems facing the family; the parents' emotional immaturity which makes it difficult for them to deal with such problems; their social isolation from potential sources of help such as relatives and neighbours; and, finally, some characteristic of the battered child that singles him out as a likely victim.

It is the last factor that is particularly relevant to us, for it illustrates once again that the way in which parents treat their children is influenced by the children themselves. There is evidence that children most likely to be battered are 'difficult': they are more likely to be sickly, or to have been born prematurely, or to have feeding and sleeping problems. Being more difficult to rear, they make extra demands that the parents are just not able to meet. The child's condition acts on the parent's inadequacy, and so the child, unwittingly, contributes to his own fate.

Mother-child mutuality

It is apparent that children do not start life as psycho-logical nonentities. From the beginning they already have an individuality that influences the adults around them. Thus a mother's initial task is not to create something out of nothing; it is rather to dovetail her behaviour to that of the child.

Such dovetailing takes many forms. Take our previous example of the non-cuddlers. If the mother herself has a preference for close physical contact with the baby which are then rejected, some mutual readjustment will need to take place. Fortunately, most mothers quickly adjust and find other ways of relating to the child. It is only when they are too inflexible, or interpret the baby's behaviour as rejection, that trouble can arise from a mismatch.

Mutual adjustment is the hallmark of all interpersonal behaviour; it can be found in even the earliest social interactions. The feeding situation provides a good example. Should babies be fed by demand or by a rigid, pre-determined schedule? Advice by doctors and nurses has swung fashion-wise, sometimes stressing the importance of exerting discipline from the very beginning and of not 'giving in', at other times pointing to the free and easy methods of primitive tribes as the 'natural way'. In actual fact each mother and baby, however they may start off, sooner or later work out a pattern which satisfies both partners. On the one hand, there are few mothers who can bear to listen for long to a bawling infant unable as yet to tell the time; on the other hand, one should not under-estimate the ability of even very young babies to adjust to the demands of their environment. An example is provided by an experiment, carried out many years ago, in which two groups of babies were fed during the first ten days of life according to a three-hour and four-hour schedule respectively. Within just a few days after birth each baby had already developed a peak of restlessness just before the accustomed feeding time, and this became particularly obvious when the three-hour group was shifted to a four-hour schedule and so had to wait an extra hour for their feed. In time, however, these babies too became accustomed to the new timetable and showed the restlessness peak at four-hourly intervals. We can see here a form of adaptation to social demands that must represent one of the earliest forms of learning.

Not surprisingly, the major responsibility for mutual adjustment lies initially with the adult. The degree of flexibility one can expect from very young children is limited. Yet the very fact that they are involved in social interactions from the very beginning of life means that they have the opportunity of gradually acquiring the skills necessary to become full partners in such exchanges. Observations of give-and-take games with babies at the end of the first year have made this point. Initially babies know only how to take: they have not learnt that their behaviour is just one part of a sequence, that they need to take turns with others, and that the roles of two participants are interchangeable (one being a giver, the other a taker). Such and other rules of behaviour they will learn in time; rules form the basis for much of social intercourse, and it is through social intercourse that children acquire them in the first place.

Socialization is sometimes portrayed as a long drawn-out battle, as a confrontation between wilful young children and irritated parents that must at all cost be resolved in favour of the latter. Goodness knows such battles occur, yet they are far from telling us everything about the process of socialization. There is a basic mutuality between parent and child without which interaction would not be possible. The sight of the mother's face automatically elicits a smile from the baby; that produces a feeling of delight in the mother and causes her in turn to smile back and to talk or tickle or pick up, in this way calling forth further responses from the baby. A whole chain of interaction is thus started, not infrequently initiated by the baby. Mother and child learn about each other in the course of these interactions, and more often than not mutual adjustment is brought about by a kind of negotiation process in which both partners show some degree of flexibility. On the mother's part, this calls for sensitivity to the particular needs and requirements of her child, an ingredient of parenthood that we return to subsequently; on the child's part, it refers to one of the most essential aspects of social living that he must learn early on.

Some conditions that foster development

If we are to promote the mental health and social integration of children, it is necessary to identify the factors that further, or on the contrary hinder, such an aim. We all have our favourite theories as to why some children do not develop in what we regard as a desirable manner: not enough parental discipline, too much violence on television, the declining influence of religion, the social isolation of today's family, and so on. It is much more difficult, however, to substantiate through objective research that any one factor does play a part. Nevertheless, there are some conclusions to which we can point.

The blood-bond: myth or reality?

Is it essential, or at least desirable, that children should be brought up by their natural parents? Is a woman who conceived and bore a child by that very fact more fitted to care for this child than an unrelated individual?

This is no academic question. Children have been removed by courts of law from the foster parents with whom they had lived nearly all their lives and to whom they had formed deep attachments, in order to restore them to their biological mother from whom they may have been apart since the early days of life, and all because of the 'blood-bond'. Yet such a thing is a complete myth. There is nothing at all to suggest that firm attachments cannot grow between children and unrelated adults who have taken over the parental role. The notion that the biological mother, by virtue of being the biological mother, is uniquely capable of caring for her child is without foundation.

Were it otherwise, the whole institution of adoption would be in jeopardy. Yet there is nothing to suggest that adoptive parents are in any way inferior to natural parents. In a study by Barbara Tizard (to which we refer again), children who had been in care throughout their early years were followed up on leaving care. One group of children was adopted, another returned to their own families. It was found that the latter did less well than the adopted children, both in the initial stages of settling in and in their subsequent progress. The reason lay primarily in the attitudes of the two sets of parents: the adoptive group worked harder at being parents, possibly just because the child was not their own. There have been a good many studies which have examined the effects of adoption, and virtually all stress the high proportion of successful cases to be found. And this despite the difficulties such children may have had to face, such as problems in the pre-adoption phase and the knowledge gained later on of the fact of their adoption. Successful parenting is a matter of particular personality characteristics that need to be identified, not of 'blood'.

Fathers as parents: more myths?

Do children have to be cared for primarily by women? Is there something about females that makes them more suitable for this task than males? What part should fathers play in the child's upbringing?

The answer is simple. There is no 'should' or 'should not'. It is a matter of what each society and each family decides about the division of roles between the parents. There have in fact been marked changes over the last few decades in the extent to which fathers participate in child care. They now do so to a far greater extent than they used to, and this trend is continuing. For instance, with increasing unemployment it is no longer uncommon to find families in which a complete role reversal has taken place: mother, having found a job, goes out to work, leaving her unemployed husband in charge of home and children. Fortunately, there is no evidence to indicate that the biological make-up of men makes them unfit for this task or even necessarily inferior to women in this respect. Parenting is unisex; the reasons for the traditional division of labour (such as the need to breast-feed the child and the importance of using men's greater physical strength for hunting and tilling the fields) are no longer applicable.

Children brought up without a father are more likely to encounter difficulties than those in a complete family. There are various reasons for this. One is that in any single-parent family the remaining parent must cope with a great multiplicity of stresses - financial, occupational, or emotional - and the strain felt by him or (more often) her is very likely to have repercussions for the child too. Again, a fatherless boy has no model to imitate, and the developmental tasks of acquiring sex-appropriate behaviour may be more difficult. And, finally, the child isolated with his mother and caught up in one all-encompassing relationship does not have the same chance of learning from the beginning about some of the complexities of the social world: having two parents helps him to learn at once that not all people are alike and that he must adapt his own behaviour according to their different characteristics and different demands.

Parenthood: full-time or part-time?

Until fairly recently there was a widespread belief among parents and professional workers that children in the pre-school period required full-time mothering, and that it was the duty of mothers to stay with the child night and day, 24 hours on end. Otherwise, it was feared, children's mental health would suffer.

We can look at this situation from both the mother's and the child's point of view. As far as mothers are concerned, a crucial consideration is the recent finding of an extremely high incidence of depression among house-bound women. With no outlet such as a job, tied to the house by the presence of several dependant children, a large proportion of mothers (especially among the working class) become isolated and hence depressed. Mothers, on the other hand, who do go out to work are far less likely to suffer from depression, anxiety and feelings of low self-esteem.

As far as the children are concerned, comparisons of those with mothers at work and those with mothers at home have not found any differences between them. Far from being adversely affected, the former may even stand to gain both intellectually and socially. The intellectual effects stem from the extra stimulation and extra provision of play materials that most children in day care obtain: a point of particular significance for those from disadvantaged back-grounds. And, socially, not only is there no evidence that the child's attachment to the mother is in some way 'dilu-ted' by a daily period of being apart, but also the child in day care has the enormous advantage of coming into contact with other children. The benefit of such experience for social development has until quite recently been overlooked; yet other children, even in the early years, can exercise a considerable socializing influence, and in addition may further the child's diversification of social behaviour. After all, the more children are encouraged to adapt to a variety of other individuals the more their repertoires of social skills will grow.

Thus a daily period away from mother may produce good rather than harm. There is, however, one important proviso, and this concerns the quality of the substitute care which the child receives. For one thing, there is a need for con-sistency: a young child continually being left with differ-ent people is likely to become bewildered and upset. And for another, we have the enormous problem of illegal child-minders, looking after an estimated 100,000 children in Britain. According to recent findings, the quality of care provided by such childminders is only too frequently of an unsatisfactory nature, being marked by ignorance and neglect that in some cases can be quite appalling. It is only in the officially provided facilities, such as nursery schools, that the care given by trained staff is such that the social and intellectual benefits can be felt.

Sensitive and insensitive parents

A child's development does not take place in a vacuum; it occurs because the people responsible for his care carefully and sensitively provide him with the kind of environment that will foster his growth. They do so not only by such conscious decisions as what toys to buy him for Christmas or which nursery school to send him to, but also quite unconsciously by the manner in which they relate to him.

Take the language which adults use in talking to a child. This is in many ways strikingly different from the language used to address another adult: it has a much more restricted vocabulary, a considerably simplified grammar, and a great deal of repetition. In addition, it is characterized by a slowing down in the rate of speech, a high pitch of voice, and the use of special intonation patterns. Not only mothers but most adults will quite unconsciously adopt this style when confronted by a young child. What is more, the younger the child the more marked is the simplification, repetition, slowing down and all the other characteristics listed. It is as though the adult is making allowance for the child's limited ability to absorb whatever one tells him, thereby showing sensitivity to the abilities and requirements of that particular child.

Such examples of (usually quite unconscious) sensitivity in relating to children are numerous. Watch how a mother hands her baby a rattle to grasp: how carefully she adjusts the manner and speed with which she offers the toy to the still uncertain reaching skills of the child. She shows thereby that she is able to see things from the child's point of view, that she is aware of his requirements and can respond to these appropriately. Sensitivity is an essential part of helping a child to develop. Children brought up in institutions, in which they are all treated the same and where care is never personalized, become developmentally retarded. While most adults show sensitivity to children quite naturally, some parents are unfortunately devoid of this vital part of parenting. Why this is so we still do not know for certain; it does seem, however, that parents who themselves had a deprived childhood and did not themselves experience sensitive care are more likely to show the same attitude to their own children.

Are the early years special?

There is a widespread belief that experience in childhood, and particularly so in the earliest years, has a crucial formulative influence on later personality. Thus the early years are said to be the most important, and special care therefore needs to be taken to protect the child during this period against harmful experiences that might mark him for life. Let us look at the evidence for this belief.

The influence of child-rearing practices

According to Freud, a child's development is marked by a series of phases (oral, anal, genital) during which he is especially sensitive to certain kinds of experience. During the oral phase, for example, the baby is mainly concerned with activities like sucking, chewing, swallowing and biting, and the experiences that matter to him most thus include the manner of his feeding (breast or bottle), the timing of feeding (schedule or demand), the age when he is weaned, and so on. When these experiences are congenial to the child he passes on to the next developmental phase without difficulty; when they are frustrating and stressful, however, he remains 'fixated' at this stage in the sense that, even as an adult, he continues to show characteristics such as dependence and passivity in his personality make-up that distinguish babies at the oral stage. In this way Freud's theory suggests that there are definite links between particular kinds of infantile experiences on the one hand, and adult personality characteristics on the other.

However, this theory has not been borne out. A large number of investigations have compared breast-feeding with bottle-feeding, self-demand with rigidly scheduled regimes, early with later weaning, and other aspects of the child's early experience that could be expected to produce lasting after-effects. No such effects have been found. The sum total of these investigations adds up to the conclusion that specific infant care practices do not produce unvarying traces that may unfailingly be picked up in later life. Whatever their impact at the time, there is no reason to believe that these early experiences mark the child for good or ill for the rest of his life.

And just as well! Were it otherwise we would all be at the mercy of some single event, some specific parental aberration, that we happened to have experienced at some long-distant point in our past. Freud's theory made little allowance for the ameliorating influence of later experience, yet the more we study human development the more apparent it becomes that children, given the opportunity, are able to recuperate from many an early misfortune. Let us consider some other examples that make this point.

Maternal deprivation

In 1951 a report was published by John Bowlby, a British child psychiatrist, pointing to the psychological ill-effects of being deprived of maternal care during the early years. The evidence, Bowlby believed, indicated that a child must be with his mother during the crucial period of the first two or three years if he is to develop the ability to form relationships with other people. Deprived of a relationship with a permanent mother-figure at that time, such an ability will never develop. Thus children in institutions and long-term hospitals, where they are deprived of this necessity, become 'affectionless characters': that is, they are unable ever to form a deep, emotionally meaningful

relationship with another person. Having missed out on a
vital experience, namely being mothered, the child is mentally crippled for life. And that experience has to happen
at a particular time, namely in the first years. No amount
of good mothering subsequently can remedy the situation.

There is no doubt about the tremendous influence on the
practice of caring for childen that Bowlby's ideas have had.
And no wonder, for so many children are thereby implicated.
Many thousands of children every year are taken into the
care of local authorities; many thousands are admitted to
hospital. Anything that can be done to improve the lot of so
many children is therefore worth considering, and there is
no doubt that in the last two decades a great deal has been
done in the UK. Children's institutions have become less
impersonal with the introduction of family group systems;
there is greater emphasis on fostering children with
ordinary families and, most important, far more stress is
placed on prevention and keeping children with their own
parents. Similarly, the psychological care of children in
hospitals has improved greatly during this period. Visiting
by parents is nowhere near as restricted as it was at one
time; mother-baby units make it possible for parents to stay
with their children; and again the emphasis on prevention
means that rather more thought is now given to the need to
admit the child in the first place.

Anyone who has ever seen a young child separated from
his mother and admitted, say, to a strange hospital ward,
where he is looked after by strangers and may be subjected
to unpleasant procedures like injections, knows the extreme
distress that one then finds. It is perhaps difficult for an
adult to appreciate the depth of a child's panic when he has
just lost his mother: a panic that may continue for days and
only be succeeded by a depressive-like picture when the
child withdraws into himself from a too painful world.
Parents also know only too well about the insecurity which
the child shows subsequently on return home, even after
quite brief absences, when he dare not let the mother out
of sight. There is no doubt about these dramatic short-term
effects, and for their sake alone the steps taken to
humanize procedures have been well worth while.

Far more problematic, however, is the question of long-
term effects: that is, the suggestion that periods of prolonged maternal deprivation in the early years impair the
child's capacity to form interpersonal relationships. What
evidence we have here suggests that things are not as cut
and dried as Bowlby indicated, and to make this point we can
do no better than to turn to the report by Barbara Tizard to
which we have already referred.

Tizard examined adopted children who had spent all their
early lives in institutions, with no opportunity to form any
stable attachments to any adult during that period. One
might have expected them to be so marked by this experience
as to be incapable of forming any emotional relationship to
their adoptive parents and to show all the signs of the

affectionless character. Yet this proved not to be the case. Nearly all these children developed deep attachments to their adoptive parents, and this included even a child placed as late as seven years of age. They did show some deviant symptoms, such as poor concentration and over-friendliness to strangers, but there was no indication that the inevitable outcome of their earlier upbringing was the 'affectionless character'. We must conclude that children's recuperative powers should not be under-estimated: given a new environment in which they receive very much improved treatment, the outlook can be good. There is no reason to believe that they will be marked for life by earlier misfortunes, just because these occurred early on.

Birth abnormalities and social class

When misfortune takes a 'physical' form, such as some abnormality of the birth process, the outcome is again not necessarily a poor one. Once more, it all depends on the child's subsequent experience.

Take such birth complications as anoxia (the severe shortage of oxygen in the brain) or prematurity. Follow-up studies of children who arrive in the world in such a precarious condition show that, on the basis of the child's condition at birth, it is impossible to predict his subsequent development. Two children coming into the world with the identical kind of pathology may develop along quite different lines. In one case, the child's condition at birth may give rise to a whole sequence of problems that continue and even mount up throughout his life; in the other, the difficulty is surmounted and the child functions normally.

The answer to this paradox lies in the different kinds of social environment in which the children develop. Where these are favourable the effects of the initial handicap may be minimized and in due course be overcome altogether. Where they are unfavourable the deficits remain and may even be amplified. The outcome, that is, depends not so much on the adverse circumstances of the child's birth as on the way in which his family then copes with the problem. And this, it has been found, is very much related to the social class to which the family belongs.

Social class is in many respects a nebulous concept. Nevertheless, it does refer to a set of factors (concerned with education, housing, health and so forth) that usually exert a continuing influence on the child throughout his formative years, and it is therefore not surprising that social and economic status turn out to have a much stronger influence on the course of development than some specific event at birth.

Thus even organic damage, just as the other aspects of a child's early experience, cannot in and of itself account for the particular course which that child's development takes. The irreversible effects of early experience have no doubt been greatly overrated. To believe in such effects is indeed dangerous for two reasons: first, because of the suggestion that during the first few years children are so vulnerable that they are beyond help if they do encounter some unfortunate experience; second, because it leads one to conclude that the latter years of childhood are not as important as the earlier years. All the evidence indicates that neither proposition is true: the effects of early experiences are reversible if need be, and older children may be just as affected by unfortunate circumstances (though possibly different ones) as younger children.

Conclusions

A child's development always occurs in a social context. Right from the beginning he is a member of a particular society, and the hopes and beliefs and expectations of those around him will have a crucial bearing on his psychological growth.

There is still a tremendous amount to be learnt about the nature of the child's development and the way that it is affected by particular features of the environment. But in the meantime we can at least make one negative statement with some very positive implications: development can never be explained in terms of single causes. Thus we have seen that isolated events, however traumatic at the time, do not preclude later influences; that the one relationship with the mother does not account for everything. For that matter, development is not simply a matter of the environment acting on the child, for the child too can act on his environment. Not surprisingly, when confronted with a specific problem such as child abuse, we invariably find that a combination of circumstances needs to be considered if one is to explain it. Simple-minded explanations of the kind, 'juvenile delin-quency is due to poverty (or heredity or lack of discip-line)' never do justice to such a complex process as a child's development. And, similarly, action taken to prevent or treat which focusses on only single factors is most unlikely to succeed.

The early years: Part IV
Questions

1. Discuss the possible implications of a first pregnancy for a couple who have already been married for ten years.
2. What steps can be taken to involve fathers in both the birth and early parenting?
3. Do you think that the way in which a birth is conducted affects the parents' acceptance of the new baby?
4. Can children be studied scientifically?
5. Are there 'experts' in child rearing? Is this process too important to be left to parents?
6. What are the main aspects of 'mothering'?
7. What principles should be used when deciding whether a child should be adopted?
8. Why are the effects of early experience not necessarily permanent?
9. What are the main developmental stages a child passes through according to (i) Piaget, (ii) Freud?
10. How can the effects of social disadvantage on the intellectual development of young children be overcome?
11. In what ways should a knowledge of social development in the early years affect the upbringing of handicapped children?
12. The parent-child relationship is said to be reciprocal. Explain what this means, and give examples.
13. What factors affect the success of substitute mothering?
14. How do young children develop a concept of their own sexual identity?
15. In what ways does a child's ability to solve problems vary with age?
16. What is known about the reasons for baby-battering, and what effect on the child could such treatment produce?
17. How would you classify different kinds of play, and what functions may they have?
18. Should education begin during the pre-school years?
19. Discuss the role of language in intellectual development, and examine the suggestion that there are class differences in the use of language.
20. What psychological principles are relevant when looking after children in residential care?
21. What are the main individual differences between children (i) in the first year of life, and (ii) in later childhood?

22. What advice would you give to the mother of a four year old who is thinking of returning to work?
23. Discuss the extent to which development during adolescence is determined by social factors.
24. Why is there greater scope for conflict between parents and older children now, compared to 50 years ago?
25. What is the role of the father in child rearing?
26. Describe the provision for play which should be made for one-year-old Annette, who is being nursed in a side room, and eight-year-old George, who is confined to bed.
27. How could you persuade a stubborn three-year-old boy to take his oral medication without a lot of mess?
28. Linda is one year old and will be immobilized for the next few months with a plaster for the reduction of a congenitally displaced hip. How will her growth and development at home be affected, and what advice given to her parents?
29. A young married woman with a five-month-old child is suffering from depression and needs to come into hospital. What are the advantages of keeping mother and baby together?
30. Mrs Yates is aged 18, and is in the early stages of her first pregnancy: what are the possible reasons for her complaints of anxiety and loss of libido?

Part five
Family Life and Old Age

14

The family and later life
John Hall

Many studies of family life concentrate on the effect that
the family has on the developing young child, yet children
equally have an effect on their parents. Similarly, many
accounts of human development dwell in great detail on the
early years of life, with perhaps some attention paid to the
middle years.

It is possible to think of both life itself, and the
life of a family, as following a cycle. There are milestones
in adult life just as in childhood. Some of the most important milestones in adulthood are indicated below together
with an indication of the ages at which they typically
occur.

Legal adulthood: the right to vote	18-21 years
Start work after completing education and training	16-25 years
Marriage	20-30 years
Death of parents	40-50 years
Grandparenthood	45-55 years
Retirement	60-65 years

The age at which these milestones occur is more predictable
earlier than later in life, since marriage - and parenthood -
may be delayed, and so the actual age at which the later
milestones are reached is highly variable. None the less,
there is a general sequence to the milestones, irrespective
of the ages at which they occur.

A corresponding model of the life cycle of the family
has been proposed, showing the milestones of family life,
which divide it up into a series of phases, as shown in
table 1.

This part of the book examines the interaction between
these two cycles, the individual's life cycle and the family
life cycle, from adulthood onwards. The subsequent chapters
look in detail at family life, ageing, and dying: it is useful to look in addition at development in the middle years
and the role of the family in sickness.

The middle years
From a health point of view, early adulthood is a period of
low morbidity. During this period most people have less

Table 1
From: World Health Organization (1976)

Phase of family life-cycle	Key events or milestones
	Marriage
Formation	
	Birth of first child
Extension	
	Birth of last child
Completed extension	
	First child leaves home
Contraction	
	Last child leaves home
Completed contraction	
	Death of first spouse
Dissolution	
	Death of survivor

contact with health care services than at any other time of their lives, with the exception of those women who are having babies.

Chemotherapy for malignant conditions can produce foetal abnormalities; this could be a problem when one member of a newly married couple is found to have cancer. Should they start a family? Accola and Summerfield (1979) discussed the general issues involved in counselling people with cancer who want to have a family. Chemotherapy may have terato-genic effects (causing abnormalities after conception), mutagenic effects (causing foetal abnormality because of a developmental defect in sperm or ovum), or may lead to sterility. These risks need to be considered, as do the implications of possible single-parenthood if one partner should die because of the malignant condition.

Early adulthood is a period when most people learn a wide range of skills relating to their work, to marriage, to domestic responsibilities and to the constructive use of leisure. Even at this age abstract mental ability is start-ing to decline slowly, but this is offset for nearly all activities by the growing availability of relevant skills and life experience. The job or work which people do is influenced by a number of factors, such as family expecta-tions and opportunities for work. Apart from the family, work is the other major source of both personal accomplish-ment and personal dissatisfaction.

While a monogamous heterosexual relationship is the most significant long-term relationship for many people during adulthood, the divorce statistics indicate that, for a con-siderable proportion of people, marriage has failed to meet their expectations. This has led to the exploration of dif-ferent ways of construing the roles of husband and wife, such as job-sharing. These explorations may, for example, change the way in which parents divide the responsibilities involved in caring for a young child, and suggest that some aspects of the presentation of health education material, for instance, may need to be changed if the aim of the material is to affect the family member most involved in caring for the child.

Others choose not to marry, and for them the family life cycle that has been outlined is irrelevant. While many single people make a positive and informed decision not to marry, it is worth noting that some people stay single because they cannot cope with the pressure of marriage, or because they lack the social skills to obtain a marriage partner. It is this latter group who contribute to the finding in some studies of psychiatric breakdown that single people are more prone to some psychological problems than married people.

The middle years of life can be interpreted in two opposing ways. One approach is to see this phase of life as the most productive period, and indeed studies of some groups of professional people have shown the period between 30 and 40 to be the most prolific in terms of productivity. Another approach is to see the period as one of crisis, precisely because of the lack of change and pressure, and because of the effect of the menopause for women and the so-called 'mid-life crisis' for men.

Difficulties that are common in this period are thought to be the consequences of children leaving home, the consequences of the menopause, and the growing realization that some financial and occupational aspirations may never be achieved. Certainly some parents will have problems in facing separation from their children, and the consequent realization that they have now to face up to relating to the spouse from whom they may have become psychologically separated. Equally, the departure of the children may confer a new financial freedom to the parents, and a greater domestic liberty evident in such matters as freer choice of holiday times. Some women may have unpleasant physical symptoms during the menopause, but equally some women are simply relieved that the long threat of possible pregnancy has now been removed. For some men the realization that further promotion is unlikely may be frustrating, and indeed embittering, but it may also lead to feelings of stability, and a greater commitment to social activities and the wider community. Enforced redundancy, when it occurs, is a problem in later middle age or beyond, and it can obviously be hard for someone to accept a new job at the age of 50 or so which is much below the status and financial level of a previous job. Yet even under these circumstances some people are glad to be out of a possibly tedious job, and relish and respond to the challenge of something new.

It is, then, a mistake to conceive of the middle years as being psychologically stagnant and unimportant. Apart from the immediate pressures of family and work, the way in which people respond to new events in their lives during

this phase depends on how they interpret those events in the
light of similar events in their own past, either at the
world level or the personal level. For example, those children who had a vivid experience of separation from their
fathers during the Second World War may, when they are
adults, be affected by that experience when contemplating
taking a job involving separation from their children in the
1980s.

There is no sudden physical transition from middle to
old age. Variations in normal physical ageing mean that some
people experience a marked decline in physical strength and
speed of movement even in their late 40s or early 50s. Two
events, however, may particularly signal a change in social
and psychological functioning not necessarily associated
with ageing.

The first of these is retirement from work. For most men
in Britain the retirement age is between 60 and 65, and for
women it is some five years earlier. There is some evidence
to suggest that anticipation of retirement occurs some time
before the actual event, characterized by changes in work
rate, and attitudes to work. Retirement from work constitutes several things: a change in the pattern of daily routine; a loss of functionally-related social contacts; a
reduction in social standing; and often a reduction in the
standard of living. Some people add to the changes imposed
by retirement by moving house and going to live in another
part of the country, which may contribute further to the
problems of adjustment to a non-working condition.

The second is widowhood. Since women have a longer
life expectancy than men, and since women in Britain are on
average two years younger than their husbands, widowhood is
a much greater possibility for women than for men. Social
expectations are reduced for the widowed, and these expectations may themselves lead to lower levels of social activity. None the less, whether retired or widowed, it is
sometimes remarkable to see how some extremely old people
retain their interests and abilities to an astounding
degree.

McGilloway (1979) reviewed the implications of the pro-
portional increase in older people for patterns of nursing
care. The review examined the health problems presented by
the elderly, and noted the frequency of multiple ailments.
The author had previously carried out a survey of 33 general
medical wards, covering 779 patients, to give an indication
of the most frequent reasons for hospitalization in the
group. The three most frequent reasons were cerebro-vascular
accidents, respiratory disease, and cardio-vascular disease,
which together contributed to 60 per cent of all reasons.
The review also looked at family circumstances of the elderly, and the 'Diogenes syndrome' exhibited by those elderly
people who, for no clear reason, live in conditions of filth
and deprivation. The relationship between patterns of disability and patterns of help offered by the personal social

services and the health services was examined. The concluding comment emphasizes that apart from professional perspectives on the elderly, there are at least three other perspectives: 'the elderly person herself ... family members,
if any ... and other persons who touch on the life of the
old person; there may be many or few'.

The number of retired people is rising both numerically
and proportionately at present. The way in which retirement
is viewed varies according to a number of different factors,
but social class, or socio-economic status, is one of the
most important. Homewood (1981) reviewed the main aspects
of retirement that are relevant to nurses, and pointed out
that real poverty can be a consequence of retirement for
those who, when working, were earning relatively little.
About 50 per cent of people about to retire would like to
carry on working, but for the poor who want to work there
may be major difficulties in gaining employment. The review
points out that many retired people - and indeed other
people who are handicapped - do not fully understand the
range of services and facilities available to them, and thus
one role of the community nurse is to help older people to
assess their own needs and implement their own individual
plans.

When a spouse dies, the nurse may often be in a position
to help support the new widow or widower. Rosenbaum (1981)
carried out a study of the way in which newly-widowed
spouses coped with their bereavement, paying particular
attention to their use of psychotropic medication and
alcohol. The study looked at 56 widowed spouses, half of
whom belonged to a widow and widower self-help group. The
study indicated an increase in the use of psychotropic
medication following bereavement, extending to the follow-up
period which was up to five years after bereavement, with
most subjects having been widowed between one and three
years. A self-rating of depression was also carried out
which showed that, as the depression score increased, the
number of subjects reporting use of medication increased.
However, there was no evidence of increased alcohol use, and
for those subjects who did report depressive feelings there
was an indication of a reduced use of alcohol. There was
some evidence in the study of inadequate monitoring by the
spouse's family doctor of the level of medication which was
taken. It was concluded that the recently bereaved should
positively seek alternatives to medication, especially to
cope with insomnia and loneliness.

The family in sickness

There are many patterns of family life apparent in different
cultures. One consequence of increased availability of travel, and of immigration from one country to another, is that
more people now have an awareness of the power that families
can have over their members in some countries. This power is
often seen as residing in the 'extended family' of a person:

the several generations of a family, together with associated brothers and sisters and their children and relatives by marriage. In nursing it is often important to know something of the general pattern of family life of patients, and considerable skill is needed to unravel the intricacies of some family networks, especially with members of some immigrant communities.

By contrast, the family unit most often presented in Britain is the 'nuclear family' of not more than two generations living together, consisting of parents and children. There may be relatively infrequent contact between the nuclear family and other relatives, so that support from the rest of the family in times of sickness is hard to obtain. The lack of an available natural extended family means that support may be sought from other friends and neighbours, so that such other people take the place of the extended family, though lacking any blood relationship.

Illness often has a considerable effect on the family of a patient. The two aspects of an illness which most affect the family are its severity and chronicity. When patients are severely ill, they are most likely to be in hospital. Relatives may then be in a position of conflict, between feeling that the sick relative ought not to be left, combined with a sense of helplessness that makes visiting particularly difficult. In particular, relatives may feel extremely guilty if they are not present with the patient at a time of crisis or at the point of death.

Visiting in hospitals is often difficult for patients and relatives alike. Many relatives are unsure how to use the visiting time, and can sometimes spend more time paying attention to staff, or to other patients, than to their own sick relative. It is often hard in hospital to be spontaneously affectionate, or to communicate in the idiosyncratic way natural to a particular family, the result being a corresponding awkwardness in ensuing conversation.

When a child goes into hospital, the effects may be positive or negative in terms of physical or medical outcome, and quite independently may be positive or negative in terms of attitudes. However, if a child needs to go into hospital again, the whole family may need support to 'detoxify' them from prior hospital experience. Johnston and Salazar (1979) described a pilot project to help both staff and families prepare for a forthcoming admission of a child. In the course of the project, they found that two of the principal concerns of mothers are that their child's individual living pattern will be disregarded, and that the mothers are afraid of being displaced as the main caregivers. The interesting point about this study is the amount of time that was directed at the family, rather than just the child, before the child was admitted.

The support available to the spouse of a critically ill patient is changing, as many of the supports afforded by an extended family are no longer available. The nursing staff in a coronary care unit were aware that the spouses of their patients had needs related to their anticipatory grief which were neither specifically identified nor met; accordingly, a research project was carried out to see what could be done. Dracup and Breu (1978) looked at 26 men and women, whose spouses had been admitted to the coronary unit. Thirteen of these men and women were offered a specific nursing intervention, based upon Hampe's research on needs of the spouses of dying patients. In accordance with this research, the intervention interviews covered such areas as the spouse's need to be helpful to the dying patient, the need to be informed of impending death, and the need for the comfort and support of family members. There was, at the end of the study, a significant difference between the 13 people who had received the nursing intervention, and the 13 who had not. In this particular project, since it was carried out on the ward where interest had originally been expressed in the topic, ward staff were receptive to the resulting information, and subsequently altered standard ward practice in accordance with the findings.

Some severely ill people may be in the long-term care of their families, with support from domiciliary nursing staff and other agencies. This is particularly likely for those who are mentally handicapped or permanently physically handicapped. Considerable family stress can result from continuous home care. There may be an unremitting physical burden of lifting and turning at night which is physically tiring, or an incessant burden of coping with an overactive or aggressive child. The demands of the patient may mean that the caring relative cannot work, and despite the availability of grants, help with assisted holidays, and so on, there may be real financial hardship. Prolonged care may lead to profound resentment by the care-giver, which may, however, be difficult to express. The degree of support and assistance which is required by the patient on medical grounds may be confounded by the desire of the care-giver to give 'smother-love' perhaps, or conversely, the care-giver may feel the patient is malingering. In the extreme case, the family may become increasingly isolated as the care-givers find it difficult to get out of the home, and friends may not want to visit.

When there is very long-term care in hospital, as with the mentally handicapped or chronically mentally ill, there is a possibility of total rejection of the patient by the family. An additional role is then placed upon ward nursing staff of being family to a patient as well, bringing with it the responsibility to remember such events as birthdays, and the need to motivate the patient to make such personal decisions as choosing clothes and holidays. There is a growing concern with this type of patient to explore ways of providing surrogate, or substitute, families for those abandoned by their natural families. In some settings it is possible to encourage patients to become the families of each other.

Coping with death

Whether or not a chronic illness intervenes, the end of both individual and family life is death. Most people now die in hospital, so that dealing with death has become an unknown problem for the large majority of people, especially as the rate of infant mortality has fallen dramatically this century. If a patient dies at home, it is quite likely that a community nurse will have to support the relatives both at the time of death and for a period of time afterwards. Because death is familiar to nursing staff, it is possible to forget the effect it has, and to forget that everyone who has repeated contact with death - including the hospital chaplain - may need support themselves.

Health care staff face death more consistently than any other major occupational group. Only recently has the reaction of staff to death been recognized as a variable in the type of care which the dying patient receives. From the available literature it might be predicted that there is an inverse relationship between death experience and anxiety about death, so that greater experience is associated with lower anxiety. Denton and Wisenbaker (1977) tested this prediction with a group of 76 nurses and nursing students. The key procedure was the use of a three-item 'experience of death' questionnaire, devised for the study, and a standard 'death anxiety scale'. The prediction was only partially supported, in that the relationship between death anxieties and experience of death varied depending on which aspect of death experience was analysed. The results were further complicated by the effect of the age and amount of work experience of the nurse. The results suggest that experience of death is not a simple linear dimension, and requires further clarification.

References

Accola, K. and Summerfield, D. (1979)
Helping people with cancer consider parenthood. American Journal of Nursing, 79, 1580-1583.

Denton, J. and Wisenbaker, V. (1977)
Death experience and death anxiety among nurses and nursing students. Nursing Research, 26, 61-64.

Dracup, K. and Breu, C. (1978)
Using nursing research findings to meet the needs of grieving spouses. Nursing Research, 27, 212-216.

Homewood, J. (1981)
When you retire. Nursing, May, 1081-1082.

Johnston, M. and Salazar, M. (1979)
Pre-admission program for rehospitalised children. American Journal of Nursing, 79, 1420-1422.

McGilloway, F.A. (1979)
Care of the elderly. Journal of Advanced Nursing, 4, 545-554.

Rosenbaum, J. (1981)
Widows and widowers and their medication use: nursing implications. Journal of Psychiatric Nursing and Mental Health Services, 19, 17-19.

World Health Organization (1976)
Statistical Indices of Family Life (WHO Technical Report
Series 587). Geneva: WHO.

15

The family
Neil Frude

Psychology and the family

The psychologist may regard the family as a background against which to view the individual, asking perhaps how the parents influence the development of a child or how families of alcoholics may help the individual to overcome his or her difficulties, or alternatively the family itself may be the unit of study. The family is a small group and we can observe the patterns of communication within it, the process of mutual decision making, and so forth. It is a system, with individuals as sub-units or elements within. Typically, psychologists have focussed their interests on the biological and social nature of the individual, but they are now becoming increasingly concerned not only with individuals or even 'individuals in relationships' but with the relationships themselves.

Clinical and educational psychologists, for example, are increasingly working within the family context and some problems which were initially identified as 'belonging' to the individual adult or child are now seen, more appropriately, as problems of the 'family system'. Also, psychologists working, for example, with handicapped children have come to recognize that the powerful influence and involvement of the parents means that they can be harnessed as highly potent sources of training, and such clinicians are increasingly using these strategies to establish a far more effective educational programme than they themselves could possibly provide. But the needs of parents, and the stresses which such a high level of involvement may place upon them, are also recognized and so the psychologists may well regard themselves as involved with the problems of the family as a whole.

So there are vital problems in the area and there are some impressive results. Let us look at some of these, choosing some of those areas which relate to major social problems and some innovations which suggest methods for their alleviation.

Family planning

Current surveys of the plans of young married couples for families have shown a high level of conscious control and active planning, a reflection of the wide availability of highly effective contraceptive techniques. The number and spacing of children are controlled with varying degrees of skill and success. The number of couples who opt for voluntary childlessness seems to be increasing. In about half of such cases the couple have planned from the start not to have children, while the other half postpone pregnancy and eventually decide to remain childless.

Contraceptive use varies greatly. Despite the numerous methods available, none is perfect, for various reasons. Some men find that the sheath reduces pleasurable sensation, the pill may have side effects on health or mood, and a number of women find methods such as the cap bothersome and distasteful. The coil may involve a painful initial fitting and an extensive gynaecological involvement which some find embarrassing and disturbing. Sterilization or vasectomy may be advisable for the older and highly stable couple, but a number of people who have undergone such surgery later change their partners. They may then request reversal surgery and in many cases successful reversal will not be possible. The solution to the contraception problem is thus by no means always simple and family planning counselling, and the tailoring of recommendations to the particular needs and life stage of the couple, is a task requiring considerable skill and insight as well as knowledge of the technical features of the particular methods.

Different couples have different 'ideal family structures', often specifying not only the number of children but also their spacing and sex. There is still some preference, overall, for boys and current research makes it likely that in the near future couples will be able, with some accuracy, to determine the sex of their baby. Many will prefer to 'leave it to nature' but others will choose one option or the other. This is likely to result in a relative excess of boys, with longer-term social results which can only be guessed.

Reactions to pregnancy range from unqualified delight to profound despair. The option of abortion is now increasingly available. Reactions to this also vary from relief to regret and while, overall, the evidence is that there are rarely long-term negative consequences for the women, several studies have suggested the need for pre- and for post-termination counselling. A number of women miscarry, some repeatedly, and again this can be a very stressful experience requiring skilled intervention.

Birth and early interaction

The process of birth is biological, but the importance of social variables is also apparent. The pregnant woman may anticipate the sex and looks of her baby, but initial acceptance is by no means inevitable. Premature babies, for example, may look very unlike the baby-food advertisements which may have conditioned the mothers' expectations.

Fathers are now often present at the delivery and there is evidence that this helps the woman in the birth process itself and also helps the couple to feel that the baby is part of both of them. The demands which the baby makes may not have been fully anticipated and the initial period with the infant may call for a difficult process of adaptation and adjustment, just as the first period of the couple living together calls for give and take and the setting-up of new norms of interaction.

Not all babies are the same: they differ in their activity level, their crying and their patterns of sleep and wakefulness. Some are not easy to care for, and may be unresponsive and difficult to soothe. Baby-care makes great demands and the mother may be totally unprepared for the energy and level of skill required. Surveys show that many of them find the period of early childhood highly stressful. They may be tired and feel inadequate and, at times, very angry. If mothers fail to understand and control their babies, their treatment of them may be poor and sometimes harsh.

The level of medical care in pregnancy and around the time of the birth may be high, but many mothers then feel isolated with the baby, unsure about such matters as feeding, toileting and weaning.

In assuming that a 'mother's instinct' will aid her in these tasks we may have seriously under-estimated the extent to which, in earlier times, the informal training opportunities offered to the young girl by larger family units and the close neighbourhood community helped her in her own parenting.

The developing child

In the early years interactions with parents form the major social background for the child. There is a good deal of informal teaching and the child learns by example. Guidance and discipline help the infant to establish a set of internal rules and encouragement and praise help to develop skills and intellectual abilities. Overhearing conversations between adults enables the child to learn about the structure of language and conversation and the rules of social interaction. Watching the parents' interactions and reactions enables children to develop their own emotional repertoire and social skills, and they will experiment and consciously imitate the behaviour of their parents. The child may identify strongly with a particular parent. Games of pretence enable youngsters to practise complex tasks and build a repertoire of interactive styles, and in collaboration with other young children they may rehearse a number of roles. In both competitive and co-operative play social interaction patterns are devised and perfected, children learn about rule-following and discover their strengths and weaknesses relative to their peers.

Different parents treat their children differently, and there are many styles of parenting. Some parents are warm and affectionate, others are more distant, and some are openly hostile. Some give the child a lot of freedom and exercise little control while others are very restrictive.

Not surprisingly, the children reared in such atmospheres develop somewhat differently. The children of highly restrictive parents tend to be well-mannered but lack independence, the children of warm parents come to have a confident high regard for themselves, and the children of hostile parents tend to be aggressive. There are various ways in which such findings can be explained. Do the aggressive children of hostile parents, for example, behave in that way because they are reacting against the pressures which their parents put on them, are they simply imitating the behaviour of the adults around them and picking up their interactive styles, or is there perhaps some hereditary biological component which makes both parents and children hostile?

Probably, as in so many cases of such overall correlations, there is a combination of such factors. It is also possible, of course, that hostility originating in the children themselves causes a parental reaction. We must be wary of the conclusion that children simply respond to the atmosphere of their home. They also help to create that atmosphere and the relationship between parents' behaviour and the child's behaviour is a fully interactive one. Children are not shapeless psychological forms capable of being moulded totally in response to their social environment, but have dispositions and levels of potential of their own which they bring into the family.

Children have certain psychological needs which the family should be able to provide. They need a certain stability, they need guidance and a set of rules to follow and the feeling needs to be conveyed to them that they are 'prized' by their parents. In the traditional system with two parents there may be a certain safeguard for the constant provision of these needs by one or other of the parents, and for the prevention of total lack of interest or of rejection. But if the natural family with two parents is ideal in many ways as an arrangement in which to provide for the child's development, this is not to say that the child's best interests cannot also be met in alternative contexts. Most children in single-parent households fare well and develop happily. For the child living apart from the natural parents adoption seems a better option than does fostering (though long-term fostering seems to share many of the positive features of adoption) and fostering seems to be better for the child than a continued stay in an institution. Even this context, however, can provide reasonably well for the child's needs if there is stability, a high level of staffing, high intimacy between staff and children and the provision of high levels of verbal and other types of stimulation.

family and stress   Just as the family is a principal source of a person's happiness and well-being, it can also be the most powerful source of stress. Research has now been done to try to establish inventories of the life stresses which people experience and in even a cursory glance through such a list it is difficult not to be struck by the extent to which the relationships within the family are bound up with personal change. Some of these events, like the birth of a handicapped child or the death of a child, happen to only a few people, but others, such as the older child leaving home, marital conflict, sexual problems, and the death of a parent happen to many or most. Stress precipitated by such life events has been shown to have a marked effect on both physical and mental health, and if illness is the result then this in turn will provide added hardship.

It is not only particular events which cause stress. The constant presence of ill-health, handicap or marital conflict can similarly take its toll over the years. On the other hand, the stability and comfort of the family setting and the constant presence of others seems to provide much that is beneficial. Marriage reduces the risk of alcoholism, suicide and many forms of psychological ill-health, and interviews with separated and widowed people reveal the elements which they feel they are now missing in their lives, and which in turn may help to explain why living in relative isolation tends to be associated with a greater risk of experiencing psychological problems. As well as providing the opportunity to discuss problems and providing stability, the presence of a spouse reduces loneliness. It also facilitates discussion of a variety of issues and so enables the partners to forge a consensus view of the world: it provides extra interest and social contact, the opportunity to give love and express concern, and provides constant feedback to the individuals about themselves, their value and their role. Practical tasks may be shared and the person may be aware of being prized by the other. This then fosters the sense of self-worth which has been found to be very important for overall well-being.

Of course, not all marital relationships are good and some may lead to far greater problems than those of living in isolation. Certainly recent family changes and conflict seem, in many cases, to be a trigger factor leading to subsequent admission to a psychiatric hospital. Overall, however, it seems that the emotional impact of an intimate relationship, in adult life as in childhood, is likely to involve many more gains for the individual than losses, that people value the protection which such relationships provide and that they often suffer when such support ends.

Schizophrenia, depression and the family

There is a popular notion that schizophrenic illness originates in family relationships, and that certain forms of family communication, in particular, may cause an adolescent or young adult to become schizophrenic. A considerable number of studies have now been carried out to establish whether or not there is a firm evidential basis for such an assumption and, at this point, it looks as if the decided lack of positive evidence should lead us to abandon the hypothesis that such relationship problems constitute the major cause of the illness. While no strong data have been forthcoming to support the family interaction claim, a great deal of evidence implicating the role of genetics in schizophrenia has been found and it now looks as if a predominantly biological explanation may eventually be given. But while there is no good evidence that family relationships are formative in schizophrenia, there is strong support for the notion that family interaction markedly influences the course of a schizophrenic illness and the pattern of relapses and remission from symptoms over the years. It seems that the emotional climate in the home and particular family crisis events often trigger renewed episodes of schizophrenic breakdown.

On the other hand, it seems that depression often has its origin in severe life events and difficulties and that the family context provides many of these. In a recent study conducted in London, Brown and Harris (1978) found that depression was more common in those women in the community who had recently experienced a severe event or difficulty. Many of the events involved loss. Women with several young children were more vulnerable than others, as were the widowed, divorced and separated. Social contact seemed to provide a protective function against the effects of severe life events and the rate of depression was lower in those women who had a close intimate relationship with their husbands. Women without employment outside the home were found to be more vulnerable and the loss of a mother in childhood also seemed to have a similar effect. Brown and Harris suggest that such early loss through the death of a parent may change the way in which the person comes to view the world and attempts to cope with the problems that arise. The study provides clear evidence that family relationship factors may make a person more or less susceptible to clinical depression, and again illustrates how the contribution of family life to personal problems is two-sided. The family may be the source of much stress, but a close supportive marital relationship will enable the individual to cope with many problems without succumbing to the threat of clinical depression.

Sexual behaviour and sexual problems

Married couples vary greatly in the frequency of their sexual contact and in the style and variety of their sexual interaction. The rate of intercourse does not seem to be related to overall satisfaction with the marriage, except that where a marriage is failing for other reasons sexual contact may be low or absent. If there is a marked discrepancy, however, between the expectations or needs of the partners then this may lead to conflict and dissatisfaction. Sex is also one of the factors which can cause problems in the early stages of adjustment to marriage.

Although several medical men and women wrote 'marriage manuals' during the nineteenth century and in the early part of this century, our knowledge of human sexuality was very limited before the studies of people such as Kinsey and Masters and Johnson. Using interviews, and later observational and physiological techniques, researchers have now provided us with extensive information about sexual practices. Masters and Johnson (1966, 1970), in particular, have supplied a thorough and detailed account of human sexual behaviour, and they have also provided insights into such questions as sexuality in the older person and sexual behaviour during pregnancy.

It has become clear that problems of sexual dysfunction affect a great many people at some stage in their marriage. Masters and Johnson have produced a range of therapies which has been shown to be highly effective, and many of these have now been adopted by other psychologists, psychiatrists and marriage counsellors. The couple, rather than the individual man or woman, is considered to be the most appropriate treatment unit, and discussion and detailed advice are followed up with 'homework assignments' which the partners carry out in the home. Anxiety about sexual performance can have a serious effect on behaviour and a vicious circle can easily form, for example, between anxiety and failure to achieve erection. Awareness of the female orgasm has increased considerably in recent years and it appears that the pattern of problems for which advice is sought has changed. Whereas the majority of sexual problems encountered by counsellors some decades ago involved a mismatch of sexual appetites, with the woman complaining about her husband's excessive demands, a dominant problem now seems to be that of the woman's dissatisfaction with her husband's ability to bring her to orgasm.

Opinions differ about how much the 'couple unit' is always the appropriate focus for treatment and how far deep-seated relationship difficulties, rather than specific sexual skills and attitudes, underlie the problems presented. It does appear that in about half of the cases seen there are other serious marital difficulties in addition to the sexual dysfunction being treated by sex therapy which is aimed at improving other aspects of the relationship.

Family conflict and violence

There is open conflict at times in most families. Sometimes the focus of disagreements is easily apparent; it may centre, for example, on matters concerning money, sex or the handling of children; but at other times the row seems to reflect underlying resentments and difficulties in the relationship. Studies have been made of how arguments start how they escalate and how they are resolved, and some research in this area has been successful in identifying patterns of conflict which seem to predict later marital breakdown. It appears that there are right ways and wrong ways to fight with other family members. In some marriages there may be constant conflict which, however, is successfully worked through and which does not endanger the basic relationship.

Inter-generational conflict is also common. In the early years the parents have the power and may use discipline to settle matters of disagreement. Again, the way in which this is done is important and it seems that parents should not use their power in such a way that the child feels rejected. Children should be made to feel that their behaviour, rather than their whole personality, is the target of the parents' disapproval. In the adolescent years, the child's struggle for power and independence is often the focus of conflict. Adolescence is frequently a period of stress and young people may have doubts about their status and future. It is also a time when peer-influence may conflict with that of the parents.

Marital conflict sometimes leads to physical assault and a number of wives have to receive medical attention for injuries inflicted by their husbands. Many such wives choose to return to the home after such an incident although some seek the haven of a women's refuge. Even where there is repeated violence, the wife often feels that her husband is not likely to treat her badly in the future; she may feel that drinking or stress triggered the assault, and such wives often report that the man is generally caring and responsible and that his violent outbursts are out of character. Jealousy and sexual failure or refusal are also associated with attacks on the wife, though it is also true that for some couples physical assault or restraint represents a modal response in conflict situations, and that in some marriages (and indeed in some sub-cultures) there are few inhibitions against the couple hitting one another.

Violence against children also occurs with alarming frequency in families, and it is estimated that about two children die each week in England and Wales as a result of injuries inflicted by their parents. The children involved are often very young, and it does not take much physical strength to seriously injure a small child or baby. Only a small proportion of the parents involved in these attacks have a known psychiatric history and, contrary to one popular image, they often provide well for the general needs of their children. Sadistic premeditated cases do occur but they are relatively rare. Generally the attack occurs when a child is crying or screaming or has committed some 'crime' in the eyes of the parent. The mother or father involved is often under considerable stress, and there are frequently severe marital difficulties. The parents involved are often young and may have little idea of how to cope with the crying child, and there is evidence that many abused children are themselves difficult to handle. They may be disturbed, over-active or unresponsive although, of course, many such problems may themselves be the result of longer-term difficulties in the family.

family therapy

There has recently been a considerable growth of interest in 'family therapy'. This is practised in a variety of ways and with a number of alternative theoretical underpinnings but it claims, in all its forms, that when there is a psychological disturbance it is useful to work with the 'family system' rather than with the individual identified client. The view is often expressed that the symptom should properly be seen as an attribute not of the individual but of the family as a whole. By focussing on the structure of the group, on the emotional climate and on the pattern of relationships and communication, an attempt is made to bring about a fundamental change which will result in a well-functioning family and an alteration in the circumstances which have maintained the symptom.

Thus a child who is truanting from school may be presented as the only problem by a family who, in fact, have a number of difficulties. By focussing on or scapegoating the child in this way, the family system may preserve itself from serious conflict between other members or between the family group and another part of the wider social system. The child's problem with school is therefore in some way 'useful' to the family and any direct attempt to deal with the truanting may be directed at reducing the underlying conflict or at changing a disordered style of communication which has led to the family 'needing' the child's symptom.

In the therapeutic sessions family members are seen together. The focus is largely on the group processes operating and involves the observations of such inter-actional elements as coalitions, stratagems and avoidances. As these are further analysed, they may be revealed to the family or they may be simply 'corrected' by the direct authoritative action of the therapist. The periods inter-vening between treatment sessions are seen as being of primary importance for the family, who may then revert to original dysfunctional patterns or may continue in the direction of therapeutic change.

The role of the therapist is varied. Some therapists regard themselves primarily as analysts and concentrate on making the family aware of its interactional style, whereas some regard themselves as mediators or referees or may take sides with one or more family members to provide a necessary balance of power. If two or more therapists work as a team then they may present their own relationship as a model of open communication and in this way try, for example, to illustrate the constructive potential of conflict.

The professional background of family therapists is highly varied and their original training may be in psychology, social work or psychiatry. The theoretical concepts used similarly cover a wide range including psychoanalysis, communications theory and behavioural analysis. Concepts have also been borrowed freely from general systems theory, which is predominantly a mathematical theory with applications in cybernetics and biology. In behavioural family therapy the focus is on the manipulation of the family consequences of individual behaviour and the attempt is made to analyse and modify social reinforcement patterns and observational learning.

Because family therapy involves a varied and often subtle set of procedures, it is very difficult to carry out satisfactory studies to measure its effectiveness. Many of the variables said to be involved are rather intangible and the processes underlying changes in social systems are highly complex. Preliminary evidence suggests that it is often useful but this can also be said of many other forms of therapy, and the 'cost-effectiveness' considerations which play a part in treatment choice sometimes make it difficult to support a strong case for the use of family therapy. Many critics would return a general verdict of 'not proven', but the level of interest by professionals is undoubtedly high and growing. One special difficulty has been the failure of those working in this area to provide an adequate means of identifying the cases which may be most appropriately treated in this way. Any attempt to treat all conditions with a uniform approach is unlikely to return a high overall rate of effectiveness. With a more limited set of identified problems this mode of treatment may in future prove to be the optimal means of effective intervention for a range of cases. At present, family therapy reflects just one aspect of the increasing awareness of the importance of understanding the social context when dealing with a presented psychological symptom.

The effects of marital breakdown

Divorce statistics represent a very conservative estimate of marital failure and a still more conservative estimate of marital unhappiness and disharmony, but the rates are high and increasing. There are various estimates of the likely divorce rate of currently made marriages but one in four is a frequently encountered figure. There are certain known predictors of marital breakdown. It is more frequent, for example, when the couple married at an early age, when they have few friends, when they have had relatively little education and when their life style is unconventional. The marital success or failure of their own parents also bears a direct statistical relationship to the couple's chances of breakdown.

Psychological studies have shown that certain measures of personality and social style are also predictors of failure. If the wife rates her husband as being emotionally immature, if the husband's self-image is lacking in coherence and stability, or if either of the partners is emotionally unstable then marital breakdown is more likely than if the reverse holds. Good communication, a high level of emotional support and the constructive handling of conflict situations are, not surprisingly, features of relationships which are associated with high levels of marital happiness and low rates of breakdown. In many of these studies it is, of course, difficult to disentangle cause and effect.

The process of adjustment to a marriage may be a long and difficult one, and some marriages never successfully 'take'. The highest rates of breakdown therefore occur in the first years, but many relationships are stable and

satisfactory for a while and are then beset with difficulties at a later stage. Divorce is usually preceded by
months or years of intense conflict and may eventually come
as a relief, but the evidence suggests that generally the
whole process is a very painful one for many members of the
family involved, both adults and children.

Research with divorcees has revealed a high degree of
stress and unhappiness which may last for a very long time.
On the whole, it appears that the experiences of women in
this situation result in rather more disturbance than those
of men, but for both sexes the status of divorce is associated with higher risk of clinical depression, alcoholism
and attempted suicide. The psychological effects of a
marriage breakdown may stem largely from lack of social
support, the absence of an intimate relationship and a loss
of self-esteem, but there are often additional pressures
relating to the loss of contact with the children or of
having to bring them up alone. There is a high rate of
remarriage among the divorced; and divorce itself, for
all the apparent risks which it brings, is still often
preferable to continuing in a marriage which has failed.

The 'broken home' is associated with increased aggres-
siveness and delinquency in children, but there seems to be
only a weak association with neurotic and other psychiatric
problems of childhood. While the rate of conduct problems in
the children of divorce is considerably higher than that for
children of stable marriages, there is apparently little
increase in such antisocial behaviour for children whose
homes have been broken by the death of a parent. This
suggests that it is the discord in the home which produces
the effect rather than the mere absence of one parent. This
is supported by the finding that conduct problems also occur
with increased frequency in homes with continual discord,
even when there is no separation or divorce.

Single-parent families

Children are raised in single-parent families when the
mother has not married, when there has been a divorce or
separation, or when one parent has died. 'Illegitimacy' is a
somewhat outmoded term and an increasing number of single
women now feel that they want to rear their child on
their own. Social attitudes against illegitimacy and
single parenthood have softened over the years and this has
encouraged more mothers to keep the baby rather than have it
adopted.

Single parenthood appears to be more stressful for the
remaining parent than sharing the responsibilities with a
partner. Lack of emotional support and of adult company are
some of the reasons for this but there are also likely to be
increased financial hardships, and the homes of single
parents have been shown to be overcrowded and often lack
both luxuries and basic amenities. During times of parental
illness there may be few additional social resources to call
upon, and the single parent is less likely to be able to
organize a social life for herself (about 90 per cent of

single parents are women). A number of self-help organizations have now been formed to fulfil some of the special
needs of the single parent.

One-parent families are viable alternatives to the more
traditional nuclear families, and most of the children
raised in such circumstances do not appear to show any signs
of disturbance or impaired development. There have been
suggestions that the boy without a father might tend to be
more effeminate but it has been found that most boys brought
up by their mothers are as masculine as the rest. If anything, they tend to make fewer sex-identity based assumptions about tasks and roles. We could say that they seem
to be less 'sexist' than other boys. Similarly, the girl
brought up with the father alone does not seem to lack
feminine identity. These findings reflect a more general
conclusion that children seem to base their own stereotypes
on the wider world around them rather than on the conditions
prevailing in their own immediate family.

The family life of old people

Old age is marked by declining health and mobility and by a
process of disengagement from several life enterprises,
notably employment. There may be low income and financial
difficulties, contemporaries are likely to die, and the old
person may find it difficult to replace such contacts with
the result that they live in a shrinking social world. The
high emphasis which some old people place on privacy may
reduce the uptake of potential neighbourhood and community
resources.

The major exception made to such concern with privacy
is with the immediate family. Typically, contacts with
children and grandchildren are highly prized and may be
a major focus of interest in their lives. While there is
likely to be an increase in dependency, however, this is
often recognized by the old and they often respect the
independence of the younger family and feel a crushing sense
of obligation if they are forced through circumstance to
accept aid from them. In some families there is an informal
'exchange of services' between generations with the older
person, for example, looking after the grandchildren while
parents are working or having a short holiday.

Recent social change has resulted in fewer three-
generation households, but with increasing age and decrea-
sing health, and perhaps the death of one of the parents,
the younger couple may want to offer the surviving partner
a place in their home. There may be doubts about how well
this will work out and conflict may be initiated between the
marital partners over how far feelings of duty should lead
to changes which might disrupt the family. As the children
become older the pressure on space may build up, and with
increasing health difficulties the burden of the older
person may become too great. Deafness may become an
irritation, there may be restricted mobility and the elderly
parent may become incontinent.

The increased strain on the family may lead to harsh feelings or even violence towards the old person as well as to a detrimental effect on the health of other members of the family. Eventually the pressure may become unmanageable and the old person may be forced to enter an institution. For many elderly people, living with a child is a halfway stage between having a home of their own and living in an old people's home. Both moves may involve their giving up possessions and pets. The quality of institutions varies greatly, but a frequent reaction is one of withdrawal, depression and depersonalization. Despite having many people around the old person may suffer from a deep sense of loneliness and isolation.

While it seems inevitable that old age will always bring unhappiness to some people, for many it is a time of contentment and fulfilment and in a number of cases the positive aspects centre on activities and memories of relationships within the family. Older women, for example, may play a major role in organizing family get-togethers and may act as a social secretary for members of the extended family, and grandmothers and grandfathers may gain great satisfaction from their relationships with their grand-children. Many of the recent social changes in housing organization and mobility, it is true, militate against a high level of interaction between the generations, and there seems as yet little awareness by policy-makers of the social costs which such changes entail.

The future of intimate life styles

Contact with intimates in the family group seems to provide the individual, overall, with considerable benefits. Significant relationships are highly potent and there may be dangers, but generally the benefits far outweigh the costs. A variety of psychological needs are very well fulfilled in the traditional family setting. The child growing in the caring and stable family setting can generally develop skills and abilities and achieve a potential for happiness better than in any other setting, and the adult can fulfil with the marital partner the needs of emotional support, freedom from loneliness, sex, stability, and the building of a mutually comfortable 'social reality'. When the basic family pattern is disturbed there can be grave consequences for each of the people involved.

There is no uniform change in western society to a single alternative life style arrangement but there is rather an increasing diversity. There are now fewer children in families, more single-parent families, more divorces and separations, and there is a high incidence of transitory relationships and less contact between generations. Several lines of evidence suggest that children are valued less than in the recent past; that women, in particular, are looking more outside the family for their role-orientation and their life satisfactions; that there is now less 'family feeling'; and that family duties and responsibilities impinge upon individual decision making less than was the case some decades ago.

We may expect this variety to increase further as ideas regarding the roles of men and women evolve, as changes in biological and 'hard' technology take place and as patterns of employment and leisure alter. It would be premature to forecast, at this stage, what effects such changes will bring to interpersonal relationships and personal life styles. What does seem certain, however, is that there will be important effects. To some extent these can be affected by direct social intervention and some undesirable effects may be prevented.

Family life, then, is a key variable in society and adverse changes may inflict an enormous social bill. For this reason the effects on individuals must be carefully monitored. Psychologists are just one of the groups which will be involved in this vitally important enterprise.

References

Brown, G.W. and Harris, T. (1978)
Social Origins of Depression. London: Tavistock Publications.

Masters, W. and Johnson, V. (1966)
Human Sexual Response. Boston: Little, Brown.

Masters, W. and Johnson, V. (1970)
Human Sexual Inadequacy. London: Churchill.

16

Ageing and social problems
Peter G. Coleman

What is it to be old?

The study of ageing and problems associated with it are now recognized as important. This is not surprising, for older people have become the major clients of the health and social services. They also have a lot of free time at their disposal. If there is to be an expansion in adult education and opportunities for creative leisure activities, the benefits should go especially to retired people.

What is surprising is that it has taken so long for the social sciences to pay attention to ageing and old age. So many young professionals are called on to devote their attention to the needs of people at the other end of the life span, yet they are likely to have received little in the way of stimulating material about the distinctive psychological features of old age.

Professional people do nevertheless have to be introduced to the subject of ageing, and it is interesting to note how that introduction has come to take on certain standard forms over the last ten years. There are two very popular, almost obligatory it seems, ways to begin talking or writing about ageing. The first way is to present the demographic data about the increasing numbers of elderly people in the population; the second way is to discuss the negative attitudes people have about working with the elderly.

The common introduction to ageing
In important respects old age as we know it today is a relatively modern phenomenon. Though there may have been individual societies in the past where a comparably large part of the population was old, it is clear that there has been a dramatic change in developed countries since the turn of the century. At that time in Britain those over the age of 65 constituted one in 20 of the population; today they constitute one in seven.

In recent years much more use is being made of the statistic 'over the age of 75', since it has become clear that this is the group in the population which makes the largest demands on the health and social services. This has highlighted the worrying news for service planners in a time of economic constraints that, while the total number of those over 65 will not increase very much in the coming

204

years, the population of those over 75 has already passed 5 per cent of the total population and will reach 6 per cent by the end of the 1980s.

However, expressing concern simply at the number of elderly people in the population is misleading. Why after all should it be a problem that 15 per cent rather than, say, 10 per cent or 5 per cent of the population is over the age of 65, or that 6 per cent rather than 4 per cent or 2 per cent is over the age of 75? A lot of the issues have to do with economics. The state must find the means to continue paying adequate and perhaps even improved pensions, and to provide welfare services to larger numbers of people.

Yet perhaps the more fundamental issues are the availability and willingness of people, whether relatives, neighbours, professionals or volunteers, to give assistance to large numbers of disabled people in the population. For ageing, as any introduction to the subject makes abundantly clear, is associated with an increasing likelihood of developing chronic disability.

Global estimates of disability in daily living (in getting around the house and providing for oneself) indicate that the need for assistance is present in 15-20 per cent of the age group 65-74, rising to 35-40 per cent in the 75-84 age group and to over 60 per cent in those above 85. If one adds on the number of people living in institutions (hospitals and old people's homes), which is about 4-5 per cent of the total elderly population, one can conclude that about 30 per cent, or nearly one in three, of all people over the age of 65 are disabled and in need of help.

A typical introduction to ageing then goes on to present further numerical data on the social position of the elderly. Almost one-third of people over 65 have been found to live alone and large numbers are lonely. Many live in poor housing, lack basic amenities and so on.

The need for a life-span perspective

Large numbers of elderly people, large numbers of disabled elderly people, and large numbers of elderly people live in deprived circumstances; such is a typical introduction to old age. But there are vitally important perspectives missing. No wonder indeed that we should be concerned with attitudes, with finding enough people prepared to work with the elderly, enough geriatricians, enough nurses, enough social workers and so on, when the only image we present of old age is a negative one. If the only perspective we emphasize is one of endless problems, often insoluble because of irremediable physical and mental deterioration, we cannot expect many people to have the courage to become involved.

Old people are people like the rest of us. What is special about them is not that they may be mentally deteriorated, disabled or isolated. The majority, after all, is none of these things and many people reach the end of their lives without suffering any disadvantages. What is special about old people is that they have lived a long time. They have had all the kinds of experience we have had and many, many more. They are moving towards the end of life it is true, but it is every bit as important how one ends one's life as how one begins it.

The perspective on ageing that is needed is one which takes into account the whole life span. The discovery any student of old age has to make is not only that old people have a long life history behind them but that their present lives, their needs and wishes, cannot be understood without an appreciation of that life history.

If we really talk to old people all this will become evident. But how often do we do this? A most eloquent testimony of our neglect is a poem (88 lines long) that was found in the hospital locker of a geriatric patient. (It can be found in full, quoted in the preface of the Open University Text, Carver, V. and Liddiard, P., 1978, 'An Ageing Population', Hodder & Stoughton.)

> What do you see nurses
> What do you see?
> Are you thinking
> When you are looking at me
> A crabbit old woman
> Not very wise,
> Uncertain of habit
> With far-away eyes
> ....
> Then open your eyes nurse,
> You're not looking at me.

The writer emphasizes the continuity between her identity as an old person and her identities at previous stages in the life cycle. She is still the small child of ten with a large family around her, still the 16 year old full of hopes and expectations, still the bride she was at 20 and the young woman of 30 with her children growing up fast. At 40 her children are leaving home, and she and her husband are on their own again. But then there are grandchildren for her to take an interest in. Years pass and she has lost her husband and must learn to live alone. She is all of these people. But the nurse does not see them.

Psychological changes with age

It is only proper to admit at the outset that the main activity of psychologists interested in ageing, with some exceptions, has not been of a life span perspective. Their work has mainly been concerned with trying to establish what psychological changes, usually changes of deterioration, occur with advancing age, with understanding the bases of such changes and finding ways of compensating for them. These are obviously important questions.

Cognitive deterioration

It would be wishful thinking to deny that there is any

deterioration with age. Physical ageing is a fact which is easy to observe, though it may occur at different rates in different people. Performance in everyday tasks in which we have to use our cognitive ability to register things we see or hear, remember them and think about them also deteriorates. Absent-mindedness is one of the most common complaints of older people in everyday life.

In more recent cross-sectional studies of the performance of different age groups on experimental tasks, psychologists have tried their best to control for obvious factors which might produce differences in their own right, like education, illness, sensory impairment and willingness to carry out the tasks in question. Of course, certain question marks remain over differences in attitude and perceived role: for instance, whether older people see the purpose of such tasks in the same way as younger people. Nevertheless, certain conclusions can be drawn about the abilities which seem to change the most as one grows older. In the first place, older people take much longer to carry out tasks and this is not only because their limb movements are slower. In tasks in which they have to divide their attention ('try to do two things at once'), decline with age is very marked and is already evident in those over 30. Ability to remember things we have seen or heard declines, as does the ability to hold associations in mind.

However, in some older people decline is not evident at all. Particular experiences, for example particular occupational backgrounds, may develop certain abilities in an individual to such an extent that they remain well developed throughout old age. Retired telephone operators who have no difficulty in dividing attention between a number of messages are a case in point. The prominence of so many older people in public life where they reap the fruit of years of experience in political dealings is also an obvious illustration. Moreover, it seems to be true that in some old people deterioration does not, in fact, occur. There are studies which indicate that the cognitive ability of a sizeable minority of elderly people, perhaps as many as one in ten, cannot be distinguished from that of younger people.

This, then, is evidence that age itself is not the important thing. Indeed it seems better to view age simply as a vector along which to measure the things that happen to people. Some things that happen with age are universal. They occur at different times, but they are unavoidable. These things we can, if we like, describe as 'age' changes. But a lot of the things we associate with old age are not due to ageing processes and are not universal. There is a great variation in the extent to which people are hit by physical and social losses as they grow old. Some people are fortunate, some people are unfortunate.

From the point of view of cognitive ability, the most unlucky are those people who suffer from the various forms of dementia or brain diseases which lead to a progressive deterioration in mental functioning. But health is by no means the only extrinsic factor influencing mental state in old age. A lot of research has been done recently on the psychological effects of such brain-washing treatments as isolation and sensory deprivation. Disorientation and confusion are common results. Yet we are often slow to recognize that old people may be living in circumstances where by any ordinary standards they are extremely isolated and deprived of stimulation. No one calls to see them, to engage them, to remind them of their names, roles and relationships. Disorientation in time and space, and confusion about identity and relationship with others, can be a natural result. From our own experience we know how time can lose meaning after one has been ill in bed for a day or two, away from the normal daily routine.

Other social and psychological factors play a role too. Motivation to recover or maintain abilities is obviously a crucial factor, and a number of studies have shown that amount of education remains one of the major factors in cognitive ability and performance throughout life.

Personality and life style

Scientific work on personality and style of life in old age does not match the amount that has been done on cognitive functioning. The evidence we do have, however, relates both to change and stability.

One clear finding from research is that introversion or interiority increases with age. This means that as people grow old they become more preoccupied with their own selves, their own thoughts and feelings and less with the outside world. This change is only relative, of course, but it is evident both from responses to questionnaires and also from projective tests, where people are asked to describe or react to stimuli they are presented with, such as pictures of family and social situations.

The term disengagement has been used to describe such a change in orientation; a decreased concern with interacting with others and being involved in the outside world and an increased satisfaction with one's own world of memories and immediate surroundings. However, critics have been quick to point out the dangers of exaggerating the extent to which disengagement is a 'natural' development in old age. Most of the decreased interaction and involvement of older people is forced upon them by undesired physical and social changes: disability, bereavement, loss of occupational roles and so on. Moreover, there is also clear evidence that old people are happier when there is a good deal of continuity between their past and present activities.

Indeed, in contrast to any change in personality that may occur, the stability that people show in their characteristics and style of life over a period of time is far more striking. Longitudinal studies show that people continue to enjoy the same interests and activities. When striking negative changes occur in a person's interests or familiar mode of activities, or ways of coping with life in old age, for no obvious reason, this is often a sign of psychiatric illness, especially depression.

Some of the most valuable studies on personality in old age are, in fact, those which have shown how important it is to take into reckoning a person's life style, for instance in explaining why people react differently to changes and losses such as retirement, bereavement and living alone, or a move to a residential home. Any research finding about old people usually has to be qualified by a reference to life style. This is mentioned again when talking about adjustment to relocation.

Growth and development

Though deterioration has been the main perspective of psychological research on ageing up to now, it is not the only one. Certainly in literature old age has been treated much more generously. The works of Nobel prize winners, such as Patrick White ('The Eye of the Storm', 1973), Saul Bellow ('Mr Sammler's Planet', 1969) and Ernest Hemingway ('The Old Man and the Sea', 1952), present vivid and compelling pictures of old age that, like King Lear, have to do with deterioration and change but also with growth in understanding and the values of existence.

Indeed, a characteristic theme in literature is of old age as a time of questioning; of one's own achievements, of the meaning of one's life, of the values one lived by and of what is of lasting value. It is as if an old person, freed from the strait-jacket of society, suffering losses in his ability to function and in his social position - perhaps indeed precisely because of them - is, somehow, let free to question life. Psychologists have only begun tentatively to approach these issues, but there is a lot in writers like Jung to consider.

Adaptation to loss in old age

From what has already been said it should be clear that old age is a time of great inequality. It is a time when losses occur, loss of physical and mental abilities, loss of people who were close to one, loss of roles and loss of activities. These losses are not inevitable; they do not occur in the same degree to everyone; but adapting to loss is a characteristic feature of old age.

Attitudes to health and well-being

Severe disability is one of the major losses of old age and its central importance in shaping the rest of an individual's life is one of the most common findings to emerge from investigations on social aspects of ageing. People who are disabled have more problems in maintaining their desired styles of life and are more dissatisfied than people who are not disabled. This is not surprising.

What is more surprising, or at least not logically to be expected, is the fact that, in general, levels of well-being do not decline with age. This is despite the fact that the incidence and severity of disability tend to increase with age and have a great influence on well-being. The key to understanding this comes from studies on subjective health.

The clear evidence from both longitudinal and cross-sectional studies is that whereas objective health and physical functioning of elderly people tend to deteriorate with age, the same is not true in regard to how they feel about their health. The most likely explanation has to do with expectations. People expect to become somewhat more disabled with old age. If they do, they accept it. But if their physical functioning remains stable they may in fact experience this as a bonus and feel better as a result. Only if their health deteriorates beyond the expected norm are they likely to feel badly about it.

This argument applies strictly only to feeling well, but it has a wider implication for well-being generally and for reactions to other losses in old age. Expectation is a very important aspect of reaction to loss. It is what people expect and what people find normal that determines how they react to things and how satisfied they feel with their situation. This kind of consideration also leads one to reflect how different things could be if old people's expectations changed. This is in fact not so unlikely. Future generations of elderly people may be far less accepting of lower standards of health and also, for instance, of income. They may expect things to be a good deal better for them. And if things are not going to be better they are going to be less happy as a result.

Adjustment to relocation

Another misfortune often following from disability is that people can find themselves being obliged to move, sometimes quite unexpectedly and against their will, to different environments, particularly institutional settings, where they often have to remain for the rest of their lives. Though this is usually done to them 'for their own good' (they are judged incapable of looking after themselves in their own homes), the end result may be much worse than leaving them alone: for instance, further deterioration and loss of interest in life.

There has been growing realization of the extent to which environmental changes can contribute to physical illness and psychiatric disorders. Even where it is voluntarily undertaken and has otherwise favourable effects, there are indications that rehousing can undermine a person's health. There is also a great deal of variation between individuals in their reactions, so it is important to discover which factors might predict the ability to adjust easily to new surroundings.

Among psychological factors cognitive ability is clearly crucial. There appear to be two major reasons why cognitively impaired old people react worse to relocation. In the first place, their lack of ability to anticipate and prepare means that they experience more stress on making the move.

Second, because of their poor short-term memory and orientation abilities it may take them a long while to understand their new surroundings.

Personality is important too. We are not sufficiently sensitive to the fact that the institutional environments we provide may be fine for one kind of elderly person but not for another. American studies have shown the importance, for instance, of rebellious and aggressive traits, as opposed to passive and compliant ones, in predicting survival and lack of deterioration after relocation to institutional settings. Vital as well, of course, are attitudinal factors concerned with what a move means to the persons concerned, whether they want to go, and how they see their own future in a new setting.

Self-esteem and its sources: the lynchpin of adjustment?

Disability and environmental change have been picked out for consideration as two of the negative changes associated with old age. There are others, of course. Bereavement requires a major adjustment which seems to follow certain definite stages. Grieving is a normal, healthy part of the process, and the support and understanding of those around in allowing bereaved people to express themselves may be very important to it. Loss of occupational role with retirement is another big change. Indeed, adjustment to it is often thought of in the same terms as adjustment to the old age role itself. Most people make good adaptations, but not all, and retirement can be a major precipitating factor in the onset of late life depression.

Then again, a very significant loss for many people as they grow older is that of income: they must adapt to making do with less. There has been almost no psychological investigation of this kind of adaptation. From what one can see it would seem that a lot of old people positively take pride in stretching their money. This, of course, may also have a lot to do with their experience of deprivation in the past.

Naturally, in all these adaptations much depends on the characteristics of the individual person involved, and one is led to ask whether there are any general ways in which one can conceptualize how a person adapts to the various losses and changes that occur with old age. Some authors talk in terms of the individual possessing particular qualities: for instance, 'coping ability'. But the most valuable index of adjustment in old age is that of self-esteem.

Maintenance of positive attitudes to oneself seems to be one of the key issues in old age. An especially important component of self-image is a sense of being in control of one's own life. Development in childhood and adulthood is associated with an increasing sense of effectiveness and of impact on the external world. In old age this sense may well be taken away.

Intrinsic to this conception of self-identity is the notion that it must have roots outside itself. Therefore, if individuals are to maintain self-esteem they have a continuing need of sources from which they can define acceptable self-images. For some people these sources can exist in past relationships and achievements or in an inner conviction about the kind of person one is, but in the main they depend on the present external circumstances of their lives; their roles in the family, in relation to other people, in work and in other activities.

When these circumstances change, as they often do in old age, individuals may have to find alternative sources to maintain positive views of themselves. Here again it is vital to understand a person's life history. A person whose sense of self has been based on one particular kind of source, for instance relationships with close family members, is going to suffer especially if such family contacts are lost through death.

One way to investigate sources of self-esteem is to ask people directly what makes them say that they feel useful or feel useless, for instance. Not surprisingly, lack of infirmity and contact with other people including the family emerge as the major sources of self-esteem. Especially in disabled people, being able to do things for oneself, and in particular to get around, appear to be key factors; also being a source of help and encouragement to others is very important.

In this context it is worth putting in a good word for residential care and other types of grouped housing schemes. In a previous part of this section it was noted that a move to an institutional setting can be damaging for certain types of individual, but a good institutional setting can also be of great benefit to certain people. This is possible when sources of self-esteem are likely to be strengthened rather than weakened by the move.

For instance, some people could be said to be 'living independently in the community'. But in reality they may be extremely isolated and totally dependent on the services being brought to them. Once they have moved to a genuine communal setting the burden of infirmity and consciousness of being alone can be diminished. Precisely because they are better able to cope for themselves in the new environment and to be of importance to others, they may gain a new lease of life.

Helping old people

Not all the loss and trauma of old age can be countered from an individual's own resources. The modern welfare state provides a range of services for the elderly; housing, health and social services. These are, of course, limited, subject to decisions about what level of services the country can 'afford'. We do not know what a perfect service for the elderly would be like, but we certainly do know that what we provide at present falls a long way short of it.

However, the achievement of the present level of services needs to be respected if we are to develop further, and it is important that people in the various caring professions who carry out these services remember their responsiblities. One of the real dangers is taking the operation of a service for granted and applying it automatically or mindlessly. The people on the receiving end then cease to be considered as individuals.

A key element in any work with elderly people is the individual assessment, and it is here that the psychological perspective has a vital role. We need a good assessment not only of people's physical condition and capabilities and of their social situations, but also of their individual needs, their abilities and interests, which should include a good picture of how they used to be.

Besides helping in assessment, psychology can also play a role in the actual provision of therapeutic interventions both to old people themselves and to those around them. Applied psychology should be able to show the best way: for example, to help recover abilities that seem to be lost or to mend social relationships that have become tense.

Maintenance of interests, activities and functioning

One of the most tragic images we have of old age is that of an old person with shoulders sunk, sitting collapsed in a chair, totally uninvolved in the world around. In a previous section the question of 'disengagement' in old age was raised, and let us repeat the point made there that, although some decline in activity may be an intrinsic part of growing old, most of such decline is the result of physical disability and environmental trauma.

When there is a dramatic decline in a person's activities for no obvious reason, we need to alert ourselves to the possibility that the person may be depressed. Loss of well-established habits and activities and lack of interest or anxiety about trying to regain them may be symptoms of the kind of depression which will respond to treatment, even though the person may not admit to having depressed feelings. But, of course, there also has to be some activity and interests for the person to go back to. Particularly if someone is disabled there may be few possibilities available, and the person is then likely to decline again. It is also quite clear that prolonged inactivity has deleterious effects both on physical and psychological functioning. Skills that are not exercised tend to atrophy.

In recent years a lot of new initiatives have been taken in geriatric hospitals in providing opportunities for patients to engage in different types of activity, arts and crafts, music discussion and so on. Generally, staff report improvements in elderly people who do take part in such activities, which can be seen in their personal appearance, in their physical and mental functioning and in their contact with others.

An even greater challenge is offered by people who are mentally deteriorated. In the first place it is very important to distinguish elderly people who really have irretrievable brain disease from those who only appear to have because they are depressed. Indeed, it may be symptomatic of someone's depression that he thinks his brain is rotting. It may be no easy matter to distinguish this, because it is difficult to motivate someone who is depressed actually to demonstrate his abilities. With the right treatment and support depressed people can be encouraged to regain their old abilities.

However, elderly people who clearly are deteriorating mentally should not be abandoned to their fate. Tests have shown that such people, given encouragement and help, can still acquire and retain new information and maintain skills. But the effort needed from outside is great. A good example is the use of so-called 'reality orientation', where people around the elderly person, either informally throughout the day or in concentrated formal classes, systematically try to help remind the person of time, place and season, of names of people, of objects, and of activities and so on.

Psychologists have a lot to do applying findings from the study of learning and memory to help old people. The trouble at present is that such people are often left alone, and this only exacerbates their condition. Dementia is a progressive illness, but what happens between its onset and death is important. If in the future we find medical means of slowing down its progress, it will become an even more urgent matter to find means as well to allow people to maintain their optimum potentialities in the time that remains left to them.

Family relationships
Another vital issue is the relationship between disabled elderly people and their families. Many more of such people are supported by their families than live in institutions for the elderly. For instance, in the case of severe dementia, there are four to five times as many suffering from such a condition living in the community as live in residential homes or hospitals. Yet often families who are doing the caring get pitifully little in the way of support services.

If they become overburdened by the stress of their involvement, both they and their elderly relatives suffer. The old person's mental condition may well be aggravated by tired and irritable relatives, and if there is a breakdown in care and there is no alternative but to take the old person into an institution, the family members are likely to suffer greatly from feelings of guilt. They often want to care for a relative until that person dies, but need help in carrying it out.

It is an important principle to accept that work with families is an integral part of work with elderly people. Family ties after all usually form a substantial part of an individual's identity. If those ties are damaged, so is the person's identity. The physical and mental deterioration that affects many people as they grow older and their ensuing state of dependency can put a strain on many relationships. Men, for instance, usually do not expect to outlive their wives. They can encounter great problems if they find instead that they have to spend their old age looking after a physically or mentally deteriorated wife, especially if in the past it was their wives who ran the household. Children too often find difficulty in taking over responsibility for ailing parents.

The actual symptoms, particularly of mental disturbance in old age, can be very disturbing. In some forms of dementia (probably dependent on the part of the brain that has been affected) the behavioural changes that can occur, caricaturing the person's old personality, increasing aggression or leading to a loss in standards of cleanliness, can be very painful for relatives to bear. It may be difficult for them to accept that the patient is not simply being difficult or unreasonable.

Families need counselling about the nature of the illness and, in the case of dementia, of its progressive nature, and preferably, too, promise of continued practical support. Group meetings held for relatives of different patients by doctors, social workers or other professionals can also be useful in allowing relatives to share common experiences and problems. Groups for the bereaved, particularly husbands or wives, can also play their part. The last years of their lives may have revolved around the care of a sick spouse and they must now find new meaning in life.

The future

In discussing ageing and social problems it may seem strange to end with a note about the future. But from what has been said it should be obvious that great improvements need to take place, both in society's provision for the elderly and in the attitudes of each and every one of us to the elderly people we live among.

For most people old age is not a particularly unhappy time, though for some it is. In part that may be, as we have suggested, because old people have low expectations. They quietly accept a society that treats them meanly and as somehow less important. In the future that may all change. We may see new generations of elderly people, foreshadowed in today's Grey Panthers in America, who will mobilize their potential power as a numerically important part of the electorate and pressurize society to give them a better deal.

On the other hand, old people may continue to remain on the sidelines. They may refuse to see their own material and other interests as being of central importance to society, in which case the rest of the population must see they are not forgotten.

The most important changes indeed are the attitudinal ones. We must recognize that old people are ourselves. They are our future selves. There is a continuity in life both between their past and present and between our present and future.

Old people remain the same people they were. Indeed, if we really want to know about a person's needs and wants and how they could be satisfied, the best introduction would be to let them tell us about their life history. Whatever new steps are taken in the future must follow on from this and make sense in relation to it.

Better provision would follow from such a recognition. If we really respected people's individuality we would provide them with choice about the circumstances and activities with which they end their days, not just enforce certain standard solutions. In short, we must allow people to grow old in ways that suit them, perhaps to explore new avenues of development in order to make the most of the years that remain. Also, when we consider those who need our help, who suffer in old age and perhaps are dependent upon us, we should not forget these wider perspectives.

Bibliography

Birren, J.E. and Schaie, K.W. (eds) (1977)
Handbook of the Psychology of Ageing. London: Van Nostrand Reinhold.

Brearley, C.P. (1975)
Social Work, Ageing and Society. London: Routledge & Kegan Paul.

Bromley, D.B. (1974)
The Psychology of Human Ageing (2nd edn). Harmondsworth: Penguin.

Carver, V. and Liddiard, P. (eds) (1978)
An Ageing Population (Open University text). Sevenoaks: Hodder & Stoughton.

Chown, S.M. (ed.) (1972)
Human Ageing. Harmondsworth: Penguin.

Dibner, A.S. (1975)
The psychology of normal aging. In M.G. Spencer and C.J. Dorr (eds), Understanding Aging: A multi-disciplinary approach. New York: Appleton-Century-Crofts.

Gray, B. and Isaacs, B. (1979)
Care of the Elderly Mentally Infirm. London: Tavistock.

Kastenbaum, R. (1979)
Growing Old - Years of Fulfilment. London: Harper & Row.

Kimmel, D.C. (1974)
Adulthood and Ageing. An interdisciplinary developmental view. Chichester: Wiley.

Miller, E. (1977)
Abnormal Ageing. The psychology of senile and presenile dementia. Chichester: Wiley.

Neugarten, B. and associates (1964)
Personality in Middle and Later Life. New York: Atherton Press.

17

Dying and bereavement
A. T. Carr

Demographic trends

If you had been born at the beginning of this century, your life expectancy at birth would have been 44 years if you were male or 48 years if you were female. If you were born today, your initial life expectancy would be 70 years or 76 years respectively. These figures reflect an ageing of the population that has occurred in all western industrial societies over the past 80 years. Although we all will die, most of us will do so at a relatively advanced age. Although we all will be bereaved, most of us will not suffer this until we are young adults or until we are in our middle years.

The fatal conditions of the present day, once hidden by the mass diseases, are those associated with longevity. In 1978, almost 590,000 people died in England and Wales and 85 per cent of these deaths were attributable to only three categories of illness: diseases of the circulatory system (heart and blood circulation), neoplasms (cancer) and diseases of the respiratory system (OPCS, 1979). Also, more than two people in every three now die in institutions of one form or another.

In the absence of any radical changes of events, the vast majority of us will die aged 65 years or over, in an institution of some sort and as a result of a disease of our circulatory system, or respiratory system, or of cancer. This underlines an important feature of dying and death at the present time: they have become unfamiliar events that take place in unfamiliar surroundings, watched over by unfamiliar people. We all know that we will die and that we may be bereaved, yet we have very little relevant experience upon which to develop our construing or anticipation of these events and states.

Telling

The majority of fatally ill people realize, at some point, that they will not recover, even if they have not been informed of the nature of their illness. However, it would appear that only about half of all fatally ill people appreciate their condition before significant changes in health force the conclusion 'I am dying'. This is almost certainly an under-estimate: there will be some people who know that they will not recover but who do not communicate this.

217

Although about one-half of terminally ill people appear
to appreciate the seriousness of their illness, this awareness is usually achieved independently, informally and
indirectly. No more than 15 per cent of terminally ill
cancer patients are told of their prognosis either by their
general practitioner or by a hospital doctor (Cartwright,
Hockey and Anderson, 1973). This contrasts markedly with the
experiences of their close relatives. Almost 90 per cent of
the close relatives of terminally ill patients are aware
that the patient's illness is terminal and most of them are
informed of this by a general practitioner or by a hospital
doctor. There are several implications of these data, the
two most obvious being that fatally ill people and their
principal carers often do not share the same information
about the illness, and that doctors usually are unwilling to
tell patients when they have a disease that will kill them.
Perhaps the most serious consequence is that one or more of
the familial participants has to cope with the demands of
this most stressful period without adequate support.

It is remarkable how little emphasis is placed upon the
wishes of the patient. Most people, including doctors,
whether they are young or old, ill or well, say they would
want to know if they had a fatal illness or that they are
glad they do know. Several studies have examined this issue
and the results are consistent in showing that more than
70 per cent of all the samples used say they would want
to be informed if they had a terminal disease. It is clear
that most people say they would want to be informed of the
seriousness of their illness and most doctors say that they
would want to be told; yet the majority of fatally ill patients are not told. Also, the existence of a real threat to
life does not reduce the very high proportion of people who
want to know if they have a fatal illness.

In general, learning that one has a fatal illness is
followed by a period of disquiet, even grief, although the
emotional response may be concealed from others. It is worth
noting that some patients do not 'hear' or at least appear
not to remember, what they have been told regarding their
prognosis. Although it has been proposed that the defence
mechanism of denial is a ubiquitous response to learning of
a fatal prognosis (Kubler-Ross, 1969), there are other more
mundane possibilities. The first is the use of terminology
that may have very precise meanings for a professional but
which may mean nothing, or something very different, to the
patient. To inform a patient of 'malignant lymphoma' or
'secondary metastases' may not constitute communication.
Even when the words that are used are understood reasonably
well, they may not convey what was intended. For some
individuals, the knowledge of their impending death will be
extremely distressing; in such cases the person may be quite
unable to accept what is plain to everybody else. They may
become distraught as their bodies show increasing signs of
impending death while they continue to deny that they are
dying. Such extreme responses, as a terminal illness

progresses, correspond to denial as elucidated by Kubler-Ross (1969). However, it would be inappropriate to regard as denial a person's failure to comprehend or to recall initial statements about prognosis. Quite apart from the communication problems mentioned above, if people have no prior suspicions that their conditions may be terminal it is probable that they will be unable to accept a fatal diagnosis. It is not that they refuse to accept such information but they are unable to accept it. It demands a radical revision of their view of the world and such a major psychological adjustment takes time. Initially, such news is not disbelieved, but on the other hand, it cannot be fitted into a person's perception of the world: it cannot be accommodated. The revised view of the world will need to be tested, amended and confirmed in the light of further information. The person will seek such information in what people say, how they behave and how his body feels. It is only when the revised view of the world 'fits', in the sense that it is not violated by new observations or new information, that the person is able fully to accommodate the 'truths' that have been offered. Individuals who have prior suspicions about the seriousness of their illnesses have already constructed, at least in part, a view of their world that includes themselves as dying individuals.

Our aim must be to maintain dignity, to alleviate suffering and to help people live as fully as possible for as long as they are able: they should be told what they are prepared to hear at a time when they are prepared to listen. The same principle might be kept in mind when dealing with relatives. There are indications that those who are told with care show improved family relationships, less tension and less desperation during their terminal illnesses than those who are not (Gerle, Lunden and Sandblow, 1960). Helping a person towards fuller awareness of, and adjustment to, a fatal prognosis is the beginning of a communication process which is itself an integral part of caring for the terminally ill.

Terminality and dying

The two words terminality and dying are being used to draw a distinction that can have important implications for the way in which fatally ill people are managed and treated. The main implication is that of regarding someone as terminally ill, but nevertheless as living and with some valuable life remaining, rather than regarding the person as dying with all the negative attitudes this provokes. Once illnesses have been diagnosed as terminal we need to regard patients as living and possibly living more intensely than the rest of us, until they clearly are dying. Terminality, then, begins when a terminal diagnosis is made but dying starts later, usually when death is much closer and when individuals are prepared to relinquish their biological life in the absence of valuable, functional life.

Sources of distress

Effective and appropriate care of the fatally ill requires an awareness of potential sources of distress so that distress can be anticipated and thus be avoided or alleviated. Of course, distress is not confined to the patient: effective care and support for those who are close to the patient is merited not only on humanitarian grounds, but also because of the exacerbation of the patient's suffering that can result from the distress of relatives and friends. Table 1 summarizes some of the most common sources of distress for patients and those who are close to them.

The listing contained in table 1 is by no means exhaustive, but it illustrates a number of points. First, given some capacity for empathy on the part of the survivor(s) there is little that the terminally ill person must endure that the survivor can avoid. This commonality of the sources of distress argues strongly for the need to attend to the welfare of survivors before they become bereaved. Second, it is clear that almost all the potential sources of distress are psychological in nature. Even some of the physical symptoms such as incontinence or smells are distressing because of our values and expectations. Also, pain itself is an experience that is subject to psychological factors rather than a sensation that is elicited by an appropriate stimulus.

Although we cannot examine in detail the physical distress of terminal illness, our discussion would be incomplete without a summary of this. Cartwright et al (1973) and Ward (1974) identified retrospectively the physical symptoms experienced by their samples of terminal cancer patients, 215 and 264 individuals respectively. These data are summarized in table 2.

It is striking that the rank order of symptoms is the same for both samples and a significant proportion of patients in each sample experienced each of the symptoms listed. Other common physical symptoms were breathing difficulties, 52 per cent; coughing, 48 per cent (Ward); and sleeplessness, 17 per cent (Cartwright et al).

Distress and coping

An examination of tables 1 and 2 points to a number of psychological processes that predispose people to react with depression and anxiety during a terminal illness. Current approaches to depression emphasize the role of loss and helplessness as aetiological factors. Loss refers to the real or imagined loss of a valued object, role, activity, relationship, etc. The individual relevance of the concept of loss lies in the individual differences of our value systems. For example, a person who highly values physical abilities, physical appearance, etc., is likely to be more at risk for depression as a result of physical debility, tiredness and deterioration in appearance, than someone for whom such attributes are low in a hierarchy of values.

Helplessness describes a state that is characterized by an awareness that one's behaviour is unrelated to the events

Table 1

Common sources of distress	
Fatally ill person (P)	Those who love P
Awareness of impending death	Awareness of impending bereavement
Anticipation of loss	Anticipation of loss
Physical sequelae of disease process, e.g. tumours, lesions, nausea, incontinence, breathlessness, unpleasant smells	Empathic concern, aversion, etc.
Frustration and help-lessness as disease progresses	Frustration and help-lessness as disease progresses
Uncertainty about the future welfare of the family	Uncertainty about the future welfare of the family
Anticipation of pain	
Empathic concern	Caring for P, night-sitting, tiredness, etc.
Changes in roles with family, friends, etc.	Changes in roles with family, friends, etc
Changes in abilities as illness progresses	Empathic concern
Changes in appearance as illness progresses	Empathic concern, aversion, etc.
Uncertainties about dying	Empathic concern
Dying	Empathic concern
	Discovery of death, directly or indirectly
	Practicalities, funeral, etc.
	Grief
	Role changes
	Reconstruction of life

Table 2

Symptoms suffered by terminal cancer patients

Symptom	Per cent in sample of Cartwright et al	Per cent in sample of Ward
Pain	87	62
Anorexia	76	61
Vomiting	54	38
Urinary incontinence	38	28
Faecal incontinence	37	20
Bedsores	24	13

which impinge upon oneself. When a person is subjected to aversive events whose occurrence, intensity, duration, etc., is quite independent of behaviour, a characteristic state may ensue. This state, which occurs in the majority of subjects tested, is known as learned helplessness. There are individual differences in susceptibility to learned helplessness, but the more aversive the events and the more frequently they are experienced as independent of behaviour the more likely it is to develop. It is a generalized state characterized by apathy, dysphoric mood, psychomotor retardation (i.e. slowness in thought and action), and feelings of hopelessness. Many clinical depressions are explained most fully in terms of the development of helplessness and there is evidence that sudden death is not an uncommon consequence of learned helplessness in laboratory animals. There can be little doubt about the relevance and importance of helplessness to our consideration of the welfare of the terminally ill.

Let us now return to the sources of distress summarized in tables 1 and 2. It is clear that some of these are intrinsically uncontrollable, and others duplicate the procedures that are used in experimental work to induce helplessness in that they are aversive, uncontrollable and repeated: for instance, urinary incontinence and vomiting. Furthermore, many patients undergo physical investigations and treatments that they do not understand, that they find unpleasant or painful and about which they feel they have little choice other than to accept them passively. It is not surprising to find that depression is commonly encountered in the terminally ill. A significant minority of fatally ill people and their next-of-kin become moderately or severely depressed (about one in five people in each group). Those most at risk are adolescents, young parents with dependents, those who have many physical symptoms and those who experience lengthy hospitalization.

The reciprocal interaction of physical and psychological processes must not be overlooked. We have already considered the depressive role of repeated, unpleasant physical symptoms. However, the interaction also proceeds in the other direction: adverse emotional states such as depression and anxiety augment pain and other physical discomforts. The essential point is that pain is not a simple response to an appropriate physical stimulus such as tissue damage: it is an experience that is compounded of the stimulation and the person's response to that stimulation. The motivational and emotional state of the person acts, as it were, to colour the sensation and to produce the experience we call pain. Without such 'colouring' and evaluation the sensation may be perceived but not experienced as painful.

It is the experience of most who work in terminal care that the relief of anxiety or depression through appropriate support, communication and practical help reduces the pain of patients and, not insignificantly, reduces the need for medication. The point is not that attention to the psychological state of the patient removes the need for relevant medication but that it reduces the dosages that may be required to bring relief. There are many obvious advantages that derive from this, not the least of which is the ability to alleviate pain without resorting to medications that render the patient confused, drowsy or comatose.

Anxiety arises when a future event is appraised as threatening. This appraisal is the evaluation of an event in terms of its harmful implications for the individual, harm being the extent to which continued physical and psychological functioning is endangered. Threat appraisal is a highly subjective process that depends upon the subjective likelihood of an event – that is, how probable the person feels the event to be – and the degree of harm that will result, this again being subjectively assessed. So terminally ill people are anxious to the extent that the events that they anticipate are both likely and harmful in their own terms: if events are not perceived as likely or harmful then they will not provoke anxiety.

Anxiety is an essentially adaptive emotion, in that it motivates us to initiate behaviours that prevent the anticipated harm being realized. To the extent that individuals accept that they are dying and are unable to reduce or eliminate the harmful consequences of this process, they are liable to remain anxious. An inspection of tables 1 and 2 reminds us that there are many potential types of harm that the fatally ill person is motivated, by anxiety, to alleviate. It is reassuring to note that the intense panic that is such a common feature of clinical anxiety states occurs rarely in terminal illness except, perhaps, in those who continue to deny the imminence of death as the end approaches and those for whom breathing is difficult. However, moderate anxiety is by no means uncommon in the terminally ill. This is not only an extra burden of suffering for the person but it also exacerbates other discomforts including pain.

There are few systematic reports of anxiety in terminal illness but from the data that do exist it is clear that moderate anxiety is experienced by between one-quarter and one-half of patients. The anxiety may be readily discerned in those people who are able to verbalize their fears, and who are given the opportunity to do so, but it may be less obvious in those who communicate less well verbally. However, the physiological and behavioural concomitants of anxiety are good indicators of the presence of unspoken fear. Often it is difficult to distinguish between physiological signs of anxiety such as gastric upset, nausea, diarrhoea, muscular pains, etc., and symptoms of the disease process or side effects of treatment. Nevertheless, the possibility that a patient might be persistently anxious should not be overlooked.

Given the subjective nature of threat appraisal, the causes of an individual's anxiety can be surprisingly idiosyncratic, but there are a few consistencies that may provide some clues. Younger adults expect to be distressed by pain and parting from the people they love, whereas the elderly fear becoming dependent and losing control of bowel and bladder functioning. Hinton (1972) reports that almost two-thirds of his patients who died aged 50 years or less were clearly anxious but this was true of only one-third of those aged 60 years and over. There is a clear and understandable trend for young parents of dependent children to be more anxious than other groups. Perhaps it is not insignificant that younger patients also tend to experience more physical discomfort during their terminal illnesses.

According to Hinton (1963), anxiety is more common in people with a lengthy terminal illness. He found more than 50 per cent of those who had been ill for more than one year to be clearly anxious, but only 20 per cent of those who had been ill for less than three months showed similar levels of anxiety. Although anxiety levels fluctuate during a patient's terminal illness, there is no general trend for anxiety to increase as the person draws closer to death. Some people become more apprehensive as their illnesses progress, but others become more calm during the last stages of their lives.

Some specific experiences of illness may be potent sources of anxiety. Prior episodes of intolerable pain can provoke great anxiety when they are recalled or when their return is anticipated. Difficulties in breathing are commonly associated with anxiety and a tendency to panic. Also, in the context of a mortal illness there are a number of sources of distress that are intrinsically uncontrollable and uncertain, such as the final process of dying, death and the nature of the world in which one's dependent survivors

will be living. When anticipated harm remains and individuals perceive it as beyond their ability to influence, they
become liable to the state of helplessness. If this is
severe they may become depressed, as we have discussed: if
less severe, then they may exhibit the resignation that has
been termed 'acceptance' (Kubler-Ross, 1969). If they
persist in their attempts to control and influence events
that are beyond their reach they are likely to remain
anxious and even to become more anxious as they approach
death.

For the fatally ill child under five or six years of
age, anxiety takes the form of separation anxiety, loneliness and fears of being abandoned. The young child does
not appear to fear death and its implications, but fears are
aroused by those aspects of illness and hospitalization
which elicit fear in most ill children who require hospital
treatment.

Between the ages of six and ten or eleven years, separation fears persist, but the child is increasingly prone to
anxiety over painful treatments and bodily intrusions. Such
fears of mutilation and physical harm are intensified in the
absence of familiar, trusted adults. Some children in this
age group, because of differing prior experiences or more
advanced cognitive development, are also aware of the
cessation of awareness and bodily functioning consequent
upon death.

Although there is some dispute as to whether the child
under ten years of age can be aware of impending death at a
conceptual level, there is little doubt that many young
children perceive that their illness is no ordinary illness. This is a frequent clinical observation and there is
a good deal of evidence that it is so whether or not the
diagnosis is discussed with the child (Spinetta, 1974). Of
course there are many cues that may indicate to the child
that something very serious and threatening is happening,
quite apart from the numerous tests, treatments and visits
to hospital. Most children are finely tuned to detect
meaningful and subtle signs in the verbal and non-verbal
behaviour of adults: the things that are not talked about,
tone of voice, eye contact, posture, etc. Also, there are
many cues that the child would find it hard to overlook:
whispered conversations, unusually frequent and intense
bodily contact, unusual generosity and freedom of choice
with regard to presents and treats, and so on.

Parents and others usually begin to grieve for the
fatally ill child soon after they accept the prognosis.
Their ability to cope with this grief is an important
determinant of their effectiveness in supporting the child.
Since familiar adults and siblings are likely to be the
child's greatest potential source of comfort and reassurance, it is important that time and attention is devoted to
these significant others for the sake of the child's welfare. There are indications of a high incidence of psychological difficulties in family members, particularly

siblings, during the terminal illness of a child. Clearly parents, who are themselves struggling with their own emotions, may have difficulty sustaining the other children in the family, let alone in providing comfort and reassurance to the one who is ill.

Adolescents and some younger children will be aware of the finality of death. Although dependent upon adults in a functional sense, they may perceive themselves as having important roles to play in the welfare of others and thus be subject to fears for the well-being of their survivors in much the same way as adults with dependents. Very young children may endure a terminal illness with striking calmness and acceptance of their lot, provided that their separation fears are allayed, but once they are past the age of six or seven years they become prone to a wide range of fears that exceed those of their 'normally ill' counterparts with severe, chronic, but non-fatal illness. Although children may be reluctant to express their fears, or may express them unclearly and indirectly, they should be anticipated in all aspects of care.

We have examined the range of potential sources of distress in terminal illness and the most common types of distress that result from these. Pain, anxiety and depression are sufficiently frequent and severe to merit attention when services are being planned and delivered. However, a majority of fatally ill people do not become severely anxious, deeply depressed or suffer from unrelieved pain. This does not minimize the awful suffering of the large minority or the pressing need for improvements in care to which this suffering testifies. It indicates only that, with whatever help they receive, most people who endure a terminal illness cope reasonably well, keeping their levels of distress within limits that are acceptable to themselves and to those who care for them.

The responses of people who are faced with impending death show sufficient uniformity to enable observers to write of stages, phases and patterns of coping (e.g. Kubler-Ross, 1969; Falek and Britton, 1974). Quite apart from doubts about the uniformity and progressive nature of stages of coping in terminal illness (e.g. Schulz and Aderman, 1974), it cannot be assumed that any particular individual needs to negotiate these stages in order to cope most effectively with impending death. The emotional responses and their dependent behaviours are indicators of the difficulties, and triumphs, experienced by people in their attempts to cope. The absence of a specific emotion does not mean that the person has omitted a necessary stage of the 'normal' coping pattern and that this omission detracts from the person's adjustment. Provided we do not equate 'typical' with 'ideal' or 'necessary', an awareness of the emotional stages or phases that are commonly encountered in terminal patients can help us to understand the problems they face, to provide the types of help and support that might be beneficial and to improve our ability to cope with the emotions that their behaviours arouse in relatives and in ourselves.

However, there are a number of general points that can be made about a stage model of terminal illness. The responses delineated, including denial, anger, bargaining, depression and acceptance (Kubler-Ross, 1969), are not specific to people who are facing death; they have been observed in many other stressful situations that involve loss and uncontrollable harm, such as bereavement, amputation and imprisonment. The generality evidenced by these observations does not confirm the progression of the stage model: it highlights the normality of disbelief, anger, sadness, etc., in the face of irretrievable and severe loss.

Often it is difficult to decide which stage or phase a person is in. Without reasonable certainty in the identification of stages, the predictive value of a stage model is severely impaired. This predictive aspect of the model is also reduced if the stages are not ubiquitous and if they are not successive. Clinical observation suggests that the emotion displayed by a person is responsive to many internal and external events. Perhaps all that can be said with any certainty is that some responses, when they occur, are likely to predominate earlier in a terminal illness, for example denial, and some are more likely to appear later, for example depression and acceptance.

We must take care not to lose sight of the individual in anticipating responses to a terminal illness. Fatally ill people bring with them their own particular views of themselves, their families, their futures, doctors, death, etc. The importance of individual differences during the terminal phase of life is well illustrated by the work of Kastenbaum and Weisman (1972). They found that their patients could be divided into two broad groups, both of which were aware of the imminence of death but which differed markedly in their behavioural styles. One group gradually withdrew from their usual activities and social contacts, remaining inactive until their final illness. The other group was characterized by involvement: patients in this group remained busily engaged in everyday activities until death occurred as an interruption in their living.

Dying

The relationship between a patient's reactions to a terminal illness and dying is not only that these are the psychological context within which the final process occurs, but also there are increasing indications that they influence the timing of death (see Achterberg and Lawlis, 1977). Whereas blood chemistries reflect on-going or current disease status, psychological factors are predictive of subsequent disease status and longevity. Poorer prognosis and shorter survival occurs in patients who, typically, show great dependence upon others, who deny the severity of their conditions, who have a history of poor social relationships and who do not have access to, or do not utilize, supportive social relationships during their illnesses. These patients tend to become more withdrawn, pessimistic and depressed as their illness progresses. Longer survival is associated with patients who maintain good personal and social relationships in the context of an existing network of such relationships. They can be assertive without hostility, asking for and receiving much medical and emotional support. They may be concerned about dying alone and seek to deter others from withdrawing from them without their needs being met. These patients also experience less pain, or at least complain less about pain and discomfort.

Dying is a process rather than an event that occurs at one point in time. This final process that constitutes the transition from life to death is usually of short duration, a matter of hours or days. For the vast majority of people it is not dramatic. Most people, both ill and well, express a desire to die peacefully or to die in their sleep. There is little doubt that this wish is fulfilled in most cases. Although there are a few people for whom pain or breathlessness may increase near the end, most slip knowingly or unawares into the unconsciousness that continues until their dying is finished.

After a terminal illness lasting some months, most patients are tired and wearied by their experiences. During their last days, apart from having their needs tended, patients may wish to be alone or to avoid news and problems of the 'outside world'. They may well become less talkative and prefer shorter visits. Communication tends to shift increasingly towards the non-verbal. In terms of interaction they may want little more than somebody to sit with them in silence, perhaps holding hands. It is clear from those who wish to talk briefly in their last hours of life that there is an experience of 'distance' from life. As Saunders (1978) so aptly puts it, 'They were not frightened nor unwilling to go, for by then they were too far away to want to come back. They were conscious of leaving weakness and exhaustion rather than life and its activities. They rarely had any pain but felt intensely weary. They wanted to say good-bye to those they loved but were not torn with longing to stay with them.'

Euthanasia

Euthanasia, meaning a gentle and easy death and the act of bringing this about, has been a source of discussion and controversy for many years. The level of current interest is evidenced by the large number of recent publications on the topic in the professional literature and the increasing support of the public for such organizations as the Voluntary Euthanasia Society in the UK and the Euthanasia Education Council in the USA.

The public support for euthanasia is probably based upon an expectation that death will come as a result of a lengthy illness, an illness that may well be prolonged unduly by the application of current medical knowledge and techniques. It is based upon fears of the physical and psychological incompetence, dependence, indignity and pain that may result from a chronic or terminal illness. Even those professionals who oppose euthanasia on ethical, religious or practical grounds readily concede that such fears are not unjustified for many people. We have already examined the potential distress of terminal illness but, for many people, support for euthanasia is prompted by thoughts of an unwanted, useless existence where biological life is maintained artificially and against their wishes in a hospital, nursing home or geriatric ward. Sadly, such thoughts are all too often reinforced by cases that Saunders (1977) rightly describes as 'truly horrendous'. As a society we cannot escape the reality that far too many elderly people end their days in loneliness, isolation and degradation. Even when the physical care provided is good, the psychological distress can be great. The prima facie case for euthanasia appears to be strong.

The many logical, philosophical and ethical arguments relating to the legalization of voluntary euthanasia, both active and passive, have been well stated several times (e.g. Rachels, 1975; Foot, 1978), and space precludes their consideration here. However, these arguments frequently take little account of relevant practical and psychological issues. In drawing up the necessary guidelines for the legalization of voluntary euthanasia there are major problems in guarding against error and potential abuse, both by relatives and professionals. Nevertheless, many of these problems could be surmounted by the use and recognition of the Living Will. This document, as distributed by the Euthanasia Educational Council, is signed and witnessed when the person is in good health. Its aim is to avoid an existence in dependence, deterioration, indignity and hopeless pain.

Doctors spend their lives preserving the lives of others and alleviating their suffering. It can be argued that, in recent years, the pendulum has swung too far in the direction of the maintenance of life at the expense of the relief of distress, but the activities of doctors make demands upon their energies and their personal time that few other professions would tolerate. This degree of commitment is consistent with, and continually reinforces, a value system that places a very high priority upon the preservation of life and actions that serve this end. For individuals in whom such values relate closely to their self-concepts, the active termination of life may be damaging to their self-regard and to their concept of their own worth as individuals. Although there is little difference between active and passive euthanasia on moral and logical grounds, for individual doctors the difference may be vast and unbridgeable in terms of their own psychology. It would be quite unjustifiable to place such men in a position where society expected them to implement active euthanasia.

From the patient's point of view, the availability of euthanasia has a wider potential than the avoidance of further suffering. People who are given control over aversive and painful stimulation, by having the facility to terminate, reduce or avoid it in some way, are better able to cope with the experience. Even though the available control is rarely exercised, the aversive stimulation is better tolerated and provokes less distress. Provided that patients are quite sure that their lives can be terminated when they wish, and only when they wish, they are likely to cope better with the effects of their illness or condition and to be less distressed.

To allow patients to die in order to release them from hopelessness and irreducible suffering, while continuing to treat their current distress, is thoroughly compatible with the humanitarian principle of care. Whether or not one wishes to describe this as passive, voluntary euthanasia is a matter of personal choice. There are grounds for a more widespread recognition of this compatibility and for more weight to be given to the wishes of patients and their families. Of course, the same grounds demand that more effort, time and resources should be devoted to improving the quality of care that is offered. All such improvements weaken the case for regarding death as a desirable release from suffering, as a release that is needed so frequently that its use should be regularized. In the long term, and certainly in the shorter term, there are likely to be some people for whom death is the preferred option. It is a problem that will become more acute as our society continues to age and as the life-preserving techniques of medicine continue to develop.

Bereavement

Bereavement is a state characterized by loss. The main focus of interest is upon the loss occasioned by the death of a significant person but people are bereaved by other losses such as loss of role, loss of status, separation and amputation. The state of loss serves as the stimulus for the bereavement response, a response that is manifested culturally and individually. The cultural response constitutes mourning and is a pattern of behaviour that is learned from and supported by one's immediate culture as appropriate following bereavement. Grief is the individual response and is the main area of concern for researchers and clinicians alike. In that grief typically follows a reasonably consistent course over time, ending ultimately in its resolution, it can be regarded as an individual process that occurs in response to individual loss.

The nature of grief

Although the major features of grief are known to most of us either intuitively or through personal experience, the chief findings of the many descriptive studies can be summarized broadly as follows:

* grief is a complex but stereotyped response pattern that includes such physical and psychological 'symptoms' as

withdrawal, fatigue, sleep disturbance, anxiety and loss of appetite;
* it is elicited by a rather well-defined stimulus situation, namely the real or imagined loss of a valued object or role, and it is resolved when new object relations are established;
* it is a ubiquitous phenomenon among human beings and appears in other social species, especially higher primates;
* it is an extremely stressful response both physically and psychologically, but grief-related behaviour is often antithetical to the establishment of new object relations and hence to the alleviation of the stress. For example, fatigue and withdrawal make it much more difficult for the bereaved person to develop new roles and new personal relationships in place of those lost through bereavement.

The complexity and stress of grief is readily appreciated when the number and nature of its components are considered. Hinton's (1972) description of grief adumbrates the most commonly observed characteristics: shock, denial, anxiety, depression, guilt, anger and a wide variety of somatic signs of anxiety. Other components include searching behaviour, suicidal thoughts, idealization of the lost person, panic, a heightened vulnerability to physical illness and to psychological disorders.

The nature of grief as a process is emphasized by the designation of stages by many observers and authors. Although there is a sequential character to the process it would be incorrect to anticipate an orderly progression through the stages in all people. As with the notion of stages in dying that was discussed earlier, the component responses of the various stages overlap and merge into one another. Also, there are frequent 'regressions' to earlier stages. Again, it is better to think in terms of components, some of which will predominate earlier in the process and others that will predominate later. In general, three stages or phases have been delineated and labelled according to inclination: perhaps the best descriptive labels are shock, despair and recovery.

Initially there may be a period of numbness and detachment depending, to some extent, on the unexpectedness of the news of the death. During this immediate response people may appear stoical and calm. Normal routines may be maintained especially where domestic or other factors structure the situation. Alternatively, people may appear dazed and quite unable to comprehend the reality of the news; they may be unresponsive to their environment and in need of care and support during this period. Whatever the specific initial reaction in a particular instance, it can last from a few minutes to two weeks or so, with the stoical reaction being the more likely to persist longer. The bereaved person is less able than the terminally ill to deny successfully the reality of the situation: sooner or later, and in many different ways, powerful and pointed signs of the reality of loss occur, such as the empty place at table, the empty bed or chair, the funeral or the silent house when friends and relatives depart. As with the news of terminal diagnosis, people need time to assimilate and to accommodate to a new state of the world. Whether the period of shock and disbelief is long or short, a sense of unreality or even disbelief is likely to return periodically for several months.

As awareness of the loss develops people may express anger at themselves, at staff or at God for not preventing the death. Whether or not anger is present, the phase of acute grieving or despair is the most painful. Lindemann (1944), in his pioneering study of bereavement, observed the following 'symptoms' as common to all individuals suffering acute grief: somatic distress lasting between 20 minutes and one hour at a time, feelings of tightness in the throat, choking with shortness of breath, muscular weakness and intense subjective distress described as tension or psychological pain. This specific response, which appears to be unique to bereavement, occurs against a background of stress, anxiety and sadness or depression, together with the somatic concomitants of these emotions.

Behaviourally, grieving persons may be unable to maintain goal-directed activity, appearing disorganized and unable to make plans. They may be restless, moving about in an aimless fashion and constantly searching for something to do. They may find themselves going, unwittingly, to the places where the dead person might be found if still alive. A preoccupation with the lost person creates a perceptual set that leads to misinterpretations of ambiguous sights and sounds as indicative of his being alive. Some grieving people report seeing the dead person with a clarity that goes beyond illusion and misperception. Such experiences can occur long after the phase of acute grieving is past. Obviously, the physical and psychological demands of this period are heavy and it is not surprising that irritability is common, especially when the person is eating and sleeping poorly. Anger, frustration and resentment may be directed at friends and neighbours irrespective of merit. Such feelings may also be directed against the dead person for abandoning the survivor.

The intense anguish of the despair phase can be unremitting, rising to peaks of distress with thoughts of the loved one who has died. Most bereaved people seem unable to prevent themselves from thinking and talking about the one who has died even though this usually exacerbates their distress. Whether this is conceptualized as 'grief-work' or as repeated exposure leading to habituation, it appears to be necessary to recovery from grief. A reduction in the frequency and intensity of periods of peak distress may be the first sign that the process of recovery is beginning. Although estimates vary, the acute despair phase of grief typically lasts for three to ten weeks.

The process of recovery from grief is a process of reconstruction. Although some aspects of the person's private and public 'self' may survive bereavement relatively unchanged, it is necessary to develop new roles, new behaviours and new relationships with others. Whatever else may or may not be changed by bereavement, the survivor must live without one important and potentially crucial personal relationship that had existed previously: the loss of this relationship is the loss of the psychological and practical advantages, and disadvantages, that it conferred. Socially, the survivor is now a widow or a widower rather than one of a married couple: he is now a boy without a father, or she is now a mother without a child, etc. Apart from the direct, personal impact of such changes, they also influence the way survivors are viewed and treated socially. The bereaved person has to develop a new private and public self that enables him to live in a changed world.

Although a reduction in the frequency and intensity of periods of extreme distress may herald the process of recovery, it cannot begin in earnest until there are periods in which the person is not overwhelmed with despair nor preoccupied with thoughts of the one who has died. Many bereaved people recall with clarity the moment when they realized that they had not been preoccupied with their loss: when, for a brief period at least, their thoughts had been directed elsewhere and their emotions had been less negative, even positive. These moments of 'spontaneous forgetting', together with improvements in sleeping and appetite, provide people with some opportunity to reconstrue and to reconstruct themselves and their futures. With less exhaustion and a lightening of mood, decisions and actions become more feasible and people can begin the active process of reviving previous relationships and activities, perhaps in a modified form, and of developing new ones. This period of active readjustment may never be complete, especially in the elderly, but it usually lasts for between six and 18 months after the phase of acute grief and despair.

Determinants of grief

Strictly speaking, it is inaccurate to talk of determinants of grief for the available data do not allow us to identify the causative factors that lead to variations in the response to bereavement. However, it makes intuitive sense to talk of determinants and is in keeping with other literature on the topic. Parkes (1972) groups the factors of potential importance according to their temporal relationship to the event of death, that is, antecedent, concurrent and subsequent determinants. Among antecedent factors, the most influential appear to be life stresses prior to bereavement, relationship with the deceased and mode of death. On the whole, an atypical grief response with associated psychological problems is more likely when bereavement occurs as one of a series of life crises, when the death is sudden, unanticipated and untimely, and when the relationship with the deceased had been one of strong attachment, reliance or ambivalence.

A number of demographic variables (concurrent) relate to the nature of grief. In particular, being young, female and married to the deceased increases the likelihood of problems arising after bereavement. Of course, these factors are not unrelated to such antecedent factors as strong attachment, reliance and untimely death. Other concurrent factors with adverse implications are susceptibility to grief, as evidenced by previous episodes of depression, an inability to express emotions, lower socio-economic status and the absence of a genuine religious faith.

The presence of religious faith might be placed more appropriately with subsequent determinants, for its role is likely to be one of supporting the bereaved person during the stressful period of grief. Also, someone with an active belief system probably will be associated with a supportive social group, and there is little doubt that a network of supportive social relationships is the most advantageous of the subsequent determinants. Other subsequent factors that have positive implications are the absence of secondary stresses during the period of grief and the development of new life opportunities at work and in interpersonal relationships, for instance. Again, these are more probable when a good network of supportive social relationships exists. It is worth recalling our earlier conclusion about the value of such relationships in a person's adjustment to impending death.

Among the wide range of factors that have implications for a person's reaction to bereavement, there is most controversy about the importance of anticipatory grief. As the term implies, this refers to grief that occurs in anticipation of an expected death, particularly the death of a child or a spouse. Overall, it can be concluded that younger widows experience more intense grief, with associated problems, than those aged 46 years or over. Sudden death exacerbates the severity of the grief response for young widows but not for the middle-aged or the elderly. For the latter two groups there appears to be a small effect in the opposite direction: that is, some symptoms of grief, especially irritability, are greater after a prolonged illness prior to death. It should be noted that the potentially beneficial effects of anticipatory grief are not confined to conjugal bereavement but also mitigate the response to other losses, such as that of a child. Also, it seems possible that there is an optimum period for the anticipation of death, perhaps up to six months, after which the lengthy duration of illness may increase stress and exhaustion and increase the likelihood of adverse reactions in subsequent grief.

Illness and death after bereavement
There are clear data that reveal an elevated mortality risk after bereavement. At all ages, bereaved persons experience a higher risk of dying than married people of corresponding

sex and age. The increase in risk is greater for bereaved males than females, and for both sexes, the increase is greater at younger ages.

The elevated risk of death is concentrated particularly in the first six months after bereavement especially for widowers, with a further rise in the second year for widows. The predominant causes of death are coronary thrombosis and other arteriosclerotic or degenerative heart diseases. Most of these causes can be seen as a result of continued stress and a lack of self-care. In general, when the data from replicated studies in the UK and the USA are taken together, the risk of dying is at least doubled for widows and widowers at all ages for a great variety of diseases.

Having briefly examined the possible psychological and physical consequences of bereavement, and having considered relevant predictive factors, it is important to remember that we are talking only of probabilities. A person may be at great risk of problems following bereavement, in the statistical sense, and yet survive the experience well. Another person with only favourable indicators may suffer badly and experience severe physical or psychological problems.

The vast majority of bereaved people, with a little help from their friends, cope well with the experience and recon- struct lives that are worth while in their own terms. There are no persuasive grounds for considering the provision of professional services for the bereaved. The most useful strategy is to maintain some form of non-intrusive follow-up after bereavement with ready access to an informal support group if this should be necessary. The bereaved need some- body who will listen when they want to talk, somebody who will not try to push them into things before they are ready: somebody who will support them emotionally and practically when appropriate and just by showing that they care. This demands an informal response rather than a professional one. However, professional care and concern should not end with the death of a patient: the newly bereaved person still has a long way to go and every effort should be made to ensure that they will have access to whatever social support may be needed.

References

Achterberg, J. and Lawlis, G.F. (1977)
Psychological factors and blood chemistries as disease outcome predictors for cancer patients. Multivariate Experimental Clinical Research, 3, 107-122.

Cartwright, A., Hockey, L. and Anderson, J.L. (1973)
Life Before Death. London: Routledge & Kegan Paul.

Falck, A. and Britton, S. (1974)
Phases in coping: the hypothesis and its implications. Social Biology, 21, 1-7.

Foot, P. (1978)
Euthanasia. In E. McMullin (ed.), Death and Decision. Boulder, Co: Westview Press.

Gerle, B., Lunden, G. and Sandblow, P. (1960)
The patient with inoperable cancer from the psychiatric
and social standpoints. Cancer, 13, 1206-1211.

Hinton, J.M. (1963)
The physical and mental distress of the dying. Quarterly
Journal of Medicine, 32, 1-21.

Hinton, J.M. (1972)
Dying. Harmondsworth: Penguin.

Kastenbaum, R. and Weisman, A.D. (1972)
The psychological autopsy as a research procedure in
gerontology. In D.P. Kent, R. Kastenbaum and S.
Sherwood (eds), Research Planning and Action for the
Elderly. New York: Behavioral Publications.

Kubler-Ross, E. (1969)
On Death and Dying. London: Tavistock.

Lindemann, E. (1944)
Symptomatology and management of acute grief. American
Journal of Psychiatry, 101, 141-148.

Office of Population Censuses and Surveys (1979)
Mortality Statistics. London: HMSO.

Parkes, C.M. (1972)
Bereavement. London: Tavistock.

Rachels, J. (1975)
Active and passive euthanasia. New England Journal of
Medicine, 292, 78-80.

Saunders, C. (1977)
Dying they live. In H. Feifel (ed.), New Meanings of
Death. New York: McGraw-Hill.

Saunders, C. (1978)
Care of the dying. In V. Carver and P. Liddiard (eds),
An Ageing Population. Sevenoaks: Hodder & Stoughton.

Schulz, R. and Aderman, D. (1974)
Clinical research and the stages of dying. Omega, 5,
137-143.

Spinetta, J.J. (1974)
The dying child's awareness of death. Psychological
Bulletin, 81, 256-260.

Ward, A.W.M. (1974)
Telling the patient. Journal of the Royal College of
General Practitioners, 24, 465-468.

Family life and old age: Part V questions

1. Consider some of the factors which might lead a couple to decide to remain childless.
2. Evaluate the evidence relating to the effect of a mother working outside the home (i) on the children, (ii) on herself, and (iii) on her husband.
3. Write an essay on the family as a source of stress.
4. Write an essay on being single as a source of stress.
5. What are the special problems of the single-parent family?
6. What problems arise in a three-generation household?
7. Is the nuclear family an institution worth preserving?
8. Is the concept of 'maturity' useful in considering middle age?
9. Write an essay on the alcoholic in the family.
10. Is there a psychological equivalent of the menopause for men?
11. What steps should be taken to prepare nurses for retirement?
12. Should the psychology of ageing be part of developmental psychology, or a separate field of study?
13. Do older people show positive developmental changes as well as deteriorating changes?
14. What problems can arise in a family as a consequence of caring for an ageing relative?
15. The natural social setting for older people is with their younger family. How true is that statement?
16. Are the problems of old age a function of the ageing process, or a function of society's attitude towards the elderly?
17. What psychological techniques are there for older people to recover interests and activities they may have lost?
18. What are the main causes of distress in the terminally ill and their families, and what are the implications of these?
19. If you could change one aspect of the care of the terminally ill, what would you change, and why?
20. How has the pattern of dying changed in Britain since 1900, and what are the causes and consequences of the changes?
21. What are the stresses of bereavement, and what can be done to help people to cope with them?

22. What factors might lead a family to reject a chronically ill relative who is likely to remain in hospital?
23. What is meant by 'quality of life' for the elderly and the dying in hospital?
24. What methods might be used to minimize the confusion of dementing patients which they may experience on admission?
25. How could you increase the rate of attendance of parents and their children at a pre-school clinic?
26. A 35-year-old single woman has made a determined attempt to kill herself. What factors could have precipitated this attempt?
27. A 40-year-old solicitor, who has two young children, is suffering from terminal cancer and asks you 'What will it be like?' What points could you cover with such a person, and the family in subsequent conversations?
28. A woman has been re-admitted in an acute phase of rheumatoid arthritis. Her husband has been caring for her at home; what steps could be taken to support the husband when she returns home?
29. A man aged 35 is dying from inoperable carcinoma of the larynx. What guidance might be appropriate for the ward staff in caring for him?
30. A 45-year-old woman, who is the mother of four children aged between six and twenty, is admitted to the ward with an associated drink problem. What effect may the admission have on relationships between the patient and her family?

Part six
Changing People

18

People, patients and change
John Hall

Psychological effects of physical illness

Nurses may not necessarily see themselves as trying to change people. It might be thought that their main role is to care for the sick by providing for immediate physical and environmental needs, or to facilitate the physical changes brought about by medical or surgical treatment.

Yet personal and psychological change is in any event imposed upon people by their illness. Several things may trigger marked psychological change: the moment of admission to hospital, the realization that a child may be handicapped, or the growing awareness that an illness may be terminal. Change may occur in circumstances where a nurse is the first person to detect it, and when a nurse is the main person, or indeed the only person, able to correct and modify harmful change.

Some personal changes arise because of non-pathological physical change in the individual. Changes in physical strength, or in physical attractiveness, or in some particular aptitude or skill, may all influence the level of acceptance of an adolescent by his peers. Some children, and indeed some adults, are extremely sensitive about aspects of their appearance. They may perceive their noses to be odd even though apparently normal, and will avoid social contact rather than run the risk of derision, or have corrective rhinoplasty performed to reduce the size of the nose.

Physical illness and medical intervention, therefore, can change people psychologically. The fit young man who suffers a spinal injury, making him permanently hemiplegic, has in a moment had all his aspirations about sporting achievement dashed. Equally, an operation to restore sight in an elderly person with cataracts can restore mobility and interest to a surprising extent. An operation to correct a cleft palate in a young child not only changes the child physically, but changes the attitude of the parents so they now communicate more positively with the child because they are encouraged by the child's clearer articulation. The psychological consequences of physical intervention and treatment can be as profound as the consequences of illness and may require an equal amount of sensitivity and skill from the nurses involved.

Any mutilating operation is likely to lead to an emotional crisis. A good example of an operation that can lead

241

to severe anxiety and apprehension is a colostomy or ileo-
stomy. Apart from the fear of impending surgery, and the
implication of the operation itself, people may worry about
their work; will they still be capable of doing their jobs?

Velangi (1980) explains how careful and lengthy counselling may be needed to help a patient through the fears
aroused by a stoma. It is usually helpful to counsel the
patient as early as possible pre-operatively, and to start
by being non-technical. A proportion of male patients may
become impotent following a colostomy, and they may then
require detailed sexual counselling and guidance. One of the
main conclusions is the importance of the psychological approach and understanding which must be given to the stig-
matized amputee.

Ways of helping

Other nurses have, as an explicit part of their job, a
clear responsibility to change people or their patients by
psychological means. Nurses working with the psychiatrically
disturbed may need to present to a patient a model of an
appropriate response to an anxiety-provoking situation, so
the patient can learn from them how to behave. Nurses working with the mentally handicapped may have to train the
residents in their ward to dress themselves, or to feed
themselves. Health visitors may want to teach an unsupported
young mother how best to care for her new baby and gradually change the baby's food as it grows. Nurse tutors need
to know how their trainee nurses can best learn a list of
drugs or parts of the body.

This part of the book introduces the main methods of
psychological intervention which have as their explicit aim
the changing of some aspect of the patient's functioning or
behaviour. Psychologists are concerned not only to describe
the process of change, but to identify ways of making change
more efficient. Some mothers of young children, for example,
are inefficient, in a psychological sense, at bringing up
their children because they do not know that learning cannot
occur until the relevant physical maturation of the nervous
system has occurred. The best example of this problem is the
mother who tries to potty-train her child too soon. A few
successes may encourage the mother, but the ensuing failures
and consequent possible resentment may be directed at the
child quite inappropriately, because the child is unable to
control the relevant sphincter muscles properly.

Some methods of change have more immediate appeal
than others because they seem 'natural' or because they have
a common-sense ring to them. From a psychological point of
view, the key question to ask of any model or method of
change is: does it work? If it works, then the reason or
reasons why it works should be established, so that the key
ingredient, as it were, can be identified and thus used more
effectively. Effectiveness can be analysed from several
viewpoints. A method of change may be preferred because
it is capable of producing the greatest degree of change.

Alternatively, the greatest rate of response may be preferred, remembering to follow-up patients to check that the
initial rate of response is related to the level of final
outcome for the patient. Or the most cost-effective method
may be preferred, because it produced the greatest overall
response for a given amount of nursing input, usually
measured in hours or work involved.

One aspect of the 'appeal' of methods for change which
deserves special mention is the ethical acceptability of the
methods used. There is a public preference for treatment
methods which do not involve physical restraint or punishment. Public opinion on some of these issues might be
thought inconsistent, as exemplified by an apparent wish for
highly custodial treatment of some groups of offenders who
perhaps pose a minimal threat to the community. There is,
however, an onus on all members of the caring professions
to ensure that the methods they use are acceptable and de-
fensible to the public and indeed to themselves. It may be
noted that a decision that a particular method is ethically
acceptable does not usually take into account knowledge of
the demonstrated effectiveness of the method for an individual problem or patient.

Another aspect of the ethics of change is the interaction between the degree of commitment of the patient to
change, and the expected direction in which change will
occur. Some patients may be coerced into a treatment programme when they have little commitment to the goal of
treatment that has been identified by the treating staff.
Although the law on homosexuality between consenting adults
has become more lenient, people may still come for 'treatment' of their homosexuality because of pressure from spouse
or parents. Some people with a chronic drinking problem may
initially accept help in a detoxification centre because of
their awareness of their debilitated condition, but may not
be prepared to make a longer-term commitment to giving up
alcohol.

It is often necessary to consider the consequence for a
patient's way of life of an apparently minor change in a
particular area of functioning. If a man who gambles com-
pulsively stops gambling he is implicitly being asked to
change a major part of his daily routine, probably affecting
his friends, the papers he reads, his spending habits, and
his use of spare time. The implications of the expected
change may need to be discussed, so that the patient is not
the passive recipient of a treatment, but an active colla-
borator in it. Indeed, the whole nature of the therapist-
patient relationship may need to be examined so that the
patient becomes as responsible and as active in the relationship as possible.

Change and hospital

Most training of nurses takes place in hospitals. While this
might seem self-evidently the best place for such training,
it has been pointed out that hospital-based training does

not produce attitudes conducive to change. Hamilton (1979) gives a pungent account of the rapidity of change in the world about us, and the failure of nursing to be prepared for change. She believes that 'Nurses have identified areas which need change, but have failed to develop a commitment to change or to promote a climate for change.' She identifies particular aspects of hospital routine which emphasize 'bureaucratic control, rigid formal routine and subordination to medical and administrative authority'. In her view, nursing practice has not followed advances of medical science, and the solution to this stagnation can only be found if nurses become 'students and teachers of planned change in nursing. Nurses can no longer afford to let change happen by chance or they will no longer meet society's expectations.'

Improvements in the care of patients may have to rely on the transformation of existing attitudes and practices, and the more effective use of available resources, rather than assuming that extra resources will become available. Towell and Dartington (1976) discussed in detail the amount of change that took place in the care of old people in a 700-bedded hospital over a four-year period. The nine wards which were studied had a relatively high proportion of untrained and other nursing staff, and levels of dissatisfaction among the nurses were high.

Over the four years there was a considerable alteration in this traditional pattern, involving changes in patterns of nursing organization. As a result of the study, a number of general principles involved in this type of change were established. These included the need for staff to have a 'protected forum' to review their own activities and consider alternative solutions, and the value of drawing on the experience of staff in other nearby hospitals.

The cost of change

Whatever the cause or direction of change, change is costly. Life is easier for all of us if we are called upon to change as little as possible. There are many pressures upon us to keep behaving the same; we may be seen by our colleagues as 'rocking the boat' if we want to change some apparently trivial ward procedure; some threats to our own method of working may arouse within ourselves feelings that our personal integrity is being challenged, so we fail to see the merits of the new suggestions. For this reason, anyone contemplating the creation of change should realize that it may be hard work. The chronic smoker does not want to give up smoking, despite a bronchial condition. The long-serving ward aides on the night shift do not want to consider a new method of getting the patients up in the morning, coming as it does for them at the end of a long shift.

Conversely, the psychological effect upon us of even apparently minor events can be minimized. Events can happen to us, or to our patients, without the potential for change implied by the event (whether positive or negative) being realized. The best example of this type of cause-effect relationship is given by what is now known as 'Life-events' research. This research approach has given a degree of precision to the commonly-held, but rather vague, belief that illnesses can be caused by everyday events which happen to us. A number of studies have examined the amount of readjustment that is required by a range of events, and attempts have been made to scale or score these events numerically. Despite the difficulties in making this type of numerical comparison, it is interesting to compare the scores, or weights, assigned to some events which happen to most of us.

Death of a spouse	100
Marriage	50
Changing jobs	36
Finishing school	26
Christmas	12

These events and their associated scores can then be added together, and combinations of particular types of event can be related in a systematic way to, for example, the differential probability of a schizophrenic or depressive breakdown. An important aspect of this example is that apparently positive or pleasant events may cause as much difficulty in adaptation as negative or unpleasant events. Not only is it costly to attempt to produce change in others, but any change in the normal pattern of an individual's life may have a cost attached to it.

Models of change
In the same way as medical and surgical interventions are selected with a specific objective in mind, so psychological interventions can be selected to achieve particular goals. There is a range of objectives which may be relevant in selecting the right method of change.

* To achieve insight: insight, or understanding, of their own condition may be a prerequisite for change to occur. For example, in a marital conflict it might be thought that no progress can be made until the husband accepts that he is actually unreasonable in some of the demands he makes on his wife.
* To encourage expression of emotion: some bereaved people are unable emotionally to accept the death of their relative, and may need help to express that emotion.
* To encourage more adaptive social behaviour: adolescents may simply not know the criteria used by potential employers in selecting people for jobs, and they may need to be taught how to conduct themselves at a job interview, even down to details of dress.
* To reduce the frequency of a distressing habit: a repetitive act, such as spasmodic torticollis, may be both embarrassing and tiring, apart from the difficulty it causes to such activities as driving a car or playing a musical instrument.

The choice of method is more likely to be informed by the nature of the psychological change that is desired, rather than by the illness or medical condition.

Indeed, some change may be sought in the absence of any illness at all. There is a growing interest in physical fitness and a regulated diet as ways of delaying or forestalling illness, over and above the changes in life style that might be indicated on strictly medical grounds. Considerable effort may be needed to encourage someone to persevere with a minor change in everyday routine, such as doing daily exercises for a few minutes. Similarly, maintaining everyday health care routines, such as brushing teeth, may have an apparently low relevance to an outcome, such as badly decayed teeth. Probably the greatest improvements in general health could arise from preventative procedures of this kind, such as the wearing of seat-belts, yet they all suffer from the psychological defect that there is usually a marked delay or apparent randomness in the harmful consequences of not conforming to the procedure.

The physical rehabilitation setting extends the length of contact between nurse and patient, so that the nurse's role is stretched beyond the alleviation of ills of the body to the relief of the problems and needs of the whole patient. Although there is plenty of theoretical literature on the psychological role of the nurse in this type of setting, Rimon (1979) considered that there was little available empirical literature on the topic. Hence she carried out a 'critical incident' technique study, using nurses as subjects rather than patients because of the difficulty of extracting negative or critical comments from patients. The study involved the collection of details of recalled incidents, from nurses working on six different wards of the hospital.

She found that eight objectives encompassed the range of general aims of the nurses in the hospital. Among these objectives were: 'explain treatment and its rationale', 'help and encourage patients to become independent' and 'use sources other than one's own observations for feedback on patients' behaviour and to create a supportive environment'.

Whether patients are or are not ill, there may be several areas of their lives where change is indicated. Thus it may be necessary to produce change in several different ways at once. A patient, previously living independently, now in a wheelchair and living at home with parents, may need help both to adapt to the physical environment and to a new role in the family. Different approaches can be used simultaneously so as to help the patient as much as possible, and these may draw upon different ways of conceptualizing the patient's multiple problems.

Alcoholism is a growing problem, and one where careful planning of treatment is necessary to help patients through the crucial first few weeks and months. Marks (1980) described a programme for alcoholics, which includes four to five weeks of in-patient treatment, and at least a year of

out-patient contact. An important part of the programme is
patient teaching, in which staff from a number of disciplines take part. A considerable range of topics are covered
in the programme, including teachin on the effects of long-
standing neglect of oral hygiene and lack of dental care.
Nutrition is included in the programme, as is the effect of
alcohol on the body's major organs. A number of psychological principles underlie the organization of the programme.
One of the most noteworthy is the recognition that material
will be forgotten, and will need to be repeated. The anticipated loss of memory retention is 65 per cent 24 hours
after presentation, and 75 per cent loss at one week, unless
there is reinforcement and repetition of the original teaching. Another point is the recognition that knowledge of
health information may be out of date: in this study it was
suggested that recovering alcoholics frequently are 15 to
20 years out of date in their information.

Some methods of change are yoked very closely to a
particular theory of personality, or learning, or social
functioning. For example, the methods of free association
used in classical psychoanalysis are supported by theoretical assumptions about the way we unconsciously reject certain associations of ideas when we think in a rational but
controlled way. It is important for nurses, in applying a
particular method of treament, to know whether it is necessary to learn the underlying theory or whether the method
can be taken on its own merits without the necessity to look
at the theory. On the one hand, it is difficult to carry out
some behaviour modification procedures without at least some
understanding of the risk of satiation, which is what happens when patients obtain so much of a 'reinforcer' or reward that they will no longer pursue a therapeutic programme
because they have had enough! Conversely, meditation and
yoga techniques are now widely taught because of the immediate perceived benefits of mental and physical relaxation, without any reference to the eastern philosophical
ideas which led to the techniques. There is a risk with some
methods that they can be tried fairly easily in a superficial way, sometimes in a 'cook-book' or routine manner.
If they then fail because they have not been carried out
properly, not only is the patient the poorer for not being
helped, but the nurse or other person who has tried out the
method will be disillusioned with the method, and will be
reluctant to try it again when it may be the method of
choice.

Suiting the method of change to the target group

The number of elderly people is increasing, yet there is
still relatively little research-based knowledge on how
best to help the elderly psychologically. Goldberg and
Fitzpatrick (1980) therefore carried out a study of 'movement therapy' to investigate the effect of the treatment on
the morale and self-esteem of a group of 30 residents in a
nursing home. The study was designed in the light of the

findings of research studies of morale and self-esteem. The residents were divided into an experimental group which participated in a series of daily movement therapy sessions, and a control group which participated in a range of other activities. The study was assessed by means of a rating scale which consisted of 17 items assigned to three sub-scales. It was found that the experimental group improved more than the control group on one of these sub-scales, called 'outlook towards own ageing', and on the total morale score. There were no significant changes in self-esteem in the experimental group. The study produced evidence to support the clinical application of movement therapy amongst institutionalized elderly people on the basis of its effect on the patients' self-concept.

Some models of change may perhaps seem to be presented in an unnecessarily complex way, so that nurses feel that an essentially straightforward technique has been surrounded by a degree of mystique and confusing jargon. Any methods of change which are presented as directly educational or as part of training thus have an advantage. In nurse training the focus is on modifying the behaviour of nursing students by an explicit process of teaching. All nurses who have been through the training course have been exposed to such pro-cesses and can thus determine for themselves how effective different methods of training have been with them. There are a number of general principles which can be usefully intro-duced into any training course. In general, learning is im-proved whenever the student is actively involved, whether by taking notes in a lecture as opposed to not taking notes, or by reciting aloud lists of terms to be learnt rather than by learning them silently. It is often better to distribute learning time over a number of sessions, rather than doing all the learning at once in a 'massed practice' way.

These various principles are often incorporated into teaching aids which can be valuable in a number of teaching settings. Programmed learning is the presentation of the material to be learnt as a series of very simple but care-fully graded steps, with the opportunity for immediate checking. It has been developing for a number of years, though perhaps it has not met the somewhat extravagant expectations initially held for it. None the less, many nurses' training programmes can be improved by the use of such aids and prepared teaching packages, some of which have been carefully produced and are excellent examples of the practical application of psychological learning theory.

Nurse therapists
One aspect of the effectiveness of a treatment is the extent to which it can be used by nurses specially trained in its use, without the necessity to involve scarcer (and often more highly-paid) members of other professions. Marks, Hallam, Connolly and Philpott (1977) have described in considerable detail a project which set out to train nurses to become specialist 'nurse-therapists', carrying out be-havioural treatment methods independently. Their report

discusses the advantages of nurses as therapists. One advantage is that, because of the large numbers of nurses relative to other disciplines, an expansion in the number of nurse therapists would represent less of a distortion of the present pattern of professional resources. Details of the effectiveness of the therapists are presented. The nurse therapists saw 196 patients, whose progress was assessed by using target problem ratings and other measures such as Fear Survey Schedules. They concluded that in their projects the nurse therapists achieved improvements in their patients of a similar order to that of other professionals treating comparable patients. The results are discussed in terms of developing advanced clinical roles for nurses.

Summary

However unwelcome change may be to patients or staff, the indications are that the rate of social change is, if anything, likely to increase. Precisely because many effective treatments are now available for a range of physical and psychological problems, the expectation of change being achieved by patients is probably growing. The result of failure to create change where it has been expected can be a disappointed and sometimes overtly hostile and resentful patient. All nurses who try to initiate change should therefore have a sound understanding of both the potentiality and limitation of the methods they use, and a willingness to persist themselves and encourage persistence in their patients.

References

Goldberg, W.G. and Fitzpatrick, J.J. (1980)
Movement therapy with the aged. Nursing Research, 29, 339-346.
Hamilton, J. (1979)
Changes in clinical nursing. International Nursing Review, 26, 75-77.
Marks, I., Hallam, R.S., Connolly, J. and Philpott, R. (1977)
Nursing in Behavioural Psychotherapy. London: Royal College of Nursing.
Marks, V. (1980)
Health teaching for recovering alcoholic patients. American Journal of Nursing, 80, 2058-2061.
Rimon, D. (1979)
Nurses' perception of the psychological role in treating rehabilitation patients: a study employing the Critical Incident Technique. Journal of Advanced Nursing, 4, 403-413.
Towell, D. and Dartington, T. (1976)
Encouraging innovations in hospital care. Journal of Advanced Nursing, 1, 391-398.
Velangi, V. (1980)
Fear fights against a stoma. Nursing Mirror, 24 January, Supplement iv-ix.

19

Counselling and helping
Barrie Hopson

Counselling today

From a situation in the mid-1960s when 'counselling' was
seen by many in education as a transatlantic transplant
which hopefully would never 'take', we have today reached
the position of being on board a band-wagon; 'counsellors'
are everywhere: beauty counsellors, tax counsellors,
investment counsellors, even carpet counsellors. There are
'counsellors' in schools, industry, hospitals, the social
services. There is marriage counselling, divorce counselling, parent counselling, bereavement counselling, abortion
counselling, retirement counselling, redundancy counselling,
career counselling, psychosexual counselling, pastoral counselling, student counselling and even disciplinary counselling! Whatever the original purpose for coining the word
'counselling', the coinage has by now certainly been de-
based. One of the unfortunate consequences of the debasing
has been that the word has become mysterious; we cannot
always be sure just what 'counselling' involves. One of the
results of the mystification of language is that we rely on
others to tell us what it is: that is, we assume that we,
the uninitiated, cannot know and understand what it is
really about. That can be a first step to denying ourselves
skills and knowledge we already possess or that we may have
the potential to acquire.

It is vital that we 'de-mystify' counselling, and to do
that we must look at the concept within the broader context
of ways in which people help other people, and we must
analyse it in relation to objectives. 'Counselling' is often
subscribed to as being 'a good thing', but we must ask the
question, 'good for what?'

Ways of helping

'Counselling' is only one form of helping. It is decidedly
not the answer to all human difficulties, though it can be
extremely productive and significant for some people, sometimes. Counselling is one way of working to help people
overcome problems, clarify or achieve personal goals. We can
distinguish between six types of helping strategies (Scally
and Hopson, 1979).

* Giving advice: offering somebody your opinion of what
  would be the best course of action based on your view
  of their situation.

* Giving information: giving a person the information he needs in a particular situation (e.g. about legal rights, the whereabouts of particular agencies, etc.). Lacking information can make one powerless; providing it can be enormously helpful.
* Direct action: doing something on behalf of somebody else or acting to provide for another's immediate needs; for example, providing a meal, lending money, stopping a fight, intervening in a crisis.
* Teaching: helping someone to acquire knowledge and skills; passing on facts and skills which improve somebody's situation.
* Systems change: working to influence and improve systems which are causing difficulty for people; that is, working on organizational development rather than with individuals.
* Counselling: helping someone to explore a problem, clarify conflicting issues and discover alternative ways of dealing with it, so that they can decide what to do about it; that is, helping people to help themselves.

There is no ranking intended in this list. What we do say is that these strategies make up a helper's 'tool-bag'. Each one is a 'piece of equipment' which may be useful in particular helping contexts. What a helper is doing is to choose from available resources whichever approach best fits the situation at the time.

There are some interesting similarities and differences between the strategies. Giving advice, information, direct action, teaching and possibly systems change recognize that the best answers, outcomes, or solutions rely on the expertise of the helper. The 'expert' offers what is felt to be most useful to the one seeking help. Counselling, on the other hand, emphasizes that the person with the difficulty is the one with the resources needed to deal with it. The counsellor provides the relationship which enables the clients to search for their own answers. The 'expert' does not hand out solutions. This does not deny the special skills of the helper, but does imply that having 'expertise' does not make a person an 'expert'. We all have expertise. In counselling, the counsellor is using personal expertise to help to get the clients in touch with their own expertise. Counselling is the only helping strategy which makes no assumption that the person's needs are known.

Teaching, systems change, and counselling are only likely to be effective if the 'helper' has relationship-making skills. Giving advice, information and direct action are likely to be more effective if he has them. Systems change is different in that it emphasizes work with groups, structures, rules and organizations.

The counsellor possibly uses most of the other strategies at some time or other, when they seem more appropriate than counselling. The other strategies would have an element of counselling in them if the 'helper' had the necessary skills. For example, a new student having difficulties making friends at school could lead to a counsellor, in addition to using counselling skills, teaching some relationship-building skills to the student, getting the staff to look at induction provision, making some suggestions to the student, or even taking the student to a lunchtime discotheque in the school club.

Who are the helpers?

Strictly speaking we are all potential helpers and people to be helped, but in this context it may be useful to distinguish between three groups.

Professional helpers

These are people whose full-time occupation is geared towards helping others in a variety of ways. They have usually, but not always, received specialist training. Social workers, doctors, teachers, school counsellors, nurses, careers officers and health visitors are a few examples. They define their own function in terms of one or more of the helping strategies.

Paraprofessional helpers

These people have a clearly defined helping role but it does not constitute the major part of their job specification or represent the dominant part of their lives, such as marriage guidance counsellors, priests, part-time youth workers, personnel officers and some managers. Probably they have received some short in-service training, often on-the-job.

Helpers in general

People who may not have any specially defined helping role but who, because of their occupational or social position or because of their own commitment, find themselves in situations where they can offer help to others, such as shop stewards, school caretakers, undertakers, social security clerks or solicitors. This group is unlikely to have received special training in helping skills. In addition to these groupings there are a variety of unstructured settings within which helping occurs: the family, friendships, and in the community (Brammer, 1973).

What makes people good helpers?

In some ways it is easier to begin with the qualities that quite clearly do not make for good helping. Loughary and Ripley (1979) people their helpers' rogue's gallery with four types of would-be helpers:

* the 'You think YOU'VE got a problem! Let me tell you about mine!' type;
* the 'Let me tell you what to do' type;
* the 'I understand because I once had the same problem myself' person;
* the 'I'll take charge and deal with it' type.

The first three approaches have been clearly identified as

being counter-productive (Carkhuff and Berenson, 1976) while the fourth one certainly deals with people's problems but prevents them ever learning skills or concepts to enable them to work through the problem on their own the next time it occurs. The only possible appropriate place for this person is in a crisis intervention. However, even this intervention would need to be followed up with additional counselling help if the needy person were to avoid such crises.

Rogers (1958) came out with clearly testable hypotheses of what constitutes effective helping. He said that helpers must be open and that they should be able to demonstrate unconditioned positive regard: acceptance of clients as worth while regardless of who they are or what they say or do; congruence: helpers should use their feelings, their verbal and non-verbal behaviour should be open to clients and be consistent; genuineness: they should be honest, sincere and without façades; empathic: they should be able to let clients know that they understand their frame of reference and can see the world as the client sees it, whilst remaining separate from it. These qualities must be not only possessed but conveyed: that is, the client must experience them.

Truax and Carkhuff (1967) put these hypotheses to the test and found considerable empirical support for what they identified as the 'core facilitative conditions' of effective helping relationships - empathy, respect and positive regard, genuineness, and concreteness - the ability to be specific and immediate to client statements. They differed from Rogers in that whereas he claimed that the facilitative conditions were necessary and sufficient, they only claimed that they were necessary. Carkhuff has gone on to try to demonstrate (Carkhuff and Berenson, 1976) that they are clearly not sufficient, and that the helper needs to be skilled in teaching a variety of life and coping skills to clients. The other important finding from Truax and Carkhuff was that helpers who do not possess those qualities are not merely ineffective, for they can contribute to people becoming worse than they were prior to helping.

The evidence tends to suggest that the quality of the interpersonal relationship between helper and client is more important than any specific philosophy of helping adhered to by the helper. This has been demonstrated to be the case in counselling, psychotherapy and also teaching (Aspy and Roebuck, 1977). A recent review of the many research studies on this topic would suggest, as one might expect, that things are not quite that simple (Parloff, Waskow, and Wolfe, 1978), but after a reappraisal of the early work of Truax and Carkhuff and a large number of more recent studies, the authors conclude that a relationship between empathy, respect and genuineness with helper effectiveness has been established. They also shed light on a number of other factors which have been discussed periodically as being essential for effective therapists (their focus was therapy, not helping):

* personal psychotherapy has not been demonstrated to be a prerequisite for an effective therapist;
* sex and race are not related to effectiveness;
* the value of therapist experience is highly questionable; that is, someone is not necessarily a better therapist because of greater experience;
* therapists with emotional problems of their own are likely to be less effective;
* there is some support for the suggestion that helpers are more effective when working with clients who hold values similar to their own.

What they do point out is the importance of the match between helper and client. No one is an effective helper with everyone, although we as yet know little as to how to match helpers with clients to gain the greatest benefits.

Helping and human relationships

Carl Rogers states very clearly that psychotherapy is not a 'special kind of relationship, different in kind from all others which occur in everyday life' (1957). A similar approach has been taken by those theorists looking at the broader concept of helping. Brammer (1973) states that 'helping relationships have much in common with friendships, family interactions, and pastoral contacts. They are all aimed at fulfilling basic human needs, and when reduced to their basic components, look much alike'. This is the approach of Egan (1975) in his training programmes for effective interpersonal relating, of Carkhuff and Berenson (1976) who talk of counselling as 'a way of life', of Illich, Zola, McKnight, Kaplan and Sharken (1977) who are concerned with the de-skilling of the population by increasing armies of specialists, and of Scally and Hopson (1979) who emphasize that counselling 'is merely a set of beliefs, values and behaviours to be found in the community at large'. Considerable stress is placed later in this chapter on the trend towards demystifying helping and counselling.

Models of helping

Any person attempting to help another must have some model in mind, however ill-formed, of the process which is about to be undertaken. There will be goals, however hazy, ranging from helping the person to feel better through to helping the person to work through an issue independently. It is essential for helpers to become more aware of the value-roots of their behaviours and the ideological underpinning of their proffered support.

The helper builds his theory through three overlapping stages. First he reflects on his own experience. He becomes aware of his values, needs, communication style, and their impact on others. He reads widely on the experience of other practitioners who have tried to make sense out of their observations by writing down their

ideas into a systematic theory ... Finally the helper
forges the first two items together into a unique theory
of his own (Brammer, 1973).

Fortunately, in recent years a number of theorists and
researchers have begun to define models of helping. This can
only assist all helpers to define their own internal models
which will then enable them in turn to evaluate their
personal, philosophical and empirical bases.

CARKHUFF AND ASSOCIATES: Carkhuff took Rogers'
ideas on psychotherapy and expanded on them to helping in
general. He has a three-stage model through which the client
is helped to (i) explore, (ii) understand and (iii) act. He
defines the skills needed by the helper at each stage of the
process (Carkhuff, 1974), and has also developed a system
for selecting and training prospective helpers to do this.
Since the skills he outlines are basically the same skills
which anyone needs to live effectively, he suggests that the
best way of helping people is to teach them directly and
systematically in life, work, learning and relationship-
building skills. He states clearly that 'the essential task
of helping is to bridge the gap between the helpee's skills
level and the helper's skills level' (Carkhuff and Berenson,
1976). For Carkhuff, helping equals teaching, but teaching
people the skills to ensure that they can take more control
over their own lives.

BRAMMER (1973) has produced an integrated, eclectic
developmental model similar to Carkhuff's. He has expanded
Carkhuff's three stages into the eight stages of entry,
classification, structure, relationship, exploration, consolidation, planning and termination. He has also identified
seven clusters of skills to promote 'understanding of self
and others'. His list of 46 specific skills is somewhat
daunting to a beginner but a rich source of stimulation for
the more experienced helper.

IVEY (1971) AND ASSOCIATES have developed a highly
systematic model for training helpers under the label
'microcounselling'. Each skill is broken up into its
constituent parts and taught via closed-circuit television,
modelling and practice.

HACKNEY AND NYE (1973) have described a helping
model which they call a 'discrimination' model. It is goal-
centred and action-centred and it stresses skills training.

KAGAN, KRATHWOHL AND ASSOCIATES (1967) have
also developed a microskills approach to counsellor training
which is widely used in the USA. It is called Interpersonal
Process Recall which involves an enquiry session in which
helper and client explore the experience they have had
together in the presence of a mediator.

EGAN (1975) has developed perhaps the next most influential model of helping in the USA after Carkhuff's and,
indeed, has been highly influenced by Carkhuff's work. The
model begins with a pre-helping phase involving attending
skills, to be followed by Stage I: responding and self-

Figure 1

Model of helping
From Loughary and Ripley (1979)

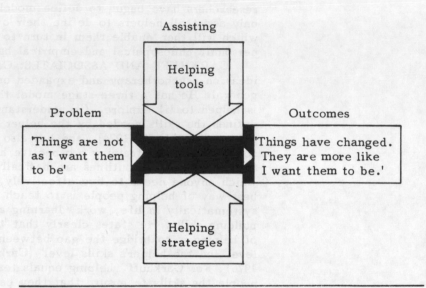

exploration; Stage II: integrative understanding and dynamic self-understanding; and Stage III: facilitating action and acting. The first goal labelled at each stage is the helper's goal and the second goal is that of the client.

LOUGHARY AND RIPLEY (1979) approach helping from a different viewpoint, which, unlike the previous theorists, is not simply on the continuum beginning with Rogers and Carkhuff. They have used a demystifying approach aimed at the general population with no training other than what can be gleaned from their book. Their model is shown in figure 1.

The helping tools include information, ideas, and skills (such as listening and reflecting dealings). The strategies are the plans for using the tools and the first step is always translating the problem into desired outcomes. Their four positive outcomes of helping are: changes in feeling states, increased understanding, decisions, and implementing decisions. Their approach does move away from the counselling-dominated approach of the other models.

The demystification of counselling

There is nothing inherently mysterious about counselling. It is merely a set of beliefs, values and behaviours to be found in the community at large. The beliefs include one that says individuals benefit and grow from a particular form of relationship and contact. The values recognize the worth and the significance of each individual and regard personal autonomy and self-direction as desirable. The behaviours cover a combination of listening, conveying warmth, asking open questions, encouraging specificity, concreteness and focussing, balancing support and confrontation, and offering strategies which help to clarify objectives and identify action plans. This terminology is more complex than the process needs to be. The words describe what is essentially a 'non-mystical' way in which some people are able to help other people to help themselves (see figure 2).

Training courses can sometimes encourage the mystification. They talk of 'counselling skills' and may, by implication, suggest that such skills are somehow separate from other human activities, are to be conferred upon those who attend courses, and are probably innovatory. In fact, what 'counselling' has done is to crystallize what we know about how warm, trusting relationships develop between people. It recognizes that:

* relationships develop if one has and conveys respect for another, if one is genuine oneself, if one attempts to see things from the other's point of view (empathizes), and if one endeavours not to pass judgement. Those who operate in this way we describe as having 'relationship-building skills';
* if the relationship is established, an individual will be prepared to talk through and explore thoughts and feelings. What one can do and say which helps that to happen we classify as exploring and clarifying skills (see figure 2);
* through this process individuals become clear about difficulties or uncertainties, and can explore options and alternatives, in terms of what they might do to change what they are not happy about;
* given support, individuals are likely to be prepared to, and are capable of, dealing with difficulties or problems they may face more effectively. They can be helped by somebody who can offer objective setting and action planning skills.

Counselling skills are what people use to help people to help themselves. They are not skills that are exclusive to one group or one activity. It is clear that the behaviours, which we bundle together and identify as skills, are liberally scattered about us in the community. Counselling ideology identifies which behaviours are consistent with its values and its goals, and teaches these as one category of helping skills.

What may happen, unfortunately, is that the promotion of counselling as a separate training responsibility can increase the mystification. An outcome can be that instead of simply now being people who, compared to the majority, are extra-sensitive listeners, are particularly good at making relationships, and are more effective at helping others to solve problems, they have become 'counsellors' and licensed to help. A licence becomes a danger if:

Figure 2

The counselling process

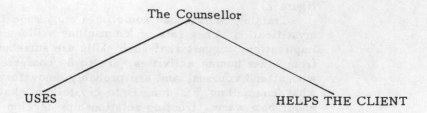

The Counsellor

USES   HELPS THE CLIENT

RELATIONSHIP BUILDING SKILLS	respect genuineness empathy	to feel valued, understood and prepared to trust the counsellor
EXPLORING AND CLARIFYING SKILLS	contracting open questions summarizing focussing reflecting immediacy clarifying concreteness confronting	to talk and explore to understand more about how he feels and why to consider options and examine alternatives to choose an alternative
	objective setting action planning problem-solving strategies	to develop clear objectives to form specific action plans to do, with support, what needs to be done

COUNSELLING IS HELPING PEOPLE TO HELP THEMSELVES

* those who have it see themselves as qualitatively
  different from the rest of the population;
* it symbolizes to the non-licensed that they are
  incap le, or inferior, or calls into question valuable
  work they may be doing, but are 'unqualified' to do.

It is important to recognize that labelling people can have
unfortunate side effects. Let us remember that whatever the
nomenclature - counsellor, client or whatever - at a
particular time or place, they are just people. All, at
some time or other, will be able to give help, at other
times will need to seek or receive help. Some are naturally
better fitted to help others; some by training can improve
their helping skills. All, through increased awareness and
skill development, can become more effective helpers than
they are now.

Counselling is not only practised by counsellors. It is
a widespread activity in the community and appears in
several guises. Its constituent skills are described
variously as 'talking it over', 'having a friendly chat',
'being a good friend' or simply 'sharing' with somebody.
These processes almost certainly include some or all of the
skills summarized in figure 2. Often, of course, there are
notable exceptions: for instance, we do not listen well; we
cannot resist giving our advice, or trying to solve problems
for our friends; we find it difficult to drop our façades
and roles. Counselling skills training can help reduce our
unhelpful behaviours and begin to develop these skills in
ourselves, making us more effective counsellors, as well as
simply being a good friend. In almost any work involving
contact with other people, we would estimate there is a
potential counselling component. There is a need for the
particular interpersonal skills categorized here as counselling skills to be understood and used by people at large,
but particularly by all people who have the welfare of
others as part of their occupational roles. Specialist
'counsellors' have an important part to play, but it is not
to replace the valuable work that is done by many who would
not claim the title. Having said that, people sometimes
think they are counselling, but in fact are doing things
very far removed: disciplining, persuading people to conform
to a system, and so on.

es of counselling

Developmental versus crisis counselling

Counselling can operate either as a response to a situation
or as a stimulus to help a client develop and grow. In the
past, counselling has often been concerned with helping
someone with a problem during or after the onset of a crisis
point: a widow unable to cope with her grief, the boy
leaving school desperate because he has no idea what job to
choose, the pregnant woman with no wish to be pregnant. This
is a legitimate function of counselling, but if this is all
that counselling is, it can only ever be concerned with

making the best of the situation in which one finds oneself. How much more ambitious to help people anticipate future problems, to educate them to recognize the cues of oncoming crisis, and to provide them with skills to take charge of it at the outset instead of running behind in an attempt to catch up! This is counselling as a stimulus to growth: developmental as opposed to crisis counselling. All successful counselling entails growth, but the distinction between the two approaches is that the crisis approach generates growth under pressure, and since this is often limited only to the presenting problem, the client's behavioural and conceptual repertoire may remain little affected by the experience. There will always be a need for crisis counselling in a wide variety of settings, but the exciting prospect of developmental counselling for growth and change has only recently begun to be tackled.

Individual counselling

As counselling was rooted in psychotherapy it is hardly surprising that the primary focus has been on the one-to-one relationship. There are a number of essential elements in the process. Clients are to be helped to reach decisions by themselves. This is achieved by establishing a relationship of trust whereby individual clients feel that the counsellor cares about them, is able to empathize with their problems, and is authentic and genuine in relating to them. Counsellors will enter the relationship as persons in their own right, disclosing relevant information about themselves as appropriate, reacting honestly to clients' statements and questions, but at no time imposing their own opinions on the clients. Their task is to facilitate the clients' own abilities and strengths in such a way that clients experience the satisfaction of having defined and solved their problems for themselves. If a client lacks information on special issues, is incapable of generating alternative strategies, or cannot make decisions in a programmatic way, then the counsellor has a function as an educator whose skills are offered to the client. In this way the client is never manipulated. The counsellor is negotiating a contract to use some skills which are possessed by the counsellor, and which can be passed on to the client if the client wishes to make use of them.

Individual counselling has the advantages over group counselling of providing a safer setting for some people to lower their defences, of developing a strong and trusting relationship with the counsellor, and of allowing the client maximum personal contact with the counsellor.

Group counselling

Group counselling involves one or more counsellors operating with a number of clients in a group session. The group size varies from four to sixteen, with eight to ten being the most usual number. The basic objectives of group and individual counselling are similar. Both seek to help the clients achieve self-direction, integration, self-responsibility, self-acceptance, and an understanding of their motivations and patterns of behaviour. In both cases the counsellor needs the skills and attitudes outlined earlier, and both require a confidential relationship. There are, however, some important differences (Hopson, 1977).

* The group counsellor needs an understanding of group dynamics: communication, decision making, role-playing, sources of power, and perceptual processes in groups.
* The group situation can provide immediate opportunities to try out ways of relating to individuals, and is an excellent way of providing the experience of intimacy with others. The physical proximity of the clients to one another can be emotionally satisfying and supportive. Clients give a first-hand opportunity to test others' perception of themselves.
* Clients not only receive help themselves; they also help other clients. In this way helping skills are generated by a larger group of people than is possible in individual counselling.
* Clients often discover that other people have similar problems, which can at the least be comforting.
* Clients learn to make effective use of other people, not just professionals, as helping agents. They can set up a mutual support group which is less demanding on the counsellor and likely to be a boost to their self-esteem when they discover they can manage to an increasing extent on their own.

There are many different kinds of group counselling. Some careers services in higher education offer counsellor-led groups as groundwork preparation for career choices; these small groups give older adolescents an opportunity to discuss the interrelations between their conscious values and preferred life styles and their crystallizing sense of identity. Other groups are provided in schools where young people can discuss with each other and an adult counsellor those relationships with parents and friends which are so important in adolescence. Training groups are held for teaching decision-making skills and assertive skills. There are also groups in which experiences are pooled and mutual help given for the married, for parents, for those bringing up families alone and for those who share a special problem such as having a handicapped child. All these types of groups are usually led by someone who has had training and experience in facilitating them. The word 'facilitating' is used advisedly, for the leader's job is not to conduct a seminar or tutorial, but to establish an atmosphere in which members of the group can explore the feelings around a particular stage of development or condition or critical choice.

Another type of group is not so specifically focussed on an area of common concern but is set up as a sort of laboratory to learn about the underlying dynamics of how people in groups function, whatever the group's focus and purpose may be. These are often referred to as sensitivity training groups (e.g. Cooper and Mangham, 1971; Smith, 1975). Yet a third category of group has more therapeutic goals, being intended to be successive or complementary to, or sometimes in place of, individual psychotherapy. This type of group will not usually have a place in work settings, whereas the other two do have useful applications there. Obvious uses for this type of group occur in induction procedures, in preparation for retirement, in relation to job change arising from promotion, or in relation to redundancy. The second type of group is employed in training for supervisory or management posts, though one hears less about their use in trade unions.

Where does counselling take place?

Until recently counselling was assumed to take place in the confines of a counsellor's office. This is changing rapidly. It is now increasingly accepted that effective counselling, as defined in this chapter, can take place on the shop floor, in the school corridor, even on a bus. The process is not made any easier by difficult surroundings, but when people need help, the helpers are not always in a position to choose from where they would like to administer it. Initial contacts are often made in these kinds of environment, and more intensive counselling can always be scheduled for a later date in a more amenable setting.

What are the goals of counselling?

Counselling is a process through which a person attains a higher stage of personal competence. It is always about change. Katz (1969) has said that counselling is concerned not with helping people to make wise decisions but with helping them to make decisions wisely. It has as its goal self-empowerment: that is, the individual's ability to move through the following stages.

* 'I am not happy with things at the moment'
* 'What I would prefer is ...'
* 'What I need to do to achieve that is ...'
* 'I have changed what I can, and have come to terms, for the moment, with what I cannot achieve'.

Counselling has as an ultimate goal the eventual redundancy of the helper, and the activity should discourage dependency and subjection. It promotes situations in which the person's views and feelings are heard, respected and not judged. It builds personal strength, confidence and invites initiative and growth. It develops the individual and encourages control of self and situations. Counselling obviously works for the formation of more capable and effective individuals, through working with people singly or in groups.

In its goals it stands alongside other approaches concerned with personal and human development. All can see how desirable would be the stage when more competent, 'healthier' individuals would live more positively and more humanly. Counselling may share its goals in terms of what it wants for individuals; where it does differ from other approaches is in its method of achieving that. It concentrates on the individual - alone or in a group - and on one form of helping. Some other approaches would work for the same goals but would advocate different methods of achieving them. It is important to explore the interrelatedness of counselling and other forms of helping as a way of asking, 'If we are clear about what we want for people, are we being as effective as we could be in achieving it?'

Counselling outcomes

This chapter has defined the ultimate outcome of counselling as 'helping people to help themselves'. A natural question to follow might be, 'to help themselves to do what?' There follows a list of counselling outcomes most frequently asked for by clients:

* increased understanding of oneself or a situation;
* achieving a change in the way one is feeling;
* being able to make a decision;
* confirming a decision;
* getting support for a decision;
* being able to change a situation;
* adjusting to a situation that is not going to change;
* the discharge of feelings;
* examining options and choosing one (Scally and Hopson, 1979).

Clients sometimes want other outcomes which are not those of counselling but stem from one or more of the other forms of helping: information, new skills, or practical help.

All of these outcomes have in common the concept of change. All counselling is about change. Given any issue or problem a person always has four possible strategies to deal with it:

* change the situation;
* change oneself to adapt to the situation;
* exit from it;
* develop ways of living with it.

To counsel or to teach?

Counselling is a process through which a person attains a higher level of personal competence. Recently, attacks have been made on the counselling approach by such widely differing adversaries as Illich (1973) and Carkhuff (Carkhuff and Berenson, 1976). They, and others, question what effect the existence of counsellors and therapists has had on human development as a whole. They maintain that, however benevolent the counselling relationship is felt to be by those involved, there are forces at work overall which are suspect. They suggest:

* that helpers largely answer their own needs, and consciously or unconsciously perpetuate dependency or inadequacy in clients;
* helping can be 'disabling' rather than 'enabling' because it often encourages dependency.

For counsellors to begin to answer such charges requires a self-analysis of their own objectives, methods and motives. They could begin by asking:

* how much of their counselling is done at the 'crisis' or 'problem' stage in their clients' lives?
* how much investment are they putting into 'prevention' rather than 'cure'?

To help somebody in crisis is an obvious task. It is, however, only one counselling option. If 'prevention' is better than 'cure' then maybe that is where the emphasis ought to be. Perhaps never before has there been more reason for individuals to feel 'in crisis'. Toffler (1970) has identified some likely personal and social consequences of living at a time of incredibly rapid change. Many, like Stonier (1979), are forecasting unparalleled technological developments over the next 30 years which will change our lives, especially our work patterns, dramatically. There are so many complex forces at work that it is not surprising that many people are feeling more anxious, unsure, pessimistic, unable to cope, depersonalized, and helpless. Helpers are at risk as much as any, but are likely to be faced with ever-increasing demands on their time and skills. Again, this requires a reassessment of approaches and priorities, which could suggest a greater concentration on the development of personal competence in our systems. We need to develop more 'skilled' (which is not the same as 'informed') individuals and thereby avert more personal difficulties and crisis. One view is that this, the developmental, educational, teaching approach, needs to involve more of those who now spend much time in one-to-one counselling; not to replace that work but to give balance to it.

Counselling in the UK

It is interesting that 'counselling' was a term rarely used in Britain until the mid-1960s. According to Vaughan's analysis (1976),

three factors gradually tended to focus more attention on this area. One was the emergence throughout this century of a wider band of 'helping' professions, such as the Youth Employment Service, the social work services, and psychotherapy, as well as other 'caring' organizations, such as marriage guidance, and more recently such bodies as the Samaritans and Help the Aged. A second was the development of empirical psychology and sociology, which began to offer specific techniques for the analysis of personal difficulties; and a third was the rapid spread from about the mid-1960s onwards of the concept of counselling as a specific profession derived almost wholly from North America, where it had undergone a long evolution throughout the century from about 1910. Thus today we have a situation comparable in some ways to that of the development of primary education in Britain before the 1870 Act. A new area of specialization seems to be emerging.

It is just because a new area of specialization is developing that people already engaged in, or about to involve themselves in, counselling need to think carefully of where and how they wish to invest their time and resources. Counselling clearly is an important way of helping people, but it is not the only way.

References

Aspy, D. and Roebuck, F. (1977)
Kids Don't Learn from People They Don't Like. Amherst, Mass.: Human Resource Development Press.

Brammer, L.M. (1973)
The Helping Relationship. Englewood Cliffs, NJ: Prentice-Hall.

Carkhuff, R.R. (1974)
The Art of Helping. Amherst, Mass.: Human Resource Development Press.

Carkhuff, R.R. and Berenson, B.G. (1976)
Teaching As Treatment. Amherst, Mass.: Human Resource Development Press.

Cooper, C.L. and Mangham, I.L. (eds) (1971)
T-Groups: A survey of research. Chichester: Wiley.

Egan, G. (1975)
The Skilled Helper. Monterey, Ca: Brooks/Cole.

Hopson, B. (1977)
Techniques and methods of counselling. In A.G. Watts (ed.), Counselling at Work. London: Bedford Square Press.

Hopson, B. and Scally, M. (1980a)
Lifeskills Teaching: Education for self-empowerment. Maidenhead: McGraw-Hill.

Hopson, B. and Scally, M. (1980b)
Lifeskills Teaching Programmes No. 1. Leeds: Lifeskills Associates.

Illich, I. (1973)
Tools of Conviviality. London: Calder & Boyars.

Illich, I., Zola, I.K., McKnight, J., Kaplan, J. and Sharken, H. (1977)
The Disabling Professions. London: Marion Boyars.

Ivey, A.E. (1971)
Microcounseling: Innovations in interviewing training. Springfield, Ill.: Thomas.

Kagan, N., Krathwohl, D.R. et al (1967)
Studies in Human Interaction: Interpersonal process
recall stimulated by videotape. East Lansing, Mich.:
Educational Publication Services, College of Education,
Michigan State University.

Katz, M.R. (1969)
Can computers make guidance decisions for students?
College Board Review, New York, No. 72.

Loughary, J.W. and Ripley, T.M. (1979)
Helping Others Help Themselves. New York: McGraw-Hill.

Parloff, M.B., Waskow, I.E. and Wolfe, B. (1978)
Research on therapist variables in relation to process
and outcome. In S.L. Garfield and A.E. Bergin (eds),
Handbook of Psychotherapy and Behavior Change: An
empirical analysis (2nd edn). New York: Wiley.

Rogers, C.R. (1957)
The necessary and sufficient conditions of therapeutic
personality change. Journal of Consulting Psychology,
21, 95-103.

Rogers, C.R. (1958)
The characteristics of a helping relationship. Personnel
and Guidance Journal, 37, 6-16.

Scally, M. and Hopson, B. (1979)
A Model of Helping and Counselling: Indications for
training. Leeds: Counselling and Careers Development
Unit, Leeds University.

Smith, P.B. (1975)
Controlled studies of the outcome of sensitivity
training. Psychological Bulletin, 82, 597-622.

Stonier, T. (1979)
On the Future of Employment. N.U.T. guide to careers
work. London: National Union of Teachers.

Toffler, A. (1970)
Future Shock. London: Bodley Head.

Truax, C.B. and Carkhuff, R.R. (1967)
Toward Effective Counselling and Psychotherapy: Training
and practice. Chicago, Ill.: Aldine.

Vaughan, T. (ed.) (1976)
Concepts of Counselling. London: Bedford Square Press.

20

Creating change
H. R. Beech

Politicians and kings have perhaps made the most distinctive and historically interesting attempts to change the behaviour of those they seek to control. Sometimes this has involved extreme measures, such as torture and execution, sometimes more subtle legal approaches to behaviour control, but these attempts perversely - and to the bafflement of the controller - have often failed to produce the desired outcome. Somehow, it seems, human nature appears to be resistant to change.

Psychologists are disposed to argue that such failures are mainly attributable to two causes. First, until recently, there was an obvious lack of the technology to effect changes with any degree of reliability: the methods which had been used before were both crude and unsystematically applied. Second, sometimes the attempts to effect change involved very fundamental aspects of human functioning and it might not be within the capacity of the species to accomplish them. Indeed, the contention of the behavioural psychologist these days might be that substantial changes can be wrought in carefully selected behaviours where the appropriate techniques can be freely applied. This is not to say, of course, that some psychologists fail to perceive in these strategies a means of acquiring very substantial or near complete control over human nature or, indeed, the means by which the very fabric of society could be altered. Of course, it would be unwise to allow psychologists (even if their techniques did permit such achievements) also to determine the types of change to be brought about. Psychologists are in no better position to decide what kind of society we should live in than is any other group.

For the most part, however, the aims and aspirations of psychologists are generally less ambitious and merely involve the deployment of strategies for change to areas where help is needed and requested. But to understand the origin of these strategies it is first useful to describe the influence exerted by Freud and Pavlov.

Freud's theories (Munroe, 1955) were important because they gave an entirely new interpretation to 'bad', 'wrong' or 'unacceptable' behaviour. Rather than seeing these behaviours as the reflection of something defective in the very substance of man, Freud argued that such conduct arose out of environmental experiences. Indeed, Freud is often thought of as a thoroughgoing psychic determinist, believing that all behaviour is determined by prior experience and, in a very real sense, is programmed to be just the way it is, free will and choice being merely illusory. In short, enormous importance is attached to the influence of the environment as a determinant of what we are.

Pavlov (1927) was also interested in how behaviour became modified (although primarily concerned with how the physiological systems of animals worked) and devised the method of classical conditioning to assist in this endeavour. The definitive experiment carried out in his laboratory was to show that, after training, the sound of a bell could produce salivation in dogs. Clearly the dog does not start life with this capacity and needs to learn this reaction, and it is the process by which such learning takes place that is called 'classical conditioning'. Briefly, the process involves presenting the new stimulus (bell) before the old stimulus (food) to the response (salivation). Repetitions of this arrangement, with only a brief (say half a second) interval between the sound of the bell and pre-sentation of food leads to the new association being formed. Instead of requiring food before salivating, the dog now has come to salivate at the sound of the bell alone.

Perhaps not of itself a particularly compelling piece of learning, but to many psychologists this type of association appeared as one of the fundamental building blocks of learn-ing; such learning could be seen as underpinning all human behaviour.

An early enthusiast of Pavlov's work, Watson, was said to have been so impressed by such demonstrations of condi-tioning that he declared that any American child might be turned into the President using these methods. Whether or not Watson accorded such power to classical conditioning, he was certainly enthusiastic to use it and has achieved an important place in psychological history through his Little Albert experiment (Watson and Rayner, 1920).

In this study Watson's aim was to investigate the acquisition of emotional responses, arguing that they are probably learned by the associative process called condi-tioning. For this demonstration he chose an 11-month-old boy called Albert and set out to create a learned emotional reaction in this child. Watson had observed Albert's fondness for a tame white rat and chose to reverse this feeling by arranging for a loud noise to be made (by crashing two metal plates together behind Albert's head) whenever the child reached out for this pet. After just a few trials of this kind, Albert's fear, occasioned by the sudden loud noise, was transferred to the white rat so that every time this animal appeared Little Albert would whimper and crawl away. Furthermore, it was noted that the new fear reaction had transferred to other objects with some similarity to the rat (e.g. a ball of cotton wool) and it appeared to be enduring over the period of observation.

This latter observation led Watson to speculate upon the fate of a more mature Albert, lying on the psychoanalyst's couch, and vainly trying to understand how he came to worry about white fluffy objects! But the conditioning process might well be the basis for all our irrational (neurotic) fears.

It is important to point out, however, that the environment is not the only contributing factor to learning since, from Pavlov on, it has been observed that not all learning opportunities are realized or, if they are, there are individual differences in the character of the learning which is affected.

The earliest experimental observations of such limitations of a purely environmentalist approach were made by Pavlov. He is said to have first formed this conclusion as a result of flood waters entering his laboratories in Leningrad, finding that this had made some of the animals very disturbed while others appeared to treat the matter with indifference. Later, experiments showed more conclusively that some animals appeared to be susceptible to disturbance and others more phlegmatic, these two types being labelled 'weak' and 'strong' nervous systems respectively. This differentiation has been repeatedly confirmed in the experimental work of other investigators and clearly shows that an opportunity to learn is not all that is involved: a major influence is the basic temperament of the organism which is doing the learning.

Another study which points to this conclusion was conducted by Rachman (1966). The problem posed by the investigator here was that of whether or not fetishistic behaviour (sexual arousal to unusual stimuli) could be acquired by a simple associative process. Briefly, three male volunteers were exposed to conditions in which pictures of boots were linked with pictures of an erotic nature to see if bonding occurred in such a way that the sight of boots alone would produce sexual excitement. Such was in fact found to be the case and establishes that fetishes can come about through associations of this kind. However, the point to be made here is that the subjects took varying numbers of trials to lose such reactions; in short, the disposition of the individual seems to be very much implicated in what we learn and how well such learning is preserved.

Generally these results are thought to reflect some permanent characteristics of the individuals concerned, but it is important to add that even temporary states of the organism can affect learning, a point which has been made by Beech and others (see Vila and Beech, 1978).

Clinical experience would tend to indicate that symptoms of distress (e.g. inability to go out of the house or to meet others socially without feeling anxious) often appear to be preceded by a period of general tension and emotional upset; it is as if such states prepare the ground for certain kinds of learning to take place: as if they put the organism on a defensive footing, ready to react adversely to relatively minor provocation. The kind of disturbance referred to here is quite commonly experienced by women in the few days prior to menstruation and has been given the name of pre-menstrual tension. If this condition is a good parallel to the situation in which abnormal fears can arise, then it should be possible to show a propensity for 'defensive' or adverse learning in pre-menstrual days which is not present at other times in the cycle. This is, in fact, what has been found. The evidence indicates that the state of the organism at the time when some noxious event is present not only determines the speed at which learning takes place but also any tendency for the learning to be preserved over time. One might be tempted to argue that this 'natural' disposition to acquire neurotic symptoms could explain why disproportionately large numbers of women complain of neurotic symptoms.

Another influence to be taken into account as limiting the scope of a purely environmentalist view of human behaviour is that of biological potential for learning. The argument here has been cogently presented by Seligman and Hager (1972), who conclude that all organisms appear to show a great readiness to acquire certain associations while other connections will be made only with difficulty or even not at all. Among the examples cited by Seligman and Hager is that of the dog which can very quickly associate the operation of a latch with its paw to escape from a box, but seems quite unable to learn to effect escape by wagging its tail. It is not that tail-wagging is a difficult action for the dog to perform or even that it is an uncommon reaction; rather it seems that the problem lies in making the connection itself. It is argued that the species has no biological propensity to make such a connection; the evolutionary history of the dog did not prepare the animal for this kind of learning.

It is not yet known to what extent humans are affected by preparedness, although it is obvious that certain connections appear to be 'natural' and made quite easily, while others are not. It has been suggested that a good example of preparedness is to be found in the prevalence of spider and snake phobia found in populations not at all at risk from these creatures. A more purely environmentalist approach might argue that one would need to be bitten by a spider or snake before a phobic reaction could be developed yet, obviously, there seems to be a great readiness in many people to display a wariness about spiders in a country such as England, while no such widespread fear is evoked by horses or hamsters. Somewhere in our evolutionary history, it can be argued, the species has acquired a readiness to respond with fear to potential dangers, including spiders and snakes. Perhaps this is why open spaces present a problem for many people; such 'exposure' was to be avoided in the interests of survival and this potential for acquiring a fear of open spaces is easily tapped.

The thoroughgoing environmentalist would want to argue that man is virtually a blank sheet, a complicated learning machine and, given the appropriate incentives and opportunities, can be moulded to any desired pattern. In the light of the limitations to learning which have been mentioned it is obviously appropriate to take a more moderate view and regard man as a creature highly susceptible to modification through learning, but far from infinitely so. As yet, we do not know quite how far the capacity to learn can take us. Can it, for example, so change human nature that one becomes entirely altruistic, greed, selfishness and other 'human failings' becoming totally alien? There are those, like Dawkins (1978) who would not think this possible but, on the other hand, Skinner (1953) and many others see almost limitless possibilities to behaviour modification with the psycho-technology currently available even now.

For Skinnerians the basic principle of change can be stated quite simply; the consequences of any piece of behaviour affects the future of that behaviour. If the consequence is rewarding then the behaviour is strengthened (i.e. rendered more likely to occur again); if it is punishing, then the same response tends to be weakened. Using this basic proposition, it is argued, far-reaching changes can be made to occur.

Of course, such a view is as profoundly hedonistic as Pavlov's or Freud's, the basic contention being that man is simply a pleasure-maximizing, pain-minimizing organism; this is as much part and parcel of his make-up as any other creature. Changing behaviour, according to this view, depends upon the nature, timing and other attributes of rewards and punishments rather than upon appeals to reason or religious precepts.

There is, understandably, considerable resistance to accepting such a stark view of man's nature; it appears to accord no place at all to free will and choice, nor does it allow man any special place in biological or other terms. Hedonism is the key mechanism in what we are; man can (and does) learn to do and to be anything, providing that the rewards and punishments are there to chart the way.

What we can now do is to examine the achievements to date; to see how far Pavlovian and Skinnerian principles of learning have been effective in producing change. It is anyone's guess how much further it is possible to go.

versive learning

Most of us subscribe to the validity of the adages that 'the burnt child dreads the fire' or 'once bitten, twice shy'. These sayings simply embody the importance of pain avoidance in our biological make-up. Clearly, deprived of such protection the species could hardly be expected to survive; we learn pretty quickly and thoroughly if the consequences of some actions are painful. Yet there appear to be some notable exceptions to such a compelling principle; martyrs and heroes often seem to subject themselves to avoidable pain while hard-bitten criminals may appear unaffected by the punishment society metes out to them. Obviously the problem is more complex than at first sight appears. Perhaps one should not be overly influenced by these exceptions, since the rule does seem to hold in general, but it is just as well to begin by recognizing that the results of punishment are unpredictable. For that matter, the outcome of rewarding behaviours shows much the same variability and such findings make fools of those who argue for simple solutions. For example, on the one hand there are those who want to create a better society by wreaking extreme retribution upon all who infringe rules while, on the other, the 'progressives' appear to think that the solution to crime is to remove all sources of discomfort and irritation. Both views, obviously, are patently absurd; crime has persisted in spite of great harshness in past years and, as is now well documented, the rate has risen dramatically as the number of social workers, leisure centres and social welfare has increased.

There are several arguments advanced to explain why punishment fails to achieve good effects in the context under discussion. In the first place it is said that its application is seldom timely: it works very well if immediate, but poorly or not at all if the crime and later court sentence are separated by lengthy intervals of time. Second, it is said that the rate of successful to unsuccessful crime is unfavourable to learning to resist temptation: numerous crimes may be rewarded before one act leads to punishment. A third argument is that the rate of criminal behaviour is inversely related to the strength of punishment, and that deterrents are not nearly strong enough to be effective. Yet another reason is said to be the temperament of the habitual criminal who, it is alleged, does not generate the kind of anxiety which most of us experience when 'wrong doing'. This last point refers to evidence that the nervous systems of individuals appear to extend over a range from the excessive 'jumpiness' of the chronically anxious at one end of the spectrum to those who appear to be 'psychopathically' resistant to showing disturbance to even strong stimulation.

There is probably something to be said for each of these points and, at least, all serve to indicate the complexities which may underlie the application of punishments.

To some extent it is possible to avoid a number of these problems when aversive consequences are part of a treatment programme; here, more of what takes place is under the control of the therapist or experimenter. Perhaps the best-known example of this is to be found in the treatment of alcoholism. With this, an attempt is made to ensure that drinking (and stimulus situations related to it) leads to aversive consequences; a convenient means of achieving this in practice has been to administer an emetic drug and, when this is beginning to take effect, the individual is permitted to sip the alcohol to which he is addicted. Unpleasant feelings of nausea and vomiting will, in this way, become associated with the particular sight, smell and taste involved (Voegtlin and Lemere, 1942).

Of course, it can be argued that simply punishing the 'wrong' response is hardly likely to lead to the adoption of a socially-acceptable reaction. What, for example, can the homosexual do with the sexual impulses he experiences after the usual way in which these are expended have been denied to him by punishment? Accordingly, more sophisticated attempts to help have included not only punishment but also opportunities to escape from punishment. In the context of treating homosexuals, for instance, the individual concerned has been allowed access to slides depicting homosexual activity only at the cost of receiving strong electric shocks, while the rejection of such slides and their sub-stitution by heterosexual material can lead to the avoidance of punishment altogether.

A perennial problem of aversive training has been that of securing appropriate levels of co-operation and motiva-tion and, no doubt, many failures are attributable to this difficulty. A simple example of this clarifies the point in practical terms. The investigation here was of a young boy whose habit of thumb-sucking was to be dealt with by capi-talizing upon his enjoyment of cartoons. The therapist arranged for the boy to sit through protracted showings of cartoon films but these showings ceased abruptly if thumb-sucking occurred, and the film would only be continued when this behaviour stopped. It took a relatively short time for the boy to control his bad habit during the film shows but it was noted that the training had no effect upon what hap-pened outside that situation! Indeed, one might reasonably argue that, in this case, the boy had learned how to control the behaviour of the psychologist, rather than the opposite!

Since aversion therapy is given only to those volun-tarily submitting themselves to this form of training, one should be able to assume a reasonable level of motivation to change. However, as we all recognize from personal experi-ence, our commitment to change can be quite ephemeral and today's resolution to give up smoking (or whatever) can disappear completely tomorrow. Perhaps this is only another way of saying that the aversive condition has not been applied sufficiently vigorously or intensively to inhibit the temptation: the associative bond between aversive feelings and the 'unwanted' action is insufficiently strongly made. Nevertheless, it is apparent that this problem is a major obstacle to the success of punishment as a means of control.

Systematic desensitization

Few doubt the power of anxiety to alter and disrupt ordi-nary behaviour patterns; anxiety can handicap our attempts to cope with a whole range of life's problems, it may prevent anything approaching an adjustment to quite ordinary events and it may totally ruin our enjoyment of relation-ships and circumstances which should be pleasurable. The capacity to deal with and eliminate anxiety can be regarded as of major importance to the effective control of our behaviour since, essentially, anxiety is a disruptive influence which erodes our capacity to control our own thought and action. In short, changing behaviour often seems to involve removing anxiety.

The behavioural strategy to resolve this problem appears to be surprisingly direct and simple. All that is needed is a gradual, step-by-step approach to the feared object or situation together with some means of inhibiting anxiety at each of these stages. The technique for accomplishing this was developed and refined by Wolpe (1969). More than 30 years earlier Mary Cover Jones (1924) had described essentially the same method in successfully eliminating the children's fears and, in a sense, there seems to be nothing particularly remarkable or novel in the method. Nevertheless, Wolpe's standardization of an effective technique for the analysis of anxiety and the application of a treatment strategy was enormously important from both practical and theoretical points of view.

The basic argument is that fear (or anxiety) has inadvertently, through a process of association, become a learned reaction to the presence of certain cues. For example, fear may be triggered by the presence of several people because, at some time in the past, the individual has been made anxious in a social setting; or anxiety is aroused by the sound of quarrelling voices because, at some time, the individual was threatened by the belligerence of others. The task of treatment, therefore, is to sever this connection: to detach anxiety from the innocuous cue.

Some years ago the author was asked for help in removing an extreme fear of spiders in a lady so incapacitated by this anxiety that she was unable to perform household chores. Any article of furniture moved or corner dusted might dislodge one of these alarming creatures and so occasion acute anxiety. Being outdoors clearly also presented problems to this lady, although she recognized that her fear was actually groundless in the sense that none of the spiders she encountered, indoors or out, could actually harm her.

Questioning revealed that the fear she experienced could be broken down into a number of separate components which, in various combinations, could evoke either more or less anxiety. Size, for example, was an important variable: the larger the spider the more fear would be experienced. Similarly, blackness, hairiness, degree of activity, and proximity all affected the amount of fear experienced. It was possible, therefore, to describe 'spider situations' which would produce little by way of upset, and others which would create a good deal. A small, light-coloured, apparently hairless spider, quite dead and at some distance away, would cause only mild apprehension, while an active, large, black and hairy spider, galloping across her body, would produce a sense of panic.

One must begin, in desensitization treatment, with the least anxiety-provoking situation and as each of these ceases to produce anxiety, so one moves on to the next step in the hierarchy. In the spider phobic case quoted, one can obviously begin with exhibiting a small, dead, pale-coloured, hairless spider in one corner of the room, while the patient sits in the opposite corner. When this condition ceases to produce anxiety, then the insect can be moved a little closer or, alternatively, some characteristic can be changed (e.g. substitution of a slightly larger specimen) so that we have moved one notch up the fear hierarchy.

What is notable here is that each step in the hierarchy appears to produce a smaller reaction than was anticipated before treatment; it is as if accomplishing each step has resulted in some small but discernible loss in the total anxiety now experienced. This kind of psychological arith-metic applies with every step taken, so that the total amount of anxiety to be eliminated becomes less and less.

So far so good, but systematic desensitization involves some means of inhibiting anxiety at each stage, for only in this way can the anxiety connection be broken. Each hierarchical step, therefore, must be capable of producing some amount of fear, but this must be sufficiently small to be extinguished by some other feeling state, and the most convenient means of achieving this is to train the indivi-dual in muscle relaxation.

It is argued that muscle relaxation is in fact an ideal counter to anxiety feelings, since it is both easy to learn and very effective. In short, there is good evidence that one cannot be anxious and completely relaxed at the same time; relaxation effectively inhibits the experience of fear. Accordingly, such training precedes the hierarchical presentation of fear stimuli; the individual is instructed to remain as relaxed as possible each time the fear-stimulus is presented so that the experience of anxiety is con-trolled. In this way a new type of association is being learnt: that in the presence of certain cues which pre-viously occasioned fear, no such feelings are present.

Understandably, while this method may work quite well it is not one which is easily put into practice in all cases. The various spider specimens needed to form the hierarchy may be easily secured, but in the case of, say, a fear of flying, there are serious practical problems. One could not, for example, easily arrange that the aeroplane merely completes the dash down the runway (as one item on the hierarchy) without actually taking off (which may occupy a very different hierarchical level). The necessary control over the situation here, and in numerous other cases, simply could not be achieved.

This problem is solved by presenting such situations as imagined scenes instead of as real-life experiences. This obviously makes it very much easier to arrange for events to accord precisely with treatment requirements and allows all the refined control over circumstances that one would wish to have. The only question to ask about this solution is that of whether or not dealing with an imagined situation is as beneficial as dealing with the real one. The evidence indicates that it is, although all therapists like to include experience of the real event (the real spider, lift, aeroplane, etc.) as a way of consolidating and affirming the new found absence of fear. Merely learning not to experience anxiety in imagined examples of fear aspects or situations, using the little-by-little approach and suppressing any worry by preserving muscle relaxation, can produce important changes in behaviour.

This approach is widely used in the treatment of major and incapacitating phobias with considerable success, but it is worth pointing out that less extreme conditions, including those commonly found in young children, respond very well to sympathetic handling along these lines. Fear of school, of being left by mother, of playing with strange children, of insects, of the car, and many others respond well to the graduated approach described and, of course, the benefit to behaviour generally of shedding such fears makes the effort well worth while.

Cognitive learning

It will be apparent from the description of the behavioural approaches given so far that they seem to depend upon a rather mechanical conception of learning. Insight, explanation, logic and other ways in which we come to modify or correct our view of things appear to count for nothing: the assumption is that we simply cannot talk anyone out of being alcoholic or experiencing acute anxiety; they must be taught to do so by a painstaking and carefully conceived programme of training which avoids any appeal to the 'mind'. Yet we are aware that cognitive learning does occur since we can behave differently as a result of being told that this or that is the case, or by receiving instructions to do something in a particular way. Indeed, if everything about our behaviour had to be acquired by trial and error or successive approximations, then learning would be tedious, slow and in many cases inefficient.

The charge often levelled at the behavioural approach is that it ignores the conceptual thinking that is so peculiarly and importantly human. But this is to misunderstand the situation since it is apparent that the kind of learning process required to effect change appears to depend upon what it is about our behaviour that we are trying to modify. Furthermore, it has been argued that mental events (cognitions, thoughts) are also behaviours and amenable to the same laws and, to an extent, the same training methods.

A good example is the technique called 'thought stopping'. Essentially this represents the attempt to produce the disruption or inhibition of a mental process in much the same way as some more overt activity might be stopped. It is usual to begin (see Wolpe, 1969) with a demonstration by the therapist that a sudden, unexpected and loud noise (banging the table, for example) can interrupt a particular focus of attention. In the same way, it is pointed out, an unpleasant and persistent idea can be interrupted and, with practice, might become permanently inhibited. By stages, the control of the interruptive signal is transferrred from therapist to patient and then from an external signal (banging on the table) to an internal one (saying 'stop' to oneself).

It is readily apparent that this strategy is direct, simple, and treats ideas or cognitions in much the same way as any reflex or motor action. There is, in the application of this technique, nothing special about mental events: they are simply regarded as internal behaviours.

A rather less rigorous behaviour approach is to be found in Rational Emotive Therapy; indeed, many hard-nosed behaviourists would reject any claim that RET derives from learning or conditioning theories and deny that there is any identifiable trace of the behavioural tradition in RET. Nevertheless, this cognitive approach has features which are 'behavioural' in character; for example, the emphasis upon the here-and-now rather than the influence of early life experiences, the parsimonious theoretical formulations, the implicit and explicit dependence upon reinforcing experiences and the directness of attack upon a clearly-identified source of malfunctioning. The main thrust of the technique (Ellis, 1962) derives from the assumption that faulty thinking is revealed in what people say to themselves; such 'self-talk' influences overt behaviours, so changing the cognitions can influence the way we act and feel.

Part of the immediate appeal of this technique lies in the very obviousness that 'self-talk' is a major preoccupation of us all when we are beset by difficulties. As a simple example, when girl informs boy that their relationship is ended a positive torrent of internal conversations is likely to be triggered: 'I am in a terrible mess ... I can't believe it ... there's no hope ... what can I do, nothing matters any more ...' etc. Such self-talk is likely to be accompanied by observable behaviour such as weeping, not eating or sleeping, refusing to socialize, failing to deal adequately with work assignments, and so on.

RET concentrates attention upon those things which are objectively true (e.g. 'she no longer loves me') and those which are not ('no one cares ... life is over ... there'll never be anyone else for me ...'). It is contended that when one is forced to examine the illogicality of deducing certain conclusions from the premise 'she doesn't love me', then shifts toward more positive emotions and behaviours have to occur. Attention is, of course, directed to all faulty ideas which serve as props for disappointment and disillusion: many of these quite commonplace errors of thinking which we are better rid of. For example, that one must always appear competent and without sign of weakness, that one must always have evidence that one is loved, needed and approved of, or that any adverse comment means that no one is to be trusted.

There is no doubt that this kind of counselling approach can help us to gain a perspective on life's bumps and abrasions and so prevent exaggerated and damaging emotional reactions. Yet there are obviously important limitations to an approach which depends so heavily upon exposing the illogicality of much self-talk; the point about such states of mind, as about prejudices of all kinds, is that they tend to be rather resistant to a logical approach. There is, it often seems, a strong desire to bring ideas into line with the feelings being experienced.

Furthermore, a cognitive strategy tends to pay little attention to the internal alterations of state which can often prompt the appearance of faulty ideas. Anyone with experience of depression will recognize that talking someone out of such a state is not just a tall order but pretty well impossible. No doubt where the pattern of gloomy thoughts and ideas arise out of what may be a purely environmental circumstance – a lost job, a failed exam, a lost love – a logical analysis of thoughts and feelings can be beneficial, but perhaps such circumstances are less common than one might at first suppose. Perhaps in part these environmental traumas are not random events but, to a degree, are visited upon those of us who are already vulnerable to an extent.

A cognitive technique which translates rather better from the traditional areas of behavioural concern to mental events is covert sensitization (Cautela, 1966). Basically, this method represents the application of aversive control to thoughts (as opposed to 'actions' such as drinking alcohol or operating a fruit machine) and involves imagined scenes of the unwanted behaviour followed by imagined noxious consequences. For example, the overweight gluttonous lady may be asked to conjure up images of a table groaning under the weight of delicious food, stuffing herself to bursting with cream cake and other goodies and then to create the mental picture of being sick: vomit spilling out over the table, over her dress, on to the food, and so on. In short, it is hoped to create the cognitive equivalent of real events with the consequences of overeating being highly unpleasant and embarrassing.

Another example comes from Foa (1976), whose male client derived sexual gratification from dressing in woman's clothing. This had brought him to the courts, where he was then referred for treatment. Covert sensitization took the form of requiring the patient to imagine that he was driving along in his car when he saw a clothes line on which desirable articles of clothing were hanging; he stops, gets out and attempts to take these clothes, but as he does so, he is overcome by intense feelings of nausea. He was then required to imagine throwing the clothes away and feeling very much better.

It is worth pointing out that in this case, as in other examples of aversive training, the unwanted habit returned again following an initially successful outcome. Generally, the therapist takes account of the need to deal with this problem by arranging 'booster' courses of treatment as and when the need arises.

Operant training

It is apparent from the accounts given that the behavioural approach to change is strongly hedonistic; organisms learn when rewarded and 'unlearn' when punished. Perhaps more than in any other technique of learning, operant training exemplifies this dependence upon the manipulation of the consequences of behaviour: a consequence which is rewarding (positively reinforcing) will strengthen some reaction or response, while one which is punishing (negatively reinforcing) will weaken and discourage further behaviour of the same kind.

It was not until B. F. Skinner's 1953 publication that there was any systematic account of the circumstances under which rewards and punishments work best. Experimenting with small animals, often rats, Skinner was able to demonstrate convincingly that if some observable piece of behaviour (response) was followed consistently by reward, the chances of the same behaviour occurring in a similar situation on subsequent occasions would increase. Similarly, if a response was punished, it would become less likely to occur. Three very important aspects of the apparently simple relationship between response and consequences arose from these animal studies. First, it is imperative that the reinforcement applied to the subject really is rewarding or punishing for them. A puff at a cigarette is obviously pleasant and rewarding to some humans but would probably prove aversive to most rats, whereas the dry food pellets enjoyed by rats would be of little interest to most humans. The second point was that, at least initially, the reinforcement (reward or punishment) must follow immediately after the target response is performed. If we wish to increase the frequency with which a rat presses a lever, it is no use providing the reward half-an-hour after the response has occurred; the necessary association between lever-pressing and, say, food reward would simply not be made. Third, as well as being immediate, the reinforcement must be applied consistently. Under all but very extreme circumstances, the rat does not learn to press a lever as a result of a single reward for doing so but needs numerous rewarded trials until lever-pressing is acquired. It is best to reward every trial initially, for although learning can take place if rewards (or punishments) are more spread out, it is very much slower. However, once learned, a response may be maintained by occasional reinforcement.

Many psychologists have been attracted by Skinnerian research and have applied the rules to the modification of human behaviour. The degree of success which has been achieved has been surprising in view of the frequent criticisms of Skinner's approach as essentially simplistic and mechanistic. Perhaps the greatest changes that have been made in order to accommodate Skinner's system to work with humans have been in response to the obvious superiority of their thinking, memory and reasoning as well as their capacity to use and to understand language. These skills have had most effect on the second aspect of reinforcement described above. As long as individual persons realize that reinforcement will be contingent upon their behaviour within a reasonable time, it may not be necessary for the reinforcement to be immediate. An individual will be able to think about or anticipate the delayed outcome. When working with children, however, some tangible reminder may be given of the reinforcement to come, such as a gold star immediately on completion of some school work as a token representing, say, extra playtime during the day.

The types of problems to which reinforcement procedures may be applied range from minor irritating habits to major disorders which threaten the well-being or even life of the sufferer. Many examples from the field of child-management may be cited to illustrate the least severe end of this scale.

Many young children go through 'phases' which are both worrying and irritating to their parents but usually not harmful in themselves. An example of this would be the temper tantrums fairly frequently observed in toddlers. In nearly all cases such episodes last a few weeks or at most months and then disappear of their own accord. In a few cases they persist much longer, or with greater severity, and perhaps begin to disrupt family life. Providing the cause is not due to some physical illness, one may attempt to modify the behaviour by applying appropriate reinforcements. Very often it is found that a great deal of attention is given when a child has a tantrum, usually because it is alarming and upsetting to the parents. On the other hand, when the child is occupied and behaving well, the parents, sighing with relief, turn their attention to other things, effectively ignoring good behaviour. Evidently the child is being rewarded for having a tantrum but is punished (as being ignored can be aversive) for being well behaved. With these contingencies it is no wonder that such behaviour becomes more frequent and good behaviour becomes rarer. Tantrums may be modified simply by reversing reward and punishment; parents leave children to their own devices when they have a tantrum but take great care to play with them and talk to them when they are being good. Applied systematically, such a straightforward alteration of reinforcements can have amazingly rapid and beneficial effects.

Even relatively minor behaviour problems in children may have more serious effects on their eventual welfare. One form of difficulty that has been tackled fairly often in this way is disruptive classroom behaviour. Children who are frequently out of their seats, moving around and making a noise, usually benefit less from their schooling than their more appropriately behaved peers and are likely to fall behind with their work. In addition they may become unpopular with their companions as they upset the others' work and interfere with their games. In busy classrooms, such children are often reprimanded by teachers when they are a nuisance but receive very little attention for being 'good' since this occurs infrequently and they rarely produce work of a high enough standard to merit praise. Relatively mild chastisements from the teacher may be more rewarding for the child (being preferred to no attention at all) so the child is rewarded for being disruptive and ignored for practically everything else. As with the younger child, the task is to reverse the contingencies. In this case it may not be possible for the teacher to ignore the bad behaviour entirely but, usually, the amount of time and effort spent in the reprimand can be reduced significantly so that the child receives a minimum of attention for each disruptive act. At the same time reward is given for appropriate behaviour and an acceptable (although possibly lower than average) standard of work. If possible, the reward is given immediately with attention and praise but may be supplemented by the use of stars or marks for good conduct, and these tokens can be exchanged for privileges at the end of the day. Usually the co-operation of not only the teacher and pupil but also of the entire class is required to make this procedure fully effective.

The much-publicized condition of anorexia nervosa is an example of a life-threatening state which may sometimes be ameliorated by the use of reinforcement procedures. Patients suffering from this disorder are most commonly girls in their mid- to late-teens who have begun to diet excessively, and now refuse to eat and sabotage attempts to feed them by hiding the food or vomiting. Many lose so much weight that they must be confined to bed. The main management problem is to reinstate eating.

There is no single acceptable account of why a girl begins to become anorexic but there is commonly evidence of considerable social reinforcement for not eating once serious dieting is under way, since serious weight loss causes friends and relatives to become increasingly concerned and respond to refusals to eat by attention and attempts to coax and persuade, and this attention contributes to the maintenance of not eating. Attempts have been made to make positive reinforcement contingent upon eating rather than not eating and, to do this, the patient has been socially isolated and denied pleasures such as radio and television in order to maximize the rewarding effect of social contact. It has been arranged that a friendly therapist will eat each meal with the patient and converse with her when, and only when, she eats a mouthful of food. Once eating a meal has been established, the reward is made less immediate by allowing the patient to earn time with the therapist or friends after the meal has been eaten. She is also allowed access to television, etc., in the same way. This kind of procedure has been found to produce important weight gain in a number of patients. When described in outline it may appear that the patient is the passive recipient of reinforcement, unaware of the contingencies that have been planned, but this is far from the case, as most patients become involved with the preparation of their programmes, the negotiation of weight targets, amounts to be eaten, planning rewards and agreeing to contingencies.

It is clear that reinforcement contingencies can be applied effectively to a wide range of behaviour problems in humans. As long as the contingencies are appropriately rewarding or punishing, and the consequences fairly immediate and consistent, the reinforcements are likely to be effective, but the chances of success will be increased if the individuals with the problems are involved in the construction and discussion of their own management programmes.

In conclusion

Behavioural approaches to change tend to lack appeal when compared to other methods. We would prefer, for example, to think that we are amenable to logic and reason and that if only the facts are made available to us we could change to be in accord with them. Or, in other contexts, we may find the dramatic aspects of psychoanalysis more compelling, with the eccentricities of human behaviour being explained as the result of mysterious and excitingly interesting forces. Certainly, behavioural approaches stand in sharp contrast and seem to inspire all the excitement of Latin conjugations!

On the other hand, while the techniques admittedly tend to apply about as well to animals as to man, their clarity and simplicity arises from sound experimental work and scientific thought, qualities which in any other context would be thought commendable. It is worth while to offer the example of bedwetting as a means of showing how such thinking offers distinct advantages over a more tortuous and complex account.

Psychoanalysts are inclined to regard bedwetting as merely the external sign of some inner turmoil. It has been regarded, for example, as a substitute for sexual gratification or a means by which a child can express aggression and resentment toward others. The behavioural formulation is starkly simple; individuals learn to be dry at night and some fail to acquire this skill. If the former view is correct, then simply removing the behaviour (bedwetting) would not cure the inner discontent; if the behavioural view is correct, however, then getting rid of the symptom would be a very useful thing.

Mowrer's simple device to unlearn bedwetting (Mowrer and Mowrer, 1938) was in fact highly successful and is very widely used today. It deals directly with the symptom and in most cases bedwetting is eliminated. No evidence exists of any underlying pathological process of the kind postulated by the psychoanalyst.

Naturally one example of a greater claim to effectiveness does not establish the general superiority of the behavioural approach, yet it does seem that such examples can be multiplied many times over. This is, in fact, what one would expect from a model constructed from painstaking laboratory experimental work and scientific formulations.

It is not, of course, that the approach or the techniques deriving from it, some of which have been briefly reviewed here, are either wildly successful or beyond criticism. There are, indeed, numerous difficulties and shortcomings and, as indicated earlier, one of the most serious of these is the partiality of the purely environmentalist viewpoint and the almost complete neglect of genetic/constitutional influences. Nevertheless, behavioural strategies now occupy a position of high importance for psychologists, and the influence of these strategies in many and diverse areas of application is still growing.

References

Cautela, J.B. (1966)
Treatment of compulsive behavior by covert sensitization. The Psychological Record, 16, 33-41.
Dawkins, R. (1978)
The Selfish Gene. Oxford: Oxford University Press.
Ellis, A. (1962)
Reason and Emotion in Psychotherapy. New York: Kyle Stewart.
Foa, E.B. (1976)
Multiple behaviour techniques in the treatment of transvestism. In H.J. Eysenck, Case Studies in Behaviour Therapy. London: Routledge & Kegan Paul.
Jones, M.C. (1924)
The elimination of children's fears. Journal of Experimental Psychology, 7, 383-90.
Mowrer, O.H. and Mowrer, W. (1938)
Enuresis: a method for its study and treatment. American Journal of Orthopsychiatry, 8, 436-59.
Munroe, R.L. (1955)
School of Psychoanalytic Thought. New York: Dryden Press.
Pavlov, I.P. (1927)
Conditioned Reflexes (Transl. Anrep). London: Oxford University Press.
Rachman, S. (1966)
Sexual fetishism: an experimental analogue. The Psychological Record, 16, 293-296.
Seligman, M.E.P. and Hager, J.L. (1972)
Biological Boundaries of Learning. New York: Appleton-Century-Crofts.
Skinner, B.F. (1953)
Science and Human Behavior. New York: Macmillan.
Vila, J. and Beech, H.R. (1978)
Vulnerability and defensive reactions in relation to the human menstrual cycle. British Journal of Social and Clinical Psychology, 17, 93-100.
Voegtlin, W.L. and Lemere, E. (1942)
The treatment of alcohol addiction. Quarterly Journal of Studies on Alcohol, 2, 717-803.
Watson, J.B. and Rayner, R. (1920)
Conditioned emotional reactions. Journal of Experimental Psychology, 3, 1-14.
Wolpe, J. (1969)
The Practice of Behavior Therapy. New York: Pergamon Press.

21

Learning and teaching
D. Fontana

Learning can be defined as a relatively persistent change in an individual's possible behaviour due to experience. It is thus clearly distinguished from those changes in behaviour which come about as a consequence of maturation (i.e. as a consequence of the individual's physical growth and development). Learning can take place either as a result of informal circumstances (e.g. parent-child relationships, interaction with friends and with the mass media), or as a result of the formal efforts of society to educate its members through schools and academic institutions. Though both are important our main concern is with the latter: that is, with the ways in which the teacher or the tutor can best monitor and assist learning within the class or lecture room.

Bruner (1973) considers that in dealing with learning activities the teacher must take account of three important variables, namely the nature of the learner, the nature of the knowledge to be learned and the nature of the learning process. Accordingly we adopt this threefold division as a way of structuring the present chapter, taking each of the variables in turn and examining the major factors associated with them.

The nature of the learner

There are a number of factors within individual learners that influence their ability to learn. Best known of these are cognitive factors such as intelligence and creativity, but there are many others of equal relevance. These include affective factors, motivation, age and sex, study habits and, above all perhaps, memory.

Affective factors

Psychologists take the term 'affective' to cover all aspects of personality. One of these aspects which has particular importance for learning is anxiety. From general experience the teacher soon discovers that a mild degree of anxiety in a pupil can be a useful aid to learning, but that too much anxiety has an inhibiting effect (particularly if the learning task is a complex one). We see this particularly in a student preparing for an important examination, or in a student fearful of the anger or ridicule that failure in a particular task may invite from unsympathetic tutors or

classmates. The anxiety consequent upon these stressful
situations interferes with both learning and performance,
and results are produced way below the individual's potential. Closely linked to anxiety as an affective factor is
the individual's self-esteem. Research studies show that
individuals with low self-esteem (i.e. with a low regard
for their personal worth and abilities) consistently set
themselves artificially depressed learning and attainment
goals, and consistently perform less well than individuals
of similar intelligence and background who enjoy high levels
of self-esteem. It appears that low self-esteem subjects are
so fearful of further blows to their self-regard that they
set themselves low goals in order to avoid the chances of
failure.

High and low self-esteem can be referred to as a dimension of personality. Another such dimension that has implications for learning is that of extraversion-introversion.
Typically the extravert is an individual who enjoys change
and variety and is orientated towards the external world of
people and experiences, while the introvert is more concerned with stability and the inner world of thoughts and
feelings. All of us find our place at some point on this
dimension, and the evidence suggests that those who incline
towards the two extremes learn best in different kinds of
learning environments. The extravert tends to favour groups
and social activities, with plenty of variety and fresh
stimuli, while the introvert generally prefers more ordered
individual activity. Thus a particular learning failure may
be due less to any lack of ability on the part of the learner than to the fact that the working environment is not
really suited to relevant aspects of that learner's personality. On occasions teachers or tutors may also tend to
favour pupils whose personalities approximate to their own,
with the extravert complaining that an introverted pupil is
too quiet, and the introvert complaining that an extraverted
pupil is too noisy.

Motivation

Satisfactory learning is unlikely to take place in the
absence of sufficient motivation to learn. We have already
mentioned one possible source of motivation, namely a degree
of anxiety, but there are many others. For convenience we
can divide these into intrinsic forms of motivation, which
come from within the individual, and extrinsic which are
imposed by the environment. Taking intrinsic first, it is
axiomatic that people work generally harder at learning
tasks that interest them than at those that do not. If we
had to say why a particular thing captures a person's
interest we would probably argue that it has some direct
relevance to the individual's daily life. It either diverts
or amuses in some way (and thus makes the person feel
better) or it enables him to cope more effectively with the
problems and achieve the ambitions in his daily life. No
matter what the subject, however, there is often the danger

that learners are asked to tackle theoretical issues whose
practical application escapes them, or to work towards goals
that are too remote or not of their own choosing. Whilst of
course students cannot be the arbiters of what they should
or should not learn, it is important that tutors who wish to
appeal to intrinsic motivation should be fully aware of the
concerns and aspirations of their students, and should
demonstrate clearly the way in which the proposed learning
relates to them.

Nevertheless, however stimulating the teacher, there
will always be occasions when intrinsic motivation is insufficient and recourse has to be made to motivation of an
extrinsic kind. Such motivation usually consists of marks,
grades, examinations, and of course tutor praise and approval. Success in these areas builds up prestige in the student's own eyes and standing is enhanced in the eyes of
others. Students find success to be rewarding, and builds up
expectations which they have to work harder and more pur-
posefully to fulfil. Thus extrinsic motivation can be highly
effective, but it raises a number of important considerations (quite apart from the obvious fear that it may raise
anxiety to an inhibiting level).

* Instead of success, some individuals experience only
  failure. This tends to produce either the low self-
  esteem to which we have already made reference, or a
  rejection of everything to do with the formal learning
  tasks offered through educational institutions. Such
  rejection is a defensive attempt to protect self-esteem
  by insisting that it is these tasks that are at fault
  rather than the individuals themselves (i.e. it is a way
  of saying 'I could do it if it was worth doing'). To
  combat the harmful effects of consistent failure the
  wise tutor provides students with opportunities for
  success at however low a level. Through such opportunities students gradually build up new self-images and
  new attitudes to work, and are encouraged progressively
  to set their sights higher.
* Sometimes motivation suffers because students are not
  supplied with prompt knowledge of results. The longer
  the gap between performance and the provision of this
  knowledge, the greater the chance that students will
  lose interest in the whole exercise.
* Competition between students is a useful extrinsic
  motivator provided they are all of a similar level of
  ability and can all experience a fair degree of success.
  Co-operation, where students adopt group norms and work
  together to achieve them, can be of even more benefit.
* Wherever the pressures of extrinsic motivation are too
  strong students may resort to strategies like feigned
  illness (or even cheating) to avoid the consequences of
  failure.

Age and sex
The ability to tackle complex learning tasks increases

throughout childhood. Both Piaget (cf. Inhelder and Piaget, 1958) and Bruner (1966) have demonstrated that children appear to go through a number of stages in the development of their powers of thinking, and that unless learning tasks are presented to them in the form appropriate to their particular stage they may be unable to understand what is required of them. For example, before children reach what Piaget calls the stage of formal operations (usually at approximately age 12) they are strictly limited in their ability to engage in abstract thinking, and can only handle concepts when they have experienced them in some practical sense (e.g. they can deal with weight and number, which can be practically experienced, but not with density and volume, which require to be defined more theoretically). On the basis of this kind of evidence it seems that the individual's powers of thinking reach maturity during adolescence, and we know that measured intelligence and memorizing abilities also appear to have reached their peak by the end of this period. Much less is known about the subsequent decline of these powers and therefore of the ability to learn. There certainly appears to be a general slowing of the rate at which the individual can learn many mental and physical skills throughout adult life, and this decline may have reached significant proportions in people not involved in academic work by the mid- and late-twenties. In those constantly using academic skills, however, the decline may be more gradual, and may be amply offset by greater self-discipline, higher motivation, and the increased ability to organize learning that comes through experience.

Just as the ability to learn is influenced by age variables, so is it influenced by sex. Girls are generally more verbal than boys at school age, and have fewer reading, speech, and general behaviour problems (Davie, Butler and Goldsmith, 1972), while boys are more advanced in number skills. These differences tend to disappear by the age of 16, however, and boys between five and ten years of age appear twice as likely to show an increase in measured intelligence as girls (Kagan, Sontag, Baker and Nelson, 1958). Throughout school life, however, girls tend to be better all-rounders, while boys are better at the subjects they enjoy and spurn those they do not. These sex-related differences could be in part genetic and in part related to the home (where girls are generally taught to be more dependent and more concerned for adult approval), but recent research in the USA suggests that they could also be due to the fact that most early school teaching is done by women, and boys therefore come to associate school with feminine values. Where such teaching is done by men, the higher rate of backwardness and school rejection shown by boys tends to disappear. Sadly, at all ages, girls tend to show lower self-esteem than boys, and may artificially depress their level of performance in conformity with an outmoded and unfortunate social conception of the inferiority of the female role.

Memory

Clearly, learning depends intimately on memory. At the
practical level psychologists recognize the existence of two
main kinds of memory, short-term and long-term. All information received by the senses and to which we pay attention
seems to enter short-term memory, but it can be held there
briefly and is either then forgotten (as when we look up a
telephone number and forget it the moment we have dialled
it) or translated to long-term memory where it can be held
more permanently (though it is still, of course, subject to
forgetting). Obviously this transfer is vital for effective
learning. Available evidence suggests it involves some form
of consolidation, typically a short pause during which the
information is held consciously in the mind. Even after an
interesting lesson or lecture students often remember
little, probably because each piece of information is so
quickly followed by the next that there is no time for
consolidation. However, a number of strategies exist for
helping consolidation and for increasing the efficiency of
long-term memory generally.

* By pausing, repeating and questioning, the lecturer can
  prompt students to dwell sufficiently upon material for
  transfer from short- to long-term to take place.
* By putting material to immediate practical use consolidation is also greatly helped. Material that is interesting, and that is properly understood, is also more
  likely to be remembered than is material which is
  perceived as dull or irrelevant.
* By practising overlearning, material is made particularly resistant to forgetting. Overlearning implies
  the continued revision of a learning task even after it
  appears to have been perfected, and is particularly
  valuable where the material has to be remembered in a
  stressful situation (e.g. in the examination room or on
  the concert platform).
* By associating new material with something that is
  already familiar, or with something that is particularly
  striking or novel in itself, the chances of its being
  remembered are greatly improved. Through the association
  with something that is already familiar the material is
  placed within context, and can be recalled readily when
  cued in by this material in future; through the association with something striking the material tends to be
  remembered when this striking stimulus is called to
  mind. This is particularly true if the stimulus is a
  visual one: hence the importance of visual aids. Such
  aids need not necessarily be closely linked in terms of
  meaning with the material to be learned (witness the
  highly successful advertisements on commercial television), but they must be presented concurrently with
  this material so that a strong association is built up.

In discussing memory, it is important to stress that there

appears to be a functional difference between recognition (where we spot as familiar some stimulus physically presented to us) and recall (where we have to retrieve some word or fact from memory itself). Recognition appears to come more readily than recall (e.g. it is easier to recognize a face than to recall a name, to recognize a work in a foreign language than to recall it from memory), and in consequence, unless we are deliberately setting out to test recall, it is of value to provide appropriate cues that bring recognition to the aid of recall.

So much for the factors that aid long-term memory. Now for those that appear to interfere with it. One of these, anxiety, has already been touched upon. Material that can readily be recalled in a relaxed state may prove elusive when one is under stress. Two others of importance are known as retroactive and proactive interference respectively. Retroactive interference occurs when recently learnt material appears to inhibit the recall of that learnt earlier. The phenomenon appears to take place at all levels of learning, and is apparent, for example, in students who cram for an examination and find that the facts they learnt the night before keep coming back when attempts are made to recall those studied earlier in the week. Proactive interference, on the other hand, occurs when earlier learning seems to block the recall of later, as when students start learning a second foreign language and find themselves unable to remember the word they want because the equivalent in the first language keeps coming to mind. We discuss ways of minimizing retroactive inhibition when we deal with study habits below, but proactive inhibition is only likely to be a problem when the two subjects being studied share certain similarities, and it tends to disappear as the new material becomes more familiar and overlearning takes place.

Finally, we come to the subject of memory training. It is often assumed that the memory can be trained, like a muscle, if we exercise it (e.g. by learning large chunks of poetry). There is no evidence, however, that this assumption is correct. The memory is improved by learning how to memorize rather than by the simple act of memorizing itself. We have already listed some of the skills relevant to this task, and reference is made to others in the next section, but we should perhaps mention here the value of mnemonic devices. These are devices created specifically to aid recall, and range from simple tricks like tying a knot in a handkerchief and short jingles like 'thirty days hath September ...' to the elaborate devices used by stage 'memory men'. One such device is the so-called peg-word system, where the digits 1-10 (or more) are each associated with a rhyming word (e.g. 1 is bun, 2 is shoe, 3 is a tree, etc.). These simple associations are learned, and then the facts to be memorized are associated with them in turn, preferably using visual imagery. Thus, for example, if we wished to learn the agricultural produce exported by New Zealand we could visualize first butter spread on a bun, second a lamb wearing shoes and so on. Such devices are remarkably effective in the learning of long lists of facts, though their use beyond this is limited.

Study habits

Much of the effectiveness of learning depends upon good study habits, particularly in older students who have to take more responsiblity for their own work. Some of these habits, like working in an environment free from distraction, are obvious while others, like overlearning, have already been covered. We can summarize the remainder as outlined below.

* REALISTIC WORK TARGETS. Realistic work targets, which the student plans in detail, are far more effective than impossibly ambitious or vague commitments. Ideally these targets should be expressed publicly (so that prestige is at stake if the student fails to stick to them!).
* REWARDS. Small rewards, built into the student's work schedule, can be very effective in helping sustain effort. These can take the form of a cup of coffee, for example, or a five-minute break at the end of each hour of solid work, with the purchase perhaps of an inexpensive though coveted treat each time weekly or monthly targets are met.
* PUNCTUALITY. Work should be started promptly at the appointed hour. This forestalls the elaborate (and plausible) strategies we each develop to delay actually sitting down at our desks and getting on with it.
* WHOLE AND PART LEARNING. A new learning task should be read through first in its entirety to get the general drift of it before being broken down into small units and learned methodically.
* ORGANIZING MATERIAL. Often textbooks (and lectures) do not present material in a way which accords best with the learner's own experience and understanding. Time spent reorganizing the material into notes that render it generally more comprehensible and assimilable is time well spent.
* REVISION. A programme of phased revision throughout the duration of a course is of far more value than an attempt to cram everything in during the final weeks before an exam. Retroactive inhibition (and increased anxiety) are the almost inevitable consequences of such cramming. Phased revision, however, leads to a growing mastery of the whole course as students work their way through it, with each new piece of knowledge being placed in its proper context. When it comes to final examination preparation the student is therefore looking back over material that has already been overlearned. Revision is best done before material has actually been forgotten. This is known as maintenance revison.

ie nature of knowledge be learnt

Obviously in any learning activity we have to consider not only the abilities of the learner but the nature of the new material. Equally obviously, this material must be organized in such a way that learning is facilitated, and in such a way that we can assess afterwards whether the desired learning has taken place or not. In considering such matters we have first of all to decide the level at which we wish learning to take place. Do we want the learner simply to learn facts, or do we want him to operate at higher levels and understand these facts, and be able to put them to use? Bloom (1956) has presented us with a comprehensive list of the various levels at which learning can take place, and this list is an indispensable aid in all matters relating to the planning and assessment of learning. The list arranges the various levels in hierarchical order, from the simplest to the most complex. Each of the higher levels subsumes those inferior to it (e.g. learning at level 3 involves learning at level 1 and 2 as well), and we can summarize them in ascending order. It will be noted that this taxonomy, as it is called, relates only to thinking skills (or skills in the cognitive domain). Other taxonomies exist which cover aspects of personality (the affective domain: see Krathwohl, 1964) and physical skills (the psychomotor domain: see Simpson, 1972), but these are of less immediate relevance for our purpose.

vels of learning in the gnitive domain (after om et al, 1956)

*   Knowledge (i.e. simple knowledge of facts, of terms, of theories, etc.).
*   Comprehension (i.e. an understanding of the meaning of this knowledge).
*   Application (i.e. the ability to apply this knowledge and comprehension in new and concrete situations).
*   Analysis (i.e. the ability to break material down into its constituent parts and to see the relationship between them).
*   Synthesis (i.e. the ability to re-assemble these parts into a new and meaningful relationship, thus forming a new whole).
*   Evaluation (i.e. the ability to judge the value of material using explicit and coherent criteria, either of one's own devising or derived from the work of others).

Having decided the level at which we intend to work, the next step (both for the tutor and for the student planning his own study programme) is to define the precise outcomes (or objectives) that our learning is intended to achieve. This is often one of the hardest parts of the exercise. Frequently learning objectives make the mistake of simply outlining what is to be done rather than concentrating upon why it is done. The best way to avoid this error is to remember that a learning objective should state the behaviour expected from a student as the result of a lesson.

Thus, for example, we would not write that our objective is 'to demonstrate a particular skill (whatever it may happen to be) to the class', but rather that at the end of the lesson the students should be able to do one or more of the following (depending upon the level at which we intend learning to take place):

* to recognize and identify the elements involved in the skill (these elements would then be specified - this is an objective at the knowledge level);
* to define these elements and to know the part they play in the skill (an objective at the comprehension level);
* to practise the skill itself (an objective at the application level);
* to describe what is happening - and why - during this practice (an objective at the analysis level);
* to utilize elements of this skill in solving a particular novel problem (an objective at the synthesis level);
* to assess the degree of success achieved in this solution and to propose improvements (an objective at the evaluation level).

It can be readily appreciated that, once a clear objective (or objectives) has (or have) been stated at the beginning of the lesson plan, the tutor is in a much better position to determine the lesson content and to keep it practical and relevant. It is also easier to assess whether learning has taken place or not at the end of the lesson, since it is specified in advance that student behaviour will provide evidence of that learning. As assessment is a major topic in itself, we now turn to it in more detail.

Assessment

Much assessment takes place simply observing student behaviours, or by directing questions at students, but often the tutor wishes to provide a class with specially devised opportunities to demonstrate whether their behaviour has changed in the desired direction or not. The tutor's choice of which opportunities to offer (i.e. of which assessment techniques to use) will be influenced by the level (in terms of the taxonomy discussed above) at which it is intended learning should take place. All too frequently, particularly in arts and social science subjects, assessment simply takes the form of a written essay, which may be appropriate for gauging progress at the more complex cognitive levels but which samples only a very limited range of knowledge and comprehension. The main alternative to the essay is the so-called objective test, each of whose items carries only a single right answer. Such items are usually of the multiple choice variety, with the student being asked which of a range of possible answers is the correct one: for example, 'The Theory of Association was first advanced by; Herbart/ William James/Francis Galton/none of these'. It will be noted that multiple choice questions test recognition; if it was desired to test recall, the question would be allowed to stand on its own without the addition of the possible answers.

It is often claimed that objective tests take the tutor longer to construct than tests of the essay type. There is no gainsaying this, but on the other hand they are quicker to mark, and teachers are left with the satisfaction of knowing that they have adequately tested the knowledge that they set out to test. Further, students are motivated to acquire this knowledge since they know that it is to be comprehensively tested, rather than fractionally sampled as in an essay. They are also left with the reassurance that good marks really do mean that they know the field and are equipped with the basic grammar of the subject.

The nature of the learning process

Having looked at the learner and at the knowledge to be learned we now come to the last major variable, namely the process (or methods or techniques) by means of which learning actually takes place. Gagné (1974) suggests that the learning act involves a chain of eight events, some internal to the learner and others external. These events are, in their usual order of occurrence:

* motivation (or expectancy);
* apprehending (the subject perceives the material and distinguishes it from the other stimuli competing for his attention);
* acquisition (the subject codes the knowledge – i.e. makes sense of it, relates it to what is already known);
* retention (the subject stores the knowledge in short- or long-term memory);
* recall (the subject retrieves the material from memory);
* generalization (the material is transferred to new situations, thus allowing the subject to develop strategies for dealing with them);
* performance (these strategies are put into practice);
* feedback (the subject obtains knowledge of results).

Where there is a failure to learn, Gagné argues, it will take place at one of these eight levels, and it is thus the task of tutors to ascertain which. It may be that the learning has failed to capture the pupils' attention, or it makes no sense to them, or they have failed to transfer it to long-term memory, or they are unable to recall it from their memory. Analysing learning failure in this way renders tutors much better able to help the pupil since it enables them to concentrate upon the specific point at which the pupil appears to be going wrong. Frequently, too, they may discover that the fault lies not simply with the pupil but with the way in which the learning task has been presented – and explained – to the pupil.

The manner in which this presentation should be effected depends again upon the level (in terms of Bloom's taxonomy) at which we intend learning to take place. Where we are concerned with levels 1-3 (knowledge, comprehension, and application) then the strategy derived from the experimental findings of Skinner (e.g. Skinner, 1969) is of most help. Skinner's work indicates that factual knowledge and its comprehension and application is normally absorbed most efficiently if it is presented to the learner in small steps, each of them within his competence; if he is then required to demonstrate this learning in some way; and if he is given immediate knowledge of results on whether his demonstration was correct or not. In the event of failure, the whole procedure is repeated. This strategy cannot only be put to efficient use by teachers in their direct dealings with pupils, it also lies at the heart of what has come to be known as programmed learning. Programmed learning uses either specially written textbooks or rolls of paper mounted in simple learning devices to present each unit of learning in turn to individual learners, to question them on it, and to inform them whether or not their answers to questions are correct. An example of an item from a programme on electrical wiring illustrates this clearly.

Stage 1 (information): In wiring a 13 amp plug the brown wire is connected to the live terminal.

Stage 2 (question): Which colour wire is connected to the live terminal of a 13 amp plug?

Stage 3 (answer): A. the blue; B. the brown; C. the green and yellow.

Stage 4 (results): The brown wire is connected to the live terminal of a 13 amp plug.

This example tests recognition in Stage 3 by offering the three possible right answers, but of course these could be omitted if we wished to test recall.

This learning procedure involves what Skinner calls operant conditioning in that at each point it involves, after the presentation of the information to be learned, a stimulus (the question), an item of behaviour (the student's answer), and a reward or reinforcement (the knowledge of results). This operant conditioning (or S-B-R) model lies behind all learning, claims Skinner, and where there is learning failure this is normally because we have omitted to present the appropriate stimulus or, more frequently, the appropriate reinforcement. For many pupils immediate and accurate knowledge of successful results (remember that Skinner advocates presenting material to pupils in small steps, each one within their competence) is sufficient reinforcement, but for others teacher approval, good marks and grades, and even small physical rewards (e.g. where the child is retarded or handicapped and cannot understand the significance of marks and grades) may have to be used. Similarly, where incorrect learning has taken place, Skinner claims this can also be due to misapplied reinforcement. The parents or teachers, for example, fail to realize that the very fact of their attention (whether angry or not) is a powerful reinforcement for some children. Thus the more scolding the adult directs at the child's misbehaviour the more persistent it may tend to become. The correct procedure would be to ignore children when they produce this behaviour and reward them with attention when they show behaviour of the opposite, desirable kind. This approach is part of a range of strategies based upon conditioning theories (and known collectively as behaviour modification techniques) which are attracting increasing attention in educational and clinical circles.

Many psychologists, however, though granting the effectiveness of Skinner's approach at the first three levels in Bloom's taxonomy, consider it an inadequate basis for prompting learning at the higher levels. Learning at these levels involves more than a mere knowledge of the facts and formulae produced by other people (the so-called middle language of the subject); it involves the ability to discover the fundamental logic underlying the subject. Bruner (1966) argues that to help students achieve such discovery we must present them with problems and challenges, with questions that contain an element of controversy and contradiction. Such questions, known as springboard questions, introduce material which does not quite fit in with the student's accepted knowledge and beliefs. A 'level 1' question, such as 'What is the population of Britain?' or 'What is the formula for water?' demands nothing from the student beyond a single answer delivered in the form in which it was first heard. A springboard question, on the other hand, such as 'The poles are equidistant from the equator, yet the south is colder than the north; why?' or 'Christianity teaches you that you should love your enemies, yet men have committed terrible massacres in its name; why?' prompts students to reflect on the subtle ways in which their subject works, on the relationship between cause and effect, on methods of procedure and enquiry. The same is true of simulation exercises, which present learners with imaginary problems designed to mimic those faced in real life by social workers, nurses and economists, for example, and ask them to produce solutions. These solutions are then compared with genuine case histories, and comparisons and contrasts are drawn which promote debate, understanding, and the efficient workings of memory.

References

Bloom, B.S. (1956)
Taxonomy of Educational Objectives. Handbook 1: The cognitive domain. London: Longmans Green.

Bruner, J.S. (1966)
Towards a Theory of Instruction. Cambridge, Mass.: Harvard University Press.

Bruner, J.S. (1973)
The Relevance of Education. New York: Norton.

Davie, R., Butler, N. and Goldsmith, H. (1972)
From Birth to Seven. London: Longmans.

Gagné, R.M. (1974)
Essentials of Learning for Instruction. Hinsdale, Ill.:
Dryden Press.

Inhelder, B. and Piaget, J. (1958)
The Growth of Logical Thinking from Childhood to
Adolescence. London: Routledge & Kegan Paul.

Kagan, J., Sontag, L., Baker, C. and Nelson, V. (1958)
Personality and IQ change. Journal of Abnormal and
Social Psychology, 56, 261-266.

Krathwohl, D.R. (1964)
Taxonomy of Educational Objectives. Handbook II: The
affective domain. New York: David McKay.

Simpson, E.J. (1972)
The classification of educational objectives in the
psychomotor domain. The Psychomotor Domain, Volume III.
Washington: Gryphon House.

Skinner, B.F. (1969)
Contingencies of Reinforcement: A theoretical analysis.
New York: Appleton-Century-Crofts.

Changing people: Part VI Questions

1. Who are the 'helpers'?
2. What characterizes effective helpers?
3. Is it possible to force people to change?
4. How can counselling and helping be demystified?
5. How large a part does counselling play in nursing?
6. What are the advantages and disadvantages of individual and group helping techniques?
7. What is the theoretical rationale underlying systematic desensitization?
8. Discuss the view that people have differing degrees of readiness to acquire particular phobias.
9. What are the implications of classical and operant conditioning for developing a policy to prevent crime?
10. What are the limitations of using punishment as a means of changing behaviour?
11. What are some of the main points of difference between a behavioural and psychodynamic approach to change?
12. Sometimes anxiety is an aid to learning and sometimes the reverse. Why?
13. Why is the experience of consistent failure so damaging to a person's readiness to learn?
14. What is overlearning, and why is it a valuable strategy?
15. What are the respective functions of the essay and the objective test in education?
16. What is the significance of cheating at academic work, whether at school, at college, or in professional training?
17. How can student nurses be helped to apply knowledge and skills that they have learnt in the classroom to the ward?
18. How can ward staff assist patients to gain insight into their problems?
19. What would be the desirable features of an occupational counselling service for nurses?
20. Outline a treatment programme designed to reduce the frequency of ritualistic behaviour.
21. Outline a treatment for enuresis.
22. Discuss the view that changing staff behaviour may be more important than changing patient behaviour.
23. What factors make a ward-wide psychological treatment programme more relevant than a series of individual programmes?

24. What practical issues need to be considered in designing a training course in behaviour modification procedures for ALL the staff of a ward?
25. What would be the main features of a health education programme designed to improve dental care in children?
26. A 13-year-old boy is in hospital for several months and is being taught by the teacher from the hospital school. What is likely to be different about the education be receives, by comparison with his normal schooling?
27. What psychological principles would guide you in retraining the speech of a 65-year-old man after a stroke?
28. A young man has become very over-active in hospital, refuses to go to bed, and wanders around the ward at night. How could the night nurse try to manage this difficulty?
29. A 30-year-old mother of two young children is excessively anxious about leaving the house. How could her husband help both to achieve and maintain some improvement?
30. Indicate some of the steps that may need to be taken when transferring an elderly man back to his home, where he lives on his own.

Part seven

The Psychology of Illness, Care and Treatment

22

People and illness
John Hall

Physical illnesses are very real to those who are suffering
from them. To most people illness is an intrusion into their
lives, an intrusion that should either be removed, or tolerated as best as possible if it will not go away.

Some people regard illness as a challenge. Young men
with spinal injuries develop their remaining functional
muscles to a level far beyond that reached before their
injury. Other people discover that with more time on their
hands they can read and think more than before, and become
more philosophical in their attitude to life.

There are, then, a range of attitudes to illness, and
people therefore differ in their response to illness. These
attitudes are themselves modified by people's past experience of the health care system, and the expectations they
may have that treatment will be successful in their particular case. One of the apparent paradoxes in health care in
Britain since the end of the Second World War is that while
many diseases, such as tuberculosis and pneumonia, have been
largely overcome, the total number of people in contact with
the health services has risen.

Some aspects of attitudes to illness have a moral quality. There is still stigmatization of some conditions, such
as venereal disease and spasticity, spilling over into colloquial terms of abuse. Others may feel that their physical
condition is a form of punishment, brought upon themselves
by some misdeed or as a result of their general style of
life.

These attitudes, or beliefs, act together with other
information the person receives so that when illness is a
possibility - when an unexplained lump is felt somewhere, or
when pain is experienced somewhere in the body - the person
is ready to develop a theory of his illness. This theory is
shaped from the patient's bodily experiences, from the information received from external sources (such as television
programmes and the family doctor), and from personal experience with illness. The way in which this theory relates to
the treatments perceived to be available from conventional
health care services will then affect whether he enters the
National Health system or alternative patterns of care, or
does not pursue treatment.

The role of 'fringe' medicine should not be underestimated. Established medicine has eschewed manipulative treatment, with a consequent increase in business for osteopaths. While some more extreme sorts of diet and herbal remedies seemed to have a weak foundation only a few years ago, the current interest in food allergies and the importance of fibre in the diet has reinforced views that particular foods should be avoided and others preferred. Given the lack of complete correlation in time between administration of a treatment and recovery, there will always be those who have a strong belief in the effectiveness of a treatment that lacks any general rational support.

One of the confusing aspects of pain research is the extent to which individuals may report pain relief from treatments or interventions that do not appear, on the surface, to be capable of helping. For example, Locsin (1981) reported a study on the effect of music on pain levels in post-operative patients. The subjects for the study were 24 women who all underwent surgery involving abdominal incision. The patients were divided into an experimental group and control group, the experimental group receiving exposure to some music which they had previously indicated they liked. The outcome of the trial was assessed by a specially constructed 'Overt Pain Reaction Rating Scale', and by gathering data on blood pressure, pulse rate, and respiratory rate.

This study is unusual, and presents some methodological problems, but has some interesting findings. The group of patients who listened to music of their own preference were better than the control patients on muscular-skeletal and verbal pain reactions during the first 48 hours after the operation. Also there were some non-significant trends, suggesting that the experimental group used less analgesics, and in addition the patients subjectively liked the music. The study offers an interesting sidelight on the value of music 'piped' to a ward which may not fit the musical preference of any patients!

The importance of all these observations is that when adults become ill, they possess a strongly structured belief system before they present any family doctor or nurse with an account of their symptoms. Their psychological reaction to illness may not be entirely unpredictable, but explicable in terms of the factors already discussed, and hence to some extent clearly predictable. One of the most interesting areas of development in medical psychology is this growth in the study of 'illness behaviour'.

The physical setting of health and illness

Important in health care is the environment which people enter when they become patients. The most significant aspects of the environment are the people they encounter within it, and the tasks those people will perform with and upon the patient. Nevertheless it is worth considering the physical aspects of the environment, as they too have an effect.

Some diseases and conditions are caused by physical aspects of the external environment. Repeated exposure to high intensity sound, as experienced by ground crew at airports, can lead to permanent hearing loss. Inhalation of certain types of mineral dust, such as asbestos fibre, causes damage to the lungs. Most of these obvious forms of environmental hazard are at least potentially preventable, and indeed the most hazardous are often minimized by legislation or other regulations specific to the industry or occupation concerned.

More diffuse but still important is the effect of poor housing: the effect of lack of heating, possibly leading to hypothermia in cold weather for the elderly; the effect of lack of piped water on the frequency of washing, both of the body and utensils and clothing; the effect of damp arising from defective roofs or damp courses. Similarly, overcrowding, and in particular overcrowded sleeping accommodation for children, may lead to lack of sleep and cross-infection. This does not necessarily mean that poor environmental conditions cause illness, but undoubtedly such conditions may make acute conditions chronic, and certainly restrict the range of recreational and social opportunities available to the families concerned.

A major concern of health visitors is with promoting the environmental health of young children. This suggests that the health visitor knows how to contact the families, and especially those families in the greatest need. This may be very difficult where a number of families are homeless, and it is dependent on the way in which a local authority deals with homeless people within its area.

Fisher reported in 1980 the results of a survey carried out in one part of London, which had inherited in 1974 a considerable number of homeless people placed in bed and breakfast accommodation. The administration of the survey indicated some of the problems of doing community surveys: the very high rate of movement in and out of temporary accommodation, and the difficulty in even initially placing families who had just moved into an area and were not yet in contact with the social services agency. Discussions arising from the surveys resulted in better placements of families with special needs (such as pregnant women), and have led to better co-operation between the various agencies. Direct benefits of the survey were the reduction of 'crisis' housing decisions and the more efficient use of nursing and other staff.

At a different level, the physical environment is important in the actual delivery of health care. There is increasing interest in the layout of hospitals, and the relationship between design of spaces and their use by patients. At the grossest level, considerable difficulties have arisen in the psychiatric services in Britain in areas where the older large psychiatric hospitals were built in remote areas, or in clusters round the largest conurbations. Travel to and from hospital then becomes both expensive and time-consuming, thus reducing the amount of contact between

patients and family. Apart from this reason, in all spe-
cialities smaller-sized units are preferred by the staff
who work in them, and the current philosophy both in building new hospitals and in refurbishing old ones is producing
smaller units of organization as far as nursing teams are
concerned.

Ahmed (1981) inherited, as a supervisory nurse, a 51-bed
acute medical unit, and was determined to change nursing
practice on the unit. When reporting what happened on the
unit, she drew attention to the need to 'stem the tide of
well-educated and creative nurses away from the hospital'.
She introduced a different system of staffing on the ward
which was patient centred, and involved dividing the ward
into three sub-units. Considerable time had to be spent in
working out all the organizational aspects of the change,
but staff enthusiasm was high. Change was not achieved
without pressure from other professions on the nursing
staff. Another feature of the changes was that unplanned
changes, beyond the original expectations of what could be
achieved, have occurred as individual nurses themselves
initiated further changes. Her conclusion was that the 'new
system is terrific, but not perfect'. However, it went a
long way towards achieving her initial objectives of closer
patient-nurse relationships, more nursing accountability for
patients' problems, and improved continuity of patient
services and communication between all the shifts.

At the individual unit or ward level, detailed design is
again important. How close to the day room are the toilet
facilities for elderly patients? Is the door to the toilet
clearly identifiable from other doors, even if you have poor
eyesight? Is the layout of the ward chairs conducive to
communication between patients, or are the chairs lined
neatly along the walls of the ward? Several writers on
environment for long-term care have emphasized the need for
'environmental personalization', or varying details of
furnishing and decorations in accordance with the wishes of
individual patients. While such personalization has a lot of
intuitive appeal, a psychologist could systematically investigate what gains are made if a previously barren ward is
decorated in such a way. There is a relative dearth of information on the specific effect of varying the physical
environment for patients, yet it is clear that both general
and immediate environmental factors are important both in
home-based and hospital-based care.

**The social setting of
health and illness**

The most important single factor in the delivery of health
care is the competence of people who deliver it, and their
ability to communicate with their patients. The skills of
communicating with patients are discussed in the last
chapter in this section, but the way in which those skills
are applied in different settings is relevant here.

In 1981 an entire issue of one nursing journal, Nursing,
was taken up with the topic of communication, starting with

a schematic presentation of the process and difficulties of communication and outlining factors such as the listener being too cold, tired, or uncomfortable which impair communication. One contribution to the issue concentrated on communication between the midwife and the pregnant mother, and was written by Crowe. Apart from the general need to develop and maintain a good relationship with the mother, the midwife needs to pay attention to different topics during contact with the family. Perhaps both parents will need to attend parent craft sessions, when a main interest of the parents-to-be will be having THEIR questions answered. If the man attends the birth, he will need to feel supported and to have a clear understanding of his role. If the child is stillborn or handicapped, the event will be perceived by parents and midwife alike as a tragedy. Examination of the role of the midwife in this setting illustrates the need for variation in the style of communication with a particular patient or family as their needs vary.

Doctors and nurses do not learn their skills in a professional vacuum, but in the setting of a carefully negotiated relationship between the professions which has taken decades to refine to its present position. The process of training as a nurse is not only a skill-learning and knowledge-acquiring process, but one of attitude-adoption and role-adoption. It has been suggested that interaction between nurses and doctors can be characterized as a 'game', using the jargon of interactional analysis. The object of the game is then for the nurse to be bold, have initiative, and be responsible for making significant recommendations, while appearing at the same time submissive so that her recommendations are accepted by the doctor.

This may be a parody of the relationship between many doctors and nurses working closely together, with mutual respect and co-operation. Yet one component of the working lives of nurses is dealing with conflict between their professional interests, and the professional interests of other groups. These conflicts are at least formally resolved by the relevant professional bodies; in Britain, these are the British Medical Association and the Royal College of Nursing (RCN). There is an institutionalized element to the positions adopted in these conflicts which may be at variance with what is going on at the hospital level. An important focus of this conflict is the question of professional responsibility. The overall responsibility of the doctor is legally or organizationally enshrined in many situations, yet in a number of those situations it is often only a nurse who is able to make a competent judgement as to what action should be taken. This outline of inter-professional conflict illustrates how necessary an understanding of some elementary organizational psychology is to many nurses, even at ward level.

Within a particular health centre or hospital, these general professional rules are supplemented by local traditions and regulations. The tendency for institutions to develop their own routines which persist in the absence of continuing need has been well documented: most experienced nurses can recall some regulation relating to their own training, or to some clinical procedure intended to reduce infection, for instance, which was not consistent with other regulations or procedure. The clearest examples of such regulations are to be found in 'total institutions', a term coined by the American sociologist Goffman (1961) to describe those institutions where the normal barriers between different areas of life have broken down. 'Total institutions' are characterized, among other things, by a clear separation between 'staff' and 'inmates', by 'initiation' or admission rituals, and by the wearing of special forms of dress not functionally related to the tasks which people perform. Goffman is not a scientific writer, in that his ideas are supported by selective quotations from his sources, some of which are literary rather than factual. However, his ideas have been extremely influential in attempts to liberalize and reform institutional practices and regulations, and are elaborated in the next chapter.

One aspect of a healing institution which can become a routine is the giving of care itself. Routines can become rigid so that patients are treated en bloc, and the time-tabling of events is arranged more for the convenience of staff than for the benefit of patients. An important element in counteracting such routines is therefore to be flexible in the use of time and facilities, to be normal in the standards of general dress and behaviour that are expected, and to allow greater autonomy to the patients in decisions which do not directly affect their care.

Another consequence of institutionalization is the suspension by staff of normal judgemental standards. Ethics may well seem to be a subject far removed from nursing. Yet there is a moral element to a number of nursing decisions, as discussed by Schröck (1980). She examined the place of value judgements in nursing, as illustrated by data gathered from a number of discussion groups with nurses, and from nurses involved in various post-basic courses.

The discussion concentrates on the stark question of whether health care professionals tell the truth! An example is given by the response of a mixed group of nurses to the question: 'If your have ever told a patient that you did not know the name or purpose of a drug that he/she was given (although you did know), why did you tell a lie or give an evasive answer?' Sixty per cent of all reasons offered could be categorized as acting under coercion (doctors' orders, ward policy), though still leaving the justification for that coercion unclear. However, 27 per cent of response appears to reflect a lack of confidence by the nurse in handling the situation if the patients had been told the truth. While recognizing that concealment, evasion, or deception may sometimes be necessary, the burden of proof lies with those who advocate it, rather than those who reject such a course.

The final elements in the social setting of health care are the characteristics of the team who together look after the patient. The term 'team' itself bears some examination. The associated concept of teamwork implies that a team has some common task to which members of the team are committed. Nothing is more demoralizing in regular team meetings than to have a team member who does not share the common task-related assumptions of the others, and who makes decisions independently of other decisions made jointly by team members. Teams generally function best if there is reasonably clear delineation of the responsibilities of different team members, and if there is differentiation between the common responsibility to reach an agreed decision, and the individual responsibility to take action dependent on the decision.

Evers (1981) has taken a detailed look at the concept of the multi-disciplinary team, particularly as it relates to care on geriatric wards and of long-stay patients. She points to the need to co-ordinate the contributions of the different professional experts in order to serve the best interests of the patients. An initial difficulty lies in defining the nature of a particular team: the term 'network' may be better in some circumstances to describe groups of staff who communicate with each other, but who do not meet face-to-face. Where the team may meet each other, one typology of teams is to consider them in terms of whether their TASKS are similar (homogeneous) or different (heterogeneous), and whether their SKILLS are of the same kind and level (homogeneous) or different (heterogeneous). A classification of this sort, together with some of the comments made on team structure, can be useful in analysing problems which arise in teamwork.

The same article goes on to consider how teams work in geriatric wards. It concludes that there has developed a 'rhetoric of teamwork', which serves a number of purposes, including coping with uncertainty in times of change, and continuing the social control over patients and subordinate professions by doctors in a medical field where there is a lot of unpopular and dirty work.

A term used to describe the effectiveness of teamwork is morale. Although the term has military overtones, it is widely used to describe several related aspects of job satisfaction and personal happiness and security. A classic study by Revans (1964) used the concept of morale in comparing the success of different hospitals, and in examining factors such as absenteeism, staff turnover, and even the number of reported accidents. Although very high morale is not necessary for good health care to be given, and indeed may be associated with complacency, low morale is easier to identify by high staff turnover, high sickness rates, and so on.

If teams are to function well, they need to be led. Lack of leadership and structure in any team or organization produces anxiety and uncertainty. The criteria by which leaders

are selected varies from one setting to another. Sometimes
leaders are self-selected by virtue of the post they hold,
and this is particularly likely to apply when a consultant
is a member of a team, or when all team members are members of one profession and a direct superior or senior
member of that profession is present. However, qualities
necessary to be a good surgeon are not necessarily those
associated with good team leadership styles. Different
leaders of the same team may sometimes be appropriate,
depending on the variability of the tasks facing the group.
A useful distinction may be made between structural authority (deriving from a post) and sapiential authority (deriving from the personal knowledge of the individual).

Leadership may appear a rather abstract quality unless
related to the group that is being led, and the nature of
the group task. It is not necessarily the case that a good
leader of a staff group would make a good leader of a patient group, since different qualities may be needed in the
two different settings.

Smith (1980) described her own experience in setting up
a patient group. After discussing some guidelines for the
selection of group members, she went on to discuss how she
dealt with her own anxieties about not being able to 'control' the group. She examined the way in which her own
leadership style developed from being initially authoritarian to being very non-directive. She then spent the
latter part of her sessions with the group achieving a
balance between these two extremes, so that leadership took
on a more 'fluid' meaning for her, with the object of finding a point of balance that shifted in response to what
happened in the group.

Different styles of leadership are required in different
settings, and some leadership skills, such as chairing or
guiding formal meetings, are not normally acquired in the
earlier stages of a career. There is some scope for the
direct training of some leadership skills, although others
are more dependent on the normal sensitivity and persuasive
ability of the person concerned.

Patients' progress

The entry of a patient into this complex social system may
be likened to the progress of either a pilgrim or a rake,
depending on eventual outcome. Following the discovery of
some symptom, the patient goes deeper and deeper into the
system. Pain is often one of the main reasons why help is
sought; pain relief is often the main goal of seeking help;
and obtaining even symptomatic relief from pain may mean
the patient falls by the wayside, and voluntarily withdraws
from the health care system. The presence of pain, and understanding of it, is thus very important in understanding
the patient's needs and responding to them.

Although pain cuts right across traditional boundaries
of medicine, there is no one central body which can give
information to nurses particularly wanting to work in pain

clinics. Fairbrother (1979) describes how nurses work in pain clinics in different parts of the country, and the problems this presents for nurses working in this way. The article discusses how emotionally draining it can be to cope with the 'hard core' of incurable patients. Work in such a unit 'is obviously not for the faint-hearted. Not is it for those who like working in a well-defined clinical area with the limits of their responsibility clearly laid down. But if you're flexible, you'll be fascinated.'

Pain is not the only reason why treatment is sought. Some people are embarrassed by their external appearance, such as the scaling produced by psoriasis. Others are motivated by fear or embarrassment of some unknown illness, in the absence of marked pain, as illustrated by an over-response to discharges from the penis. Others are concerned about loss of function, whether motor or intellectual function, for no apparent reason. The threshold level of each motivating factor which maintains their attendance is variable and is not necessarily related to objective assessment of the severity of their conditions.

The first point of contact with the health care system is the family doctor. It has been shown that the average consultation time of patients with their family doctor is of the order of ten minutes. Many patients are quite satisfied with this amount of time, but it is clearly inadequate to explore problems of any complexity. The family doctor's response to the patient at this stage is crucial: an over-willingness to prescribe medication for psychological problems both delays appropriate treatment, and may confirm the patient's view that there is an illness to be treated. If a repeat visit to the family doctor does not lead to improvement, then the patient may be sent on to the next stage: the out-patient department.

The first out-patient attendance is extremely important for anyone who is likely to continue in care, for two reasons. It constitutes the first contact with the nursing, medical and other staff who are likely to be responsible for care for a period of time. It is also likely to offer patients a considerable amount of intended and unintended information relevant to their developing theory of their disease. Repeated visits to the out-patient department may be necessary. This often entails meeting a series of different junior doctors on each occasion, who repeat basic standard questions, so possibly irritating the patient. Coupled with the long period of waiting, out-patient attendances often do not generate the conditions suggested for good communication.

The patient may then need to be admitted. Careful preparation for admission is indicated wherever possible for children, and should not be neglected for adults. Many patients are apprehensive on admission: they are entering a new environment which is strange and confusing, and they are leaving behind their normal social supports, and personal status and identity. They may respond to this uncertainty by 'testing' the nurse, in the same way as a child tests a new adult: 'What is allowed, what can I do?' Other patients may very readily relinquish all responsibility, yielding to the nurse on even minor decisions.

The final stage which is possible is permanent hospitalization. This is only relevant to the most seriously physically handicapped and mentally impaired patients, and the number of new psychiatric patients becoming long-stay residents has dropped dramatically in recent years. Even so, there are still people who have been continuously in hospital for 50 years or more. Their families have usually died or abandoned them, and they may have little apparent awareness of outside life, or even evidence of enjoying social relationships within hospital. Yet these severely handicapped people are in one sense the most deserving of good nursing care and support, since they are so handicapped that no one else can act as their advocate. The recent development of a World Health Organization (1980) classification of disabilities and handicaps serves as a reminder of the increasing burden of chronic and disabling conditions. Such a burden will place a new responsibility on many nurses, but one that is even more full of psychological implications.

References

Ahmed, M.C. (1981)
Taking charge of change in hospital nursing practice. American Journal of Nursing, 81, 540-543.

Crowe, V. (1981)
The midwife and the family. Nursing (July), 1171-1173.

Evers, H.K. (1981)
Multi-disciplinary teams in geriatric wards: myth or reality. Journal of Advanced Nursing, 6, 205-214.

Fairbrother, C. (1979)
Working in a pain relief clinic. Nursing (May), 104-107.

Fisher, E. (1980)
Homeless families: a scheme of notification to ensure effective care. Nursing Times, July (Occasional Papers), 77-80.

Goffman, E. (1961)
Asylums. New York: Doubleday.

Locsin, R.G.R.A.C. (1981)
The effect of music on the pain of selected postoperative patients. Journal of Advanced Nursing, 6, 19-25.

Revans, R.W. (1964)
Standards for Morale: Cause and effect in hospitals. Oxford: Nuffield Provincial Hospitals Trust, Oxford University Press.

Schröck, R.A. (1980)
A question of honesty in nursing practice. Journal of Advanced Nursing, 5, 135-148.

Smith, L.L. (1980)
Finding your leadership style in groups. American Journal of Nursing, 80, 1301-1303.

World Health Organization (1980)
  International Classification of Impairments, Disabilities and Handicaps. Geneva: WHO.

23

Institutional climates
Jim Orford

A person's behaviour is influenced by the surrounding
environment, as well as by attributes which the person
brings to that environment, such as personality, abilities
and attitudes; behaviour is a function of person and
environment. Many people either live or work in institutions
of one kind or another. For such people, the institution
constitutes an important part of their environment. For some
people it constitutes almost their total environment. Those
who work in an institutional setting cannot fail to notice
how the institution influences its members, either for good
or ill. Many will have felt frustrated by the values which
the institution seems to embody, or by the practices which
are prevalent within it, feeling that members could be
helped more if things were otherwise, or even that members
are being harmed by the institution. The great importance of
these matters has begun to be recognized in psychology and
there is a growing psychological literature on the organization of institutions and how to change them. The study of
institutions holds wider lessons for social psychology too.
An institution is a social psychological laboratory. The
experiments which take place there are naturally occurring
experiments in the psychology of social interaction, social
roles, intergroup attitudes, conflict and cohesiveness. The
study of institutions is of vital significance for both
theoretical and applied psychology.

Much of the literature on the subject concerns health
care or social service institutions such as mental hospitals
and hostels or homes for children, the elderly, or the
disabled. Although many of the examples upon which this
chapter draws are taken from such institutions, the chapter
attempts to build up a general picture of institutional life
which is equally as relevant, for example, to educational
institutions such as schools and colleges, and to penal institutions such as prisons and detention centres. These different institutions have a great deal in common. Each is a
collection of people, gathered together in a special building or group of buildings. These people are not normally
linked by family ties, but are there because of the special
'needs' (for education, care, treatment, rehabilitation, or
punishment) of inmates, users, or 'clients' (pupils, members, patients, residents). It is the responsibility of

another group of people, the staff, to provide for the clients' needs. This they are in a position to do on account of their special training, skills, or occupation (as teacher, prison officer, warden, doctor or nurse). Usually the institution has been set up by, and is part of, a larger organization which is responsible for managing the institution. Penal institutions in Britain are governed by the complex machinery of the Home Office; hospitals by the Department of Health and its network of Regional, Area and District Authorities, each with a complex system of members, officers and management teams; local authority schools and homes by committees and sub-committees of elected and co-opted representatives, the Authority's officers and the institution's committee of governors or managers; and institutions run by voluntary bodies by their trustees and management committees. Institutions are almost always influenced by people, often a large number of them, who have control over the institution but who are not involved in day-to-day work with the institution's clients. It is more than purely academic to consider some of these defining features of human service institutions. They immediately suggest ways in which an institution differs from a person's own home, and hence they indicate where some problems with institutions are to be expected. The small family home provides the clearest contrast to the large residential institution. People are not gathered together in the former on account of their special needs or their special qualifications, there is no demarcation between staff and clients, and the influence of outside organizations is minimal. It is no wonder that a great deal of thought and effort has been devoted to the goal of making institutions as normal and home-like as possible. Many other comparisons and contrasts between organizations and groups could be made, and there is no absolute definition of an institution.

Ideal types: the total institution and the therapeutic community

It is important to be clear what is meant by a 'total institution' and by the term 'therapeutic community'. They are important ideas which have had much influence but as terms they are liable to be used loosely, and hence may obscure rather than reveal the true facts about institutional climates. In a much-read and often-quoted collection of essays, Goffman (1961) noted that it is normal in modern society for people to conduct different aspects of their life, for example sleeping, playing and working, in different places, with different people, and under different authorities. Total institutions, in contrast, are places where these barriers between different spheres of life are broken down. All aspects of life are conducted in the same place and, most importantly, under the same single authority. It is quite likely that activities are tightly scheduled by those in authority in accordance with an overall plan. He noted that many penal and caring institutions were total institutions in this sense. So were a number of

places, with which this chapter is less concerned, such as
army barracks, ships and monasteries. On the other hand,
certain places with which we are concerned, such as day
schools and day hospitals or centres, would not qualify as
total institutions.

It is also important to recognize the variety of climates which exist even within total institutions. Tizard,
Sinclair and Clarke (1975) point out the danger of general-
izing from studies of single institutions, such as Goffman's
study of an American mental hospital. Used loosely, the
expression 'total institution' can give rise to a misleading
stereotype. There is now ample evidence, some of which is
considered later in this chapter, that institutions vary
greatly, and furthermore that individual institutions can be
changed.

Nevertheless, the harm that institutions may do has
increasingly been recognized. Barton (1959) has gone so far
as to say that the symptoms of institutionalization are so
well marked that they constitute a disease entity which he
called 'institutional neurosis'. He has written:

> Institutional Neurosis is a disease characterized by
> apathy, lack of initiative, loss of interest ...,
> submissiveness, and sometimes no expression of feelings
> of resentment at harsh and unfair orders. There is also
> lack of interest in the future ..., a deterioration in
> personal habits ..., a loss of individuality, and a
> resigned acceptance that things will go on as they are.

The concept of the 'therapeutic community' is an important
one because it represents one type of ideal contrasting
markedly with the most inhumane or least therapeutic institutional climates. The model therapeutic community was the
Henderson Unit at the Belmont Hospital in Surrey. The unit,
described by Maxwell Jones (1952) and studied by Rapoport
(1960), was principally aimed at helping young adult psychiatric patients, many of whom had problems of repeated
antisocial conduct and who were difficult to accommodate
elsewhere. Amongst the ideals of the therapeutic community
are an emphasis on active rehabilitation as opposed to
custodialism; democratization, namely that decision making
about the unit's affairs should be shared amongst staff and
patients alike; permissiveness, that is, that distressing or
deviant behaviour should be tolerated rather than repressed
in the interests of institutional conformity; communalism,
that is, that the climate should be informal without the
development of highly specialized roles, and that relationships should be close but never exclusive; and reality
confrontation, that is, that patients should be continually given interpretations of their behaviour as other
members of the unit see it. It is important to appreciate
that the Henderson model is a very specific one. Struc-
turally it was a total institution and although its climate
was undoubtedly in contrast to that of many large impersonal

institutions, in some ways it was rather formal, with a detailed programme of therapeutic and administrative groups, work assignments and other activities. Units are often self-styled 'therapeutic communities', but they are rarely aiming to recreate the type of therapeutic community unit described by Jones and Rapoport.

Structural features of institutions

There are many separate features of institutions which contribute to climate and a number of these are considered in turn.

Size

There is considerable evidence that people prefer, and are more active socially in, small units of organization. One explanation for these findings is based on the idea of 'manning'. Where there are relatively few patients, pupils or residents, there are relatively many tasks and activities for them to undertake. There is much scope for involvement in activity; the setting may be said to be relatively under-manned. In contrast, settings with relatively many indivi-duals may be over-manned, with relatively less opportunity for involvement for all.

This is perhaps why efforts are often made to break up an institution into smaller, more manageable, groups such as classes, houses or year groups in schools, and wards and small units within hospitals. Unfortunately, the overall institution may continue to exercise a strong influence on the smaller units that comprise it. One recent study (reported in Canter and Canter, 1979) found that staff working in institutions for handicapped children adopted more institution-orientated as opposed to child-orientated practices in looking after the children when their unit was part of a larger overall institution. The size of the unit itself was unimportant. Individual units within institutions are rarely fully autonomous but continue to be dependent on the larger institution in many ways. This notion of auto-nomy is an important one to which this chapter returns.

Location

Location is of both symbolic and concrete significance. The isolated mental hospital symbolizes community attitudes to the mentally ill, for example. Other features of institu-tions may symbolize a similar relationship between insti-tution and community. Prisons are often located in cities but their isolation is ensured by their high walls and impenetrable, fortress-like entrances; they are in the community, but not of it. It is important to consider what factors are operating to promote closeness of contact between an institution and its local community, and what factors are operating to inhibit it. It is interesting to speculate, for example, on whether a prominent sign announcing that a house is a home for the elderly eases visiting by members of the community or makes it more difficult? Certainly many small residential caring units such as hostels and halfway houses pride themselves on carrying no such institutional signboard.

Ease of access to community facilities may be crucial for those who must remain in an institution for a long time. A lack of interest in, or desire to return to, life outside are considered by Barton and others to be amongst the main features of institutionalization, and he lists loss of contact with the outside world, loss of personal friends, and loss of prospects outside as three of its main causes.

The issue of location illustrates an important point about the psychology of social organizations. The point is that no single variable is independent of others, and consequently it is almost impossible to impute causal significance to single features of institutions. In this case, it is very unlikely that the location of an institution is independent of the philosophy or ideology under which it operates, or the attitudes of staff who work in it. A rehabilitation philosophy is likely to be associated with close community contacts, either because the institution was located close to the community in the first place, or because means had been found to overcome an unsatisfactory location.

Internal design

Large rooms with high ceilings, glossy interior wall paint in drab colours, no change of decor from one area to another, lack of personalization by the use of pictures, photographs and ornaments, lack of privacy, even sometimes extending to a bathroom and toilet, absence of individual-ized sleeping accommodation, few personal possessions or places to keep them, and generally an absence of opportunity to express individuality; these are amongst the internal design features of an institution which contribute to an institutional as opposed to homely atmosphere.

Once again, however, it is important to avoid over-simple ideas of cause and effect. Two examples from Canter and Canter's book (1979) on the influence of design in institutions illustrate this point. One example concerns the first several years' operation of a purpose-built unit for disturbed children. A number of features, such as outside play facilities, were designed by the architect with the express purpose of reducing institutional climate. Others, such as doors for bedrooms, were strongly advocated by the director and were eventually installed. Observation of the day-to-day life of the unit, however, led to the view that the overwhelming ideology of the unit, which placed emphasis on the children's disturbance and on the need for staff control and surveillance, undermined the use of these design features. Play facilities were rarely spontaneously used, bedroom doors were hardly ever closed, and rooms which were designed for personal use were used as seclusion rooms for punishment. The second example concerns a purpose-built forensic unit where it was possible to show, by a process of behaviour mapping (a procedure whereby a map of who does what and where is produced by observing samples of behaviour in different places at different times), the use to which different spaces were put and the meanings that became attached to them. Certain areas were clearly designated as staff offices, and others as patient lounges. As a result, segregation of staff and patients was the rule rather than the exception.

One small-scale feature of physical layout which is relatively easily manipulated is that of seating arrangement. The terms 'sociopetal' (meaning encouraging interpersonal relationships) and 'sociofugal' (discouraging relationships) have been used to describe possible seating arrangements in institutions. Seats in the lounge areas of old people's homes and other institutions are often arranged around the edge of the room or in some other sociofugal pattern, such as in rows facing a television set. Sociopetal patterns, on the other hand, have been found to lead to more interaction, more multi-person interaction, and more personal conversations. Once again, it is important to appreciate other, more human, aspects of the environment. It is often found, when attempts have been made to rearrange furniture in a more sociopetal fashion, that there is a tendency for the seating to revert to its former arrangement. It is as if the institution has a will of its own and is in some way resistant to change. Exploring how this reversion to type comes about, and making a diagnosis of what is to blame, may provide vital insights into the nature of the institution.

It is worth speculating on the function which may be served by furniture arrangement in different types of institution. For example, why is the seating arrangement of pupils in a primary school often very different from, and usually more sociopetal in design than, that to be found in a secondary school? Is this difference accidental, or does it say something about the expected relationship between teacher and pupils, and perhaps thereby about the whole underlying philosophy of education?

Rules, regulations and routines

Studies of institutional practices

Considerable progress has been made in describing the variety which exists within health and social care residential institutions. Similar variety exists within educational establishments, and within penal settings.

Studies have compared hostels and hospitals for mentally handicapped children, and have found the latter to be much more institutional in their handling of the children: routine is more rigid, children are more likely to be treated en bloc, treatment is less personalized, and social distance between staff and children is greater. Wide variation is found in the degree of 'ward restrictiveness' in adult mental hospitals. Similar variation exists in halfway houses for ex-psychiatric patients. On average, hostels are less institutional than mental hospitals, the former having between one-half and two-thirds the number of 'restrictive practices' found in the average hospital ward in one study. However, considerable variation is found in both types of facility and there is an overlap between them. Some of the hostels, whilst being small in size, and designed to provide a link between the large institution and the community, nevertheless retain a number of institutional practices. In one instance a hostel had more institutional practices than the hospital rehabilitation ward from which most of its residents came.

A key idea linking these studies is that of clients' decision making freedom. Table 1 provides an indication of some of the major areas of decision making considered in such studies. The list could be expanded greatly to include a large range of day-to-day activities over which most people are able to exercise personal choice. Whether an institution allows this exercise of choice to continue for its clients or whether these decision-making freedoms are curtailed is crucial in determining whether an institution creates a therapeutic climate or institutionalization.

Table 1

A range of decisions which may be allowed or restricted in institutions and which are illustrative of those considered in studies of institutional practices

What time to get up and go to bed
What to wear
What to eat for breakfast and other meals
Planning future meals
Whether to make a drink or snack
Whether to visit the local shops
Whether to go to work
Whether to go to the pictures
How to spend own money
When to have a bath
When to have a haircut
Whether to have medicine
Deciding arrangement of own room
Deciding decoration of own room
Whether to smoke
Whether to play the radio or TV
When to invite friends in
Whether to have a sexual relationship with a friend
Planning decoration or repair of the place
Deciding how to care for or control other members
Deciding policy

Staff autonomy
Reference has already been made, when considering the size of an institution, to the importance of a unit's autonomy

within the larger institution. Decision-making freedom may
be limited not only for clients but also for those staff who
have the closest dealings with them. The advantages of the
informality which can occur in a truly independent small
unit are illustrated by an incident which occurred at
Woodley House, an American halfway house for the mentally
ill. It concerned a dispute between pro- and anti-television
factions in the house. The former decided to convert part of
the basement of the house for their use, leaving the living
room to the others. A staff member took them in her car to
buy paint and other materials and later the same day the
newly-decorated television room was in use. Such an incident
could not easily occur in that way in a larger and more
formal institution. There are a number of reasons for this,
one being that the staff member at Woodley House was not
limited to a prescribed professional role, and there were no
other members of staff upon whose role territory she was
trespassing.

It is this variable of staff autonomy which Tizard et al
(1975) considered to be one of the strongest influences upon
the quality of staff-client interaction in an institutional
setting. The firmest evidence for this hypothesis is
contained in a chapter of their book written by Barbara
Tizard. It concerns residential nurseries run by voluntary
societies. She observed 13 such units, all of which had been
modernized in recent years to provide 'family group' care.
Mixed-age groups of six children each had their own suite of
rooms and their own nurse and assistant nurse to care for
them. Despite this effort at 'de-institutionalizing', marked
differences existed in the degree to which nurses were truly
independent agents. Nurseries were divided by the research
team into three classes on the basis of the amount of unit
autonomy. The first group, it was felt, was in effect run
centrally by the matron:

> Decisions were made on an entirely routine basis or else
> referred to the matron. Each day was strictly time-
> tabled, the matron would make frequent inspections of
> each group, and freedom of the nurse and child was very
> limited. The children were moved through the day 'en
> bloc' ... The nurse had little more autonomy than the
> children, e.g. she would have to ask permission to take
> the children for a walk or to turn on the television
> set. As in hospital each grade of staff wore a special
> uniform, and had separate living quarters, and the
> nurse's behaviour when off duty was governed by quite
> strict rules.

At the other extreme was a group of nurseries which more
closely approximated a normal family setting:

> The staff were responsible for shopping, cooking, making
> excursions with the children and arranging their own
> day. The children could move freely about the house and
> garden and the staff rarely referred a decision to the

matron. The nurse-in-charge did not wear uniform, and her off-duty time was not subject to rules. Her role, in fact, approximated more closely to that of a foster-mother. Since she could plan her own day and was not under constant surveillance she could treat the children more flexibly.

A third group of nurseries was intermediate in terms of independence. As predicted, the more autonomous staff were observed to spend more time talking to children, and more time playing, reading and giving information to them. Furthermore, children in units with more autonomous staff had higher scores on a test of verbal comprehension. The difficulty of teasing out what is important in complex social situations, such as those that exist in institutions, is illustrated by Barbara Tizard's findings. Autonomy was correlated with having a relatively favourable staff-to-child ratio and hence we cannot be certain that autonomy is the crucial variable.

Nevertheless, an effect of staff hierarchy was noticed which could explain the apparent importance of autonomy. When two staff were present at once, one was always 'in charge'. This had an inhibiting effect on a nurse's beha-viour towards children: she would function in a 'notably restricted way, talking much less and using less "informa-tive talk" than the nurse in charge'. This might explain differences between autonomous and less independent units, as staff in the latter type of unit would be much more likely to feel that someone else was in charge whether that person was present or not.

Flexible use of space, time and objects

Inflexible routine is one of the major charges brought against the institution by such writers as Barton and Goffman. Institutional life can be 'normalized' as much as possible by allowing flexible use of different areas of buildings and grounds, by varying time schedules, and by allowing flexible use of objects such as kitchen and laundry equipment, televisions, radios and record players. Resi-dential institutions usually deprive adult inmates of the opportunity to take part in 'complete activity cycles'. Instead of taking part in a complete cycle of shopping for food, preparing it, eating, clearing away and washing up after it, residents may simply be required to eat what others have purchased and prepared, rather like guests in a hotel.

Staff attitudes and behaviour

Ideology
The influence of an institution's ideology or philosophy is pervasive, although its significance can be missed altogether by those taken up in the day-to-day activities of the place. Many examples could be given. The philosophy of a progressive school such as Summerhill, with its emphasis

on personal development, is distinct from that of a regular secondary school with its emphasis on academic learning. The rehabilitation philosophy of Grendon Underwood prison is distinct from that of most closed penal establishments with their emphasis on custody. Many institutions have mixed and competing ideologies. These frequently give rise to conflict within the institution, the different ideologies often being represented by different cadres of staff. For example, educational and child care philosophies compete within institutions for handicapped children, as do educational and disciplinary philosophies within institutions for young delinquents. Important shifts may take place gradually over time. For example, a general shift from a custodial philosophy to a more therapeutic ideology has occurred in mental hospitals over the last several decades. Quite recently some of those working in British prisons have detected a move in the opposite direction in response to the call for tighter security.

Words such as 'open' to describe penal institutions, 'progressive' to describe educational facilities, and expressions such as 'therapeutic community' to describe an institution for residential care, all serve as public announcements of ideology and intended behaviour. However, it has already been noted that terms such as 'therapeutic community' are frequently used loosely, and sufficient is known about the absence of a strong correlation between attitudes and behaviour to make us doubtful that ideal philosophies will always be perfectly borne out in practice.

Staff attitudes

Nevertheless, no one who has worked in an institution for very long can have failed to notice what appear to be marked individual differences in staff attitudes. In the mental hospital setting questionnaires have been devised to detect staff attitudes of 'custodialism' or 'traditionalism'. The matter is by no means simple, however, and attitudes vary along a number of dimensions. For example, one study distinguished between 'restrictive control' and 'protective benevolence'. Staff high on restrictive control tended to be described as 'impatient with others' mistakes' and 'hardboiled and critical', and not 'sensitive and understanding' and 'open and honest with me'. Those high on protective benevolence, on the other hand, were described as 'stays by himself' and 'reserved and cool', and not 'lets patients get to know him' and 'talks about a variety of things'. Staff members high on this attitude scale expressed attitudes that appeared to suggest kindliness towards patients and yet they appear to have been seen by the latter as basically aloof, distant and non-interacting.

A study of hostels for boys on probation also illustrates the complexity of the matter. This study examined the relationship between failure rate, based on the percentage of residents leaving as a result of absconding or being reconvicted, and the attitudes of 16 different wardens. Two components of attitude were identified, each positively associated with success: strictness as opposed to permissiveness; and emotional closeness, which included warmth and willingness to discuss residents' problems with them, versus emotional distance. However, the two components, each separately associated with success, were negatively associated with one another. Hence wardens who displayed more warmth and willingness to discuss problems were also likely to be over-permissive, whilst those who were relatively strict tended to be lacking in emotional closeness. The ideal combination of warmth and firmness was a combination relatively rarely encountered.

Individual staff attitudes can partly be explained in terms of individual differences in general attitudes or personality: members of staff who are more generally authoritarian in personality tend to hold more custodial attitudes. This alone, however, cannot explain differences that are found between different institutions. Although the correspondence is far from complete, it has been found to be the case that where the prevailing policy is custodial, staff subscribe to a custodial view and tend to be generally authoritarian in personality. This raises the fascinating question of how such relative uniformity comes about. It can be presumed that the same three main processes are at work as those that operate to produce consensus and similarity of attitude in any social group or organization. The three processes are (i) selection-in, (ii) selection-out, and (iii) attitude change. Selection of new staff will most likely operate in a way that increases uniformity of attitude, both because certain people are more attracted than others by the prospect of working in a particular institution, and also because certain potential staff members are thought more suitable by those responsible for the selection (selection-in). Staff remain in one place for a variable length of time, and the institution may retain for longer periods those members whose attitudes are in conformity with the prevailing ideology (selection-out).

As social psychological experiments on conformity show so clearly, it is difficult to maintain a non-conformist position in the face of combined opinion, and the third process - attitude change - is likely to be a strong factor.

Staff behaviour and staff-client social distance

Although research leads us to expect none too close a correspondence between attitudes and behaviour, a number of studies in institutions suggest that philosophy and attitudes can be conveyed to residents via staff behaviour. Studies of units for handicapped children, for autistic children, and for the adult mentally ill, suggest that staff behaviour towards clients is more personal, warmer and less rejecting or critical when management practices are more client-orientated and less institution-orientated. Large differences have also been detected in the amount of time which staff members in charge of hostel units spend in face-to-face contact with their residents. Sharing space and activities together, and spending relatively more time in contact with one another, may be the most important factors in reducing social distance.

Social distance between staff and clients was an important concept in Goffman's and Barton's analyses of institutions. Avoidance, or reduced time in contact, is a fairly universal indication of lack of affection and often of prejudiced and stereotyped attitudes. There are numerous means of preserving social distance including designation of separate spaces, such as staff offices. A clearly designated staff office makes staff and client separation easier, but such a space may be used in a variety of different ways. The door may be kept open, or closed, or even locked with a key only available to staff.

Controversy often surrounds the wearing of staff uniform in institutions. There are arguments for and against, but inevitably the uniform creates or reinforces a distinction and may therefore increase social distance. A movement away from the traditional institutional organization is very frequently accompanied by the abandonment of uniforms where these previously existed. The use of names and titles in addressing different members of a community is another indication of the presence or absence of social distance. Forms of address are known to be good signs of both solidarity and status within social groups. The reciprocal use of first names is a sign of relative intimacy, and the reciprocal use of titles (Mr, Mrs, etc.) a sign of distance. Non-reciprocal forms of address, on the other hand, are indications of a status difference, with the person of higher status almost always using the more familiar form of address (say a first name or nickname) in addressing the person of lower status, and the latter using title and surname towards the former, or even a form of address which clearly indicates the former's superior status (sir, boss, etc.). If forms of address change as people get to know one another better, it is usually the person of higher status who initiates the use of familiar forms of address first.

Hence an examination of a particular institution in terms of designated spaces for staff and others, uniforms and other visual indications of role or rank, and of forms of address, can give useful clues to status divisions and social distance within the institution. However, it is of the utmost importance to keep in mind that social distance, like all of the social psychological features of institutions considered here, is a highly complex matter. It has been suggested, for example, that there are at least two distinct forms of social distance, namely status distance and personal distance. If these aspects of social distance are relatively independent, as has been suggested, it follows that status distance need not necessarily preclude the formation of a personally close relationship.

Institutions as complex systems

The client contribution

Staff may be crucial determinants of climate, particularly senior staff, but so too are the institution's users or clients. The climate in an institution is the product of a bewildering complexity of factors which interact in ways that are far from straightforward. No simple theory which attempts to explain what goes on inside an institution in terms of physical design alone, of the attitudes of senior staff alone, or of management practices alone, can do justice to them. It would be as faulty to ignore the personalities, abilities and disabilities of the users as it would be to ignore the philosophy of the institution or the design of its buildings. This point is forcefully brought home in Miller and Gwynne's (1972) account of homes catering for people with irreversible and severe physical handicaps where the most likely termination of residence is death. They contrasted two ideologies which they believed existed in such institutions: the 'warehousing' philosophy, with its emphasis upon physical care and the dependence of residents; and the 'horticultural' philosophy, with its emphasis on the cultivation of residents' interests and abilities. They stress that each has dangers – the one of dependence and institutionalization, the other of unrealistic expectations being set – and that each is a response to the serious nature of the residents' handicaps.

There are a number of studies of social behaviour on the wards of mental hospitals which prove the point that social climate depends upon the mix of patients who are residing there. A clear instance was provided by Fairweather's (1964) study which is described more fully below. Introducing changes of a progressive nature on a hospital ward increased the level of social interaction generally but significant differences between different patient groups still persisted, with non-psychotic patients interacting most, acute psychotic patients an intermediate amount, and chronic psychotic patients the least. The mix of clients is especially crucial where group influence is considered to be one of the principal media of change (whether the change desired be educational, therapeutic or rehabilitative). Even in the relatively permissive climate of the Henderson therapeutic community, those with particularly socially disruptive personalities cannot be tolerated and, if accidentally admitted, may have to be discharged.

Under circumstances where group influence operates, it is particularly important that the client group exerts its main influence in a manner consistent with the overriding philosophy espoused by staff. This is always in danger of going wrong in secondary schools where the 'adolescent sub-culture' may exert a countervailing force, and in prisons where the 'inmate code' has to be contended with. In Canadian schools and centres for juvenile delinquents a procedure known as the 'Measurement of Treatment Potential' (MTP) has been in use to assess this aspect of climate. Where clients choose as liked fellow clients the same members as those whose behaviour is approved of by staff, then treatment potential is considered to be high. When there is a mismatch between residents' and staff choices, treatment potential is said to be low.

Climate

Many factors contributing to climate have been considered in this chapter and there are many others which it has not been possible to consider. Repeatedly emphasized has been the complex way in which these factors interact to influence the climate of an institutional unit. 'Climate', a word used here to cover any perceptions of, or feelings about, the institution held by those who use it, work in it or observe it, is not the same thing as success, effectiveness, or productivity. However, the latter are notoriously difficult to define, let alone measure, whereas people's perceptions of atmosphere can be collected and their relationships with features of the institution analysed. A massive programme of research along these lines has been conducted by Moos (1974). He has devised a series of questionnaires to tap the perceptions of members of various types of institutions and organizations. The most thoroughly tested of these scales is the Ward Atmosphere Scale (WAS), which assesses perceptions along the ten dimensions shown in table 2. This list was based upon earlier research by others as well as a great deal of preliminary work of Moos' own. He claims that dimensions 1-3 (the relationship dimensions) and 8-10 (the system maintenance and system change dimensions) are equally relevant across a wide range of institutions including schools, universities, hospitals and penal institutions. Dimensions 4-7 (the personal development dimensions), on the other hand, need modification depending upon the setting.

Amongst the many findings from research based upon the WAS and similar scales are the following. First, when staff and patient perceptions are compared in hospital treatment settings, average staff scores are regularly found to be higher on all dimensions except Order and Organization (no difference between staff and patients), and Staff Control (patients scoring higher than staff). Second, when scores are correlated with size of unit and with staff-to-patient ratio, it has been found that Support and Spontaneity are both lower and Staff Control is higher where patient numbers are greater and staff-to-patient ratios are poorer (MTP has also been found to correlate with smallness of size and favourability of staff to pupil ratios). Third, where patients have greater 'adult status' (access to bedrooms, television, unrestricted smoking, less institutional admission procedure, etc.), Spontaneity, Autonomy, Personal Problem Orientation, and Anger and Aggression are all higher and Staff Control is lower. Fourth, all scales correlate positively with ratings of general satisfaction with the ward and with ratings of liking for staff, with the exception of Staff Control which correlates negatively with both.

Table 2

The 10 dimensions measured by Moos' Ward Atmosphere Scale

RELATIONSHIP DIMENSIONS

1. Involvement measures how active and energetic patients are in the day-to-day social functioning of the ward. Attitudes such as pride in the ward, feelings of group spirit, and general enthusiasm are also assessed.

2. Support measures how helpful and supportive patients are towards other patients, how well the staff understand patient needs and are willing to help and encourage patients, and how encouraging and considerate doctors are towards patients.

3. Spontaneity measures the extent to which the environment encourages patients to act openly and to express freely their feelings towards other patients and staff.

PERSONAL DEVELOPMENT DIMENSIONS

4. Autonomy assesses how self-sufficient and independent patients are encouraged to be in their personal affairs and in their relationships with staff, and how much responsibility and self-direction patients are encouraged to exercise.

5. Practical orientation assesses the extent to which the patient's environment orients him towards preparing himself for release from the hospital and for the future.

6. Personal problem orientation measures the extent to which patients are encouraged to be concerned with their feelings and problems and to seek to understand them through openly talking to other patients and staff about themselves and their past.

7. Anger and aggression measures the extent to which a patient is allowed and encouraged to argue with patients and staff, and to become openly angry.

SYSTEM MAINTENANCE AND SYSTEM CHANGE DIMENSIONS

8. Order and organization measures the importance of order on the ward; also measures organization in terms of patients (do they follow a regular schedule and do they have carefully planned activities?) and staff (do they keep appointments and do they help patients follow schedules?)

9. Programme clarity measures the extent to which the patient knows what to expect in the day-to-day routine of the ward and how explicit the ward rules and procedures are.

10. Staff control measures the necessity for the staff to restrict patients: that is, the strictness of rules, schedules and regulations, and measures taken to keep patients under effective control.

Changing institutions   A knowledge of the factors discussed in this chapter should enable those involved in policy, planning and management to generate ideas for constructive change, and those in relatively junior positions to try and bring about change in their practice within the prevailing limits of autonomy. However, major changes may require innovations or interventions from outside and it is these that are now discussed in the remainder of this chapter.

Innovative programmes

One of the best documented programmes of institutional change in the mental health care system is the work reported in a series of publications by Fairweather and his colleagues. The first report (Fairweather, 1964) described dramatic differences in patient social behaviour between an experimental 'small group' ward and a physically identical 'traditional' ward in a mental hospital. In the traditional ward, staff members made final decisions on all important matters. By contrast, on the small group ward it was the responsibility of a group of patients to orient new fellow patients to the ward, to carry out work assignments, to assess patient progress, and to recommend privileges and even final discharge. The total experiment lasted for six months, and staff switched wards halfway through. Social activity was at a much higher level on the small group ward, and the climate in the daily ward meeting was quite different with more silence and staff control on the traditional ward, and more lively discussion, less staff talk, and many more patient remarks directed towards fellow patients on the small group ward. Nursing and other staff evaluated their experience on the small group ward more highly, and patients spent significantly fewer days in hospital.

In a further report, Fairweather, Sanders, Cressler and Maynard (1969) compared the community adjustment of ex-patients who moved together as a group from a small group ward in the hospital to a small hostel unit in the community (the 'lodge'), and others who moved out of the hospital in the normal way. The results were quite dramatic, with the lodge group surviving much better in the community in terms of the prevention of re-admission to hospital, the amount of time in work (much of which was organized by the ex-patient group as a consortium), and residents' morale and self-esteem. This is a particularly good example of the setting-up from scratch of a new small institution designed to avoid many of the most disagreeable features of large institutions.

Changes in the philosophies and modes of practice in institutions mostly take place over a period of years as a result of the slow diffusion of new ideas. A third report by Fairweather, Sanders and Tornatsky (1974) was concerned with this process. Having established the value of the lodge programme, they set out to sell the idea to mental hospitals throughout the USA. They were concerned to know the influence of a number of variables upon the diffusion process, and consequently adopted a rigorous experimental approach. First, they varied the degree of effort required on the part of the hospital contacted in order to accept the initial approach offered. Of 255 hospitals contacted, one-third were merely offered a brochure describing the lodge programme (70 per cent accepted but only 5 per cent finally adopted the lodge programme), one-third were offered a two-hour workshop about the programme (80 per cent accepted and 12 per cent finally adopted), and one-third were offered help with setting up a demonstration small group ward in the hospital for a minimum of 90 days (only 25 per cent accepted but 11 per cent finally adopted the lodge). A second variable was the position in the hospital hierarchy of the person contacted with the initial approach offer. One-fifth of initial contacts were made to hospital superintendents and one-fifth to each of the four professions, psychiatry, psychology, social work and nursing. This variable turned out to be relatively unimportant: contacts were just as likely to result in the adoption of the lodge programme when they were made to people in nursing as to superintendents or those in psychiatry.

Much more important than the status of the person who initiates an idea is, according to Fairweather et al, a high level of involvement across disciplines, professions, and social status levels within the institution. When change did occur there was most likely to exist a multi-disciplinary group which spearheaded the change, led by a person who continuously pushed for change and attempted to keep the group organized and its morale high. The disciplinary group to which this person belonged was of little importance. Nor was change related to financial resources. The need for perseverance is stressed. The need to keep pushing for change despite 'meetings that came to naught, letters that stimulated nothing, telephone calls unreturned, and promises unkept' is a necessary ingredient of institutional change.

Action research
Fairweather's studies concerned the setting-up of new facilities or units. If, on the other hand, constructive change is to be brought about in existing institutions and their units, the total climate of the institution, and particularly the autonomy of the individual staff members, are limiting factors. A number of schemes have been described for providing helpful intervention from outside in the form of a person or team who act as catalysts or change agents. Several of these involve the process known as Action Research. For example, Towell and Harries (1979) have described a number of changes brought about at Fulbourne psychiatric hospital in Cambridgeshire with the help of a specially appointed 'social research adviser'.

The process begins when the interventionist(s) is invited to a particular unit to advise or help. It is stressed that the initiative should come from the unit and not from the interventionist, although it is clearly necessary for the latter to advertise the service being offered, and Moos (1974), for example, has argued that feeding back research data on social climate can itself initiate a change process. After the initial approach there follows a period during

which the action researcher gets to know the unit, usually
by interviewing as many members as possible individually, by
attending unit meetings, and by spending time in the unit
observing. Then follow the stages which give 'action
research' its name. With the help of the action researcher,
members of the unit (usually the staff group collectively)
decide upon a piece of research which can be quickly mounted
and carried through and which is relevant to the matter in
hand. The results of this research are then used to help
decide what changes are necessary. The action researcher
remains involved during these phases and subsequently as
attempts are made to implement changes and to make them
permanent.

For example, one of the Fulbourne projects concerned a
long-stay ward which had adopted an 'open door', no-staff-
uniforms policy and which was designated as suitable for
trainee nurses to gain 'rehabilitation experience'. The
staff, however, felt 'forgotten' at the back of the hospital, felt that scope for patient improvement was not often
realized, and that they were unable to provide the rehabilitation experience intended. The social research adviser
helped the staff devise a simple interview schedule which
focussed on such matters as how patients passed their time,
friendships amongst patients, and feelings patients had
about staff and their work. Each member of staff was responsible for carrying out certain interviews and for writing
them up and presenting them to the group. All reports were
read by all members of staff and discussed at a special
meeting. The group reached a consensus that patients were
insular, took little initiative, expected to be led by
staff, had no idea of 'self-help', saw little treatment
function for the nurses, saw little purposeful nurse-patient
interaction, and had only negative feelings, if any, towards
fellow patients.

Although there were no immediate or dramatic changes,
a slow development over a period of 18 months was reported
in the direction of a much increased 'counselling approach
to care'. The research interview was incorporated into
routine care. This itself involved the setting-up of a
special contact between individual nurse and individual
patient, a factor which is mentioned in other projects
described by Towell and Harries and by many other writers
who have described constructive changes in institutions. At
first the social research adviser took a leading role in
groups in helping to understand the material gathered in
interviews. This role was later taken over by the ward
doctor and later still by a senior member of the nursing staf
At this point the social research adviser withdrew. Later on
patients read back interview reports and there were many
other signs of reduced staff and patient distance. Over the
three-year period during which these changes came about, the
number of patients resettled outside the hospital increased
from two in the first year to eight in the second and eleven
in the third.

It is stressed by those who have described 'action research' and schemes like it, such as 'administrative consultation' and the type of social systems change facilitated by a consultant described by Maxwell Jones (1976), that staff of a unit must be fully involved and identified with any change that is attempted. It is relatively easy to bring about acceptance of change on an attitudinal level, largely through talking, but to produce a behavioural commitment to change is something else. Those who have written of the 'action research' process talk of the importance of 'ownership' of the research activity. The aim is to get the unit's members fully involved and to make them feel the research is theirs.

Resistance to change

We should expect such complex social systems, whose mode of operation must have been arrived at because it serves certain needs or produces certain pay-offs for those involved, to be resistant to change. Particularly should we expect it to be resistant to change when this threatens to involve change in status and role relationships. Unfortunately, it is just such changes for which we so frequently search. The themes of decision-making autonomy and social power have been constant ones throughout this chapter; they lie at the heart of what is wrong with many of the worst institutions. Maxwell Jones (1976) believes it is almost always the required task of the social systems facilitator to 'flatten' the authority hierarchy, and to support lower status members in taking the risks involved in expressing their feelings and opinions, whilst at the same time supporting higher status members in the belief that they can change in the direction of relinquishing some of their authority.

As in most earlier sections of this chapter, examples of attempts to change institutions or parts of institutions have been taken from the mental health field. Nevertheless, the processes and problems involved can be recognized by those whose main concern is with other types of institution such as the educational and penal. In particular, those who have in any way, large or small, attempted to change such institutions can recognize the problem of resistance to change. Nothing illustrates better the need to add to our understanding of how institutions work. In the process of finding out more on this topic we learn more of man in a social context, which is part of the central core of the study of psychology.

References

Barton, R. (1959; 3rd edn, 1976)
Institutional Neurosis. Bristol: Wright.
Canter, D. and Canter, S. (eds) (1979)
Designing for Therapeutic Environments: A review of research. Chichester: Wiley.
Fairweather, G.W. (ed.) (1964)

Social Psychology in Treating Mental Illness. New York: Wiley.

Fairweather, G.W., Sanders, D.H., Cressler, D.L. and Maynard, H. (1969)
Community Life for the Mentally Ill: An alternative to institutional care. Chicago, Ill.: Aldine.

Fairweather, G.W., Sanders, D.H. and Tornatsky, L.G. (1974)
Creating Change in Mental Health Organizations. New York: Pergamon.

Goffman, E. (1961)
Asylums: Essays on the social situation of mental patients and other inmates. New York: Anchor Books, Doubleday.

Jones, Maxwell (1952)
Social Psychiatry: A study of therapeutic communities. London: Tavistock. (Published as The Therapeutic Community, New York: Basic Books: 1953.)

Jones, Maxwell (1976)
Maturation of the Therapeutic Community: An organic approach to health and mental health. New York: Human Sciences Press.

Miller, E.J. and Gwynne, G.V. (1972)
In Life Apart: A pilot study of residential institutions for the physically handicapped and the young chronic sick. London: Tavistock.

Moos, R.H. (1974)
Evaluating Treatment Environments: A social ecological approach. New York: Wiley.

Rapoport, R.M. (1960)
Community as Doctor: New perspectives on a therapeutic community. London: Tavistock.

Tizard, J., Sinclair, I. and Clarke, R.V.G. (eds) (1975)
Varieties of Residential Experience. London: Routledge & Kegan Paul.

Towell, D. and Harries, C. (1979)
Innovations in Patient Care. London: Croom Helm.

24

Pain
Colette Ray

Pain may be defined as an unpleasant sensation which is
focussed upon the body, and is often but not always
associated with tissue damage. While it may be generally
true that physical injury produces pain and that pain occurs
as a result of injury, this is by no means always the case.
There are many syndromes for which a somatic explanation
is not easily available, and the source of the disorder can
be attributed either to an abnormality in the way in which
normal sensory inputs are processed or to psychological
factors. Similarly, people may meet with injury but fail to
experience pain as a consequence. This will sometimes happen
if the damage occurs suddenly in a compelling situation,
such as in battle or on the sportsfield, where attention and
emotions are directed elsewhere. It is difficult, therefore,
to determine in a priori terms when pain should and should
not be experienced, and we must rely primarily upon the
individual's own self-report to indicate whether it is present or absent and the intensity of his feelings. Given a
similar degree of pain, however, any two people will react
to this in different ways. They may vary in their evaluation
of the symptom's significance; in their emotional reactions
and expression of these; in the extent to which they complain verbally about the pain and the kinds of remedies they
seek; and in the effect that the pain has upon their family,
occupational and social activities. Such reactions to symptoms are distinct from the symptoms themselves and are
generally referred to as 'illness behaviour' (Mechanic and
Volkart, 1960). A number of factors will influence these
behaviours, including the individual's personality and
cultural background and the rewards and expectations
associated with pain.

Personality and culture

It has been widely argued that pain will in some cases have
a psychodynamic significance: that is, a psychological
meaning and function. Freud regarded it as a common con-
version syndrome, representing the transformation of a repressed drive into physical symptoms; the pain need not be
created to achieve this end, but may be selected from a
background of 'possible' pain as that which best fulfils a
specific symbolic function. A state of emotional disturbance

can also influence pain in a less specific way, if the person fails to recognize the true nature of the disturbance and seeks instead an explanation in terms of everyday physical symptoms which might otherwise be ignored. An individual who is generally over-preoccupied with physical concerns would be most likely to misattribute psychological distress to somatic symptoms in this manner. Engel (1959) has suggested that there is a 'pain prone personality', characterized by feelings of guilt which can be in part relieved by pain; other relevant characteristics he lists are a family history of violence and punishment, a personal history of suffering and defeat, a state of anger and hostility which is turned inwards rather than outwards and conflict over sexual impulses. The immediate 'trigger' for pain in the case of such a personality may be the loss of someone valued, and several writers have seen physical pain as a symbol of real or imagined loss.

People show consistency in their response to pain over time, while there are distinct differences between people. Generally speaking, women are more responsive than men, and the young more than the old. The relationship between pain responses and personality traits has been extensively studied, particularly with respect to neuroticism and extraversion. There is some tendency for the former to be related to pain proneness, but many inconsistent findings have been obtained both in the laboratory and in natural settings. Extraverts under some conditions tolerate pain better than introverts, but may in some situations report more pain because of a greater readiness to brave the possibility of social disapproval. Many studies have looked at pain in psychiatric patients, and at the personality profiles of pain patients compared with those of control samples. A relatively high incidence of pain is found in psychiatric groups and pain patients have a more 'neurotic' profile than control groups (see Sternbach, 1974). It is, however, unclear to what extent personality disturbance predisposes to pain and to what extent the experience of pain causes emotional difficulties. The relative importance of these two different effects will depend upon whether the context is that of psychiatric patients who experience pain, or pain patients without a psychiatric history; in the former case maladjustment is likely to give rise to physical pain rather than the reverse, while in the latter emotional difficulties will generally be a consequence, rather than a cause, of pain.

Responses to pain differ not only between individuals and groups within a society, but also between cultures. All groups develop norms or expectations of how one should perceive and react to any particular situation, and individuals will adopt these to the extent that they are part of or identify with the group. Some norms are prescriptive: that is, there is a certain pressure upon the individual to conform with expectations in this respect, and deviation will meet with disapproval. An example of such a norm relevant to pain behaviour would be the expectation that one should not evade one's obligations by faking or 'malingering'. Descriptive norms, in contrast, do not imply an obligation to conform, but merely describe the behaviour which is characteristic or typical of the group. Cultural stereotypes suggest the existence of differences between nationalities in their expression of pain, and there is empirical evidence for such differences. Zborowski (1969) studied a group of American male patients and compared reactions for those of Jewish, Irish, Italian and Old American descent. Both Old Americans and Irish Americans were inhibited in the expression of pain, while the Italians and Jewish patients were more reactive. These latter groups both sought to draw attention to their pain by this expressive behaviour, but their underlying aims were different. The Italians were primarily concerned with obtaining relief from pain, while for the Jewish patients the primary concern was to discover the cause of the symptom. These cultural differences appear quite reliable, since Zborowski's findings were supported by those of a study in which the responses of similar groups were compared, but in a very different laboratory setting (Sternbach and Tursky, 1965).

Rewards and expectations   Learning theorists make a distinction between a respondent behaviour which is closely linked with the occurrence of a particular stimulus or situation and does not require any other support for its establishment or maintenance, and an operant behaviour which is not directly elicited by the stimulus but can become associated with it given appropriate conditions of reinforcement. Reinforcement is defined as any event which strengthens a behaviour; rewards will generally operate as reinforcers, as will the termination of an aversive stimulus, while punishment generally weakens behaviour. This kind of analysis may be applied to pain behaviour (Fordyce, Fowler, Lehmann and de Lateur, 1968). We can assume that certain responses to pain will be directly elicited by the experience, withdrawal or crying for example, while others may be prompted by the experience but depend effectively upon the outcomes which they produce. An individual may thus adopt and maintain a number of pain behaviours because they bring rewards such as sympathy and nurturance, and enable him to avoid activities or obligations which he finds unpleasant.

Behaviour will not only be influenced by the rewards associated with different kinds of response, but also by an awareness of how other people react in a similar situation. The experience of pain may involve considerable uncertainty, and when faced with uncertainty people often look to others as guides to determine both how the experience should be interpreted and the norms governing behaviour in that situation. This process has been described as one of 'social comparison' (Festinger, 1954). We compare our own interpretations and reactions with those of others to decide whether or not they are valid or appropriate in the circumstances, and may seek a lead from another before making our own interpretation and response. Thus the presence of a calm individual to act as a model may reduce the response to a painful stimulus, and the presence of one who appears distressed may intensify the response. Such effects have been demonstrated in the laboratory, in studies where the experimenter recruits a confederate who supposedly under-goes electric shocks similar to those to which the subject is indeed exposed, and instructs him to react to these with or without expression of pain and distress. Both 'tolerant' and 'intolerant' models in such studies can change subjects' reports of the intensity of the pain they experience and their willingness to tolerate shocks of various intensities. Similar effects can be observed in clinical settings; pa-tients with problems or treatments in common will observe each other, develop expectations about pain intensity and the course of recovery, and learn the norms of pain ex-pression within that group. Modelling processes will occur within the family but over a longer period of time. Child-ren's reactions to pain will be influenced by their obser-vations of their parents' behaviour, and the child whose parents focus upon his or their own pain symptoms and react strongly to these may come to react in the same way. This effect would initially operate with respect to specific situations but could then generalize to pain behaviour in general.

heory and research

Early theories regarded pain as arising from the relatively direct transmission of signals from 'nociceptors' to pain centres in the brain, and the receptors, pathways and centres involved were thought to be specific to pain. The assumption of specificity does not, however, seem justified, and this simple model cannot account for many common pain phenomena, including the known effects of psychological factors such as experience, motivation, attention and emo-tionality. A recent theory which has attracted much interest is the gate-control theory (see Melzack, 1973). The gate referred to is a hypothetical mechanism at the level of the spinal cord, which is assumed to modulate signals from the periphery before they are centrally processed. It is sug-gested that this mechanism is situated in the substantia gelatinosa and has its effect by inhibiting or facilitating the transmission of signals from the dorsal horns to the adrenolateral pathways of the spinal cord. Activity in peripheral fibres will not only influence the transmission of pain signals directly but also affects the operation of the gate, as can central brain processes. Three distinct psychological dimensions of the pain experience have been related to these neurophysiological concepts. These are the sensory-discriminative, the motivational-affective and the cognitive-evaluative dimensions respectively. The first is associated with the rapidly conducting spinal systems pro-jecting to the thalamus, the second with reticular and limbic structures, and the third with neocortical processes.

The model is a complex and dynamic one, and can hence explain many diverse phenomena.

Some areas of research focus upon physiological aspects of pain, while others are more directly concerned with identifying those factors which can modify the experience. These investigations are carried out both in laboratory and in clinical settings. Experimental laboratory studies may be criticized on the grounds that the kinds of pain that can be induced and the conditions in which it is experienced are rather different from those that apply under natural conditions. They do, however, allow the researcher to control and monitor carefully the variables under study. Various methods of inducing pain have been developed for this purpose. These include application of heat or pressure; administration of electric shocks; the cold pressor test for which the subject has to immerse his hand in ice-cold water; and the sub-maximal tourniquet technique which produces ischaemic pain. Using such methods experimenters can study the effects of various manipulations upon pain measures such as the threshold, or the point at which the subject first reports pain, and tolerance level or the point at which he requests that the painful stimulus be terminated. Threshold and tolerance levels are not appropriate for use in the context of naturally occurring pain, and measures in clinical situations are primarily concerned with the assessment of subjective intensity. Estimates of this may be obtained by asking the patient to rate the symptom on a scale which is gradated by numbers or by verbal descriptions representing different levels of pain from mild to severe. The experience of pain does, however, vary in quality as well as in degree. Melzack and Torgerson (1971) have thus developed a questionnaire which enables patients to describe their symptoms in terms of a wide range of adjectives such as sharp, tugging, aching, piercing, nagging and so on. These descriptions can be related to the three dimensions of pain described earlier.

Somatic therapies

The chemical agents used in the treatment of pain are numerous and varied in their nature. They include, first, narcotic drugs such as opium, morphine and their derivatives; these act centrally and produce both pain relief and a state of tranquillity. There is, however, a risk of establishing a dependency and this obviously places constraints on the way in which they may be employed. A second category comprises the psychotropic drugs or minor tranquillizers and anti-depressants; these are directed at the reduction of emotional distress rather than the pain experience per se. Third, there are agents which act peripherally and not centrally; examples are the salicyclates and analine derivatives, including aspirin and phenacetin. These have anti-pyretic and anti-inflammatory properties which can reduce pain, although not as effectively as the narcotic agents. They can have physical side effects if taken in large

quantities or over long periods of time. Recent developments in the study of the brain's chemistry may provide new
directions in the psychopharmacological treatment of pain.
Opiate-binding sites have been discovered in the dorsal
horns and in the central nervous system, and there is much
interest currently in substances such as encephalin and the
endomorphins which are naturally occurring morphine-like
peptides. It seems that morphine and similar substances may
produce their effects by mimicking the action of these
endogenous peptides. However, we are still far from fully
understanding the properties of these compounds and the
way in which they interact with the complex anatomical
structures involved in the transmission of pain.

In many cases chemical therapies provide insufficient
relief, or cannot be used in the quantities required for
adequate relief because of their side effects, and other
forms of physical treatment may then be demanded. Surgical
procedures designed to interrupt the nervous system's
transmission of pain signals have been carried out at many
different sites from the periphery to the centre, but the
general effectiveness of such procedures is disappointing.
There have been some encouraging results, but in many cases
where relief is obtained it may only be temporary. This
outcome, in the context of the irreversibility of the procedures employed, has focussed attention on less drastic
forms of treatment. One of these is to 'block' sensory input
by injecting alcohol or a local anaesthetic agent such as
procaine into the nerve root. Another is to increase this
input by peripheral stimulation. This practice is conceptually similar to the 'counter-irritation techniques' that
have been commonly used throughout history. These have
included hot fomentations, vigorous massage, and the raising
of blisters and dry cupping. For the latter a cupping glass,
with the air partly withdrawn from it by means of an air
pump or flame, was drawn across the skin, thus raising a
painful red weal. Both nerve blocks and peripheral stimulation can be very effective in the treatment of appropriate
syndromes. Not only may they have an immediate effect
through restoring normal sensory inputs, but they can disrupt abnormal patterns of central nervous system activity
and thus permanently affect the way in which pain is
processed.

A method that may comprise important psychological
as well as physical factors is acupuncture. This has only
recently been applied to the control of pain and is most
often used in the context of surgery. The procedure involves
inserting needles into one or several skin areas, and these
needles are then stimulated either manually or electrically.
The successes claimed may be in part attributable to effects
associated with peripheral stimulation, but Chaves and
Barber (1974) have proposed a number of psychological bases
for its apparent efficacy. These include the fact that a low
level of anxiety is looked for in those selected for treatment by this method; the expectation among these patients

that the experience will be pain free; a thorough preparation before surgery with a strong suggestion of pain relief, and exposure to models who have successfully undergone the experience; and the distractions associated with the general procedure which should draw attention away from the operation itself. These authors also suggest that the pain of surgery may be generally exaggerated, and point out that acupuncture is not generally used in isolation but in combination with sedatives and analgesics. The apparent success of acupuncture may then depend upon the existence of such physical and psychological supports, but as yet the relative contribution of these factors and of any direct somatic effects of the technique is unknown.

Psychological approaches to therapy

We cannot have direct access to another's experience and must make inferences about this on the basis of overt behaviours, such as motor activity, autonomic reactions, verbal descriptions, and so forth. Some psychologists argue from this that any distinction between experience and behaviour will be unproductive, and that the psychological analysis of pain and treatments for its relief should be directed at the behavioural level (Fordyce, Fowler, Lehmann, de Lateur, Sand and Trieschmann, 1973). With respect to therapy, typical goals would then be the reduction of help-seeking and dependent behaviour, a decrease in the medications taken, and an increase in physical and social activity. The therapist would first identify those behaviours thought to be undesirable within this framework, and would then seek the co-operation of the individual's family and friends in withdrawing the presumably rewarding conditions which serve to maintain these. For example, they might be advised to meet unreasonable requests for assistance with disapproval and reluctance, and to respond to legitimate demands or complaints helpfully but without the accompanying expressions of sympathy and concern which serve to reinforce these. At the same time, alternative desirable behaviours would be met with attention, approval and encouragement. This approach is most obviously appropriate where changes have occurred as a response to suffering, and have been maintained in spite of the removal of the pain source because they are found to fulfil other needs. It may also help in cases where the underlying condition cannot be alleviated, in this context by motivating the individual to lead as normal a life as possible in the circumstances, and to avoid the temptation of making a 'career of suffering'. A behavioural approach may not alter the intensity of the pain experienced, and pain may even intensify during therapy as physical activity increases. Nevertheless, a change at this level can have a positive impact on emotional adjustment and can improve the general quality of life for both the individual and his family.

Other psychological therapies attempt to modify the underlying experience of pain rather than the behaviours associated with this. One such approach is to provide training in the use of cognitive strategies which either direct attention away from pain or restructure the experience so that it is no longer distressing. The sufferer may be instructed to counter the pain when it occurs by attending to distractions in the environment rather than to his sensations, or by constructing fantasies and concentrating on thoughts which are incompatible with these. He may, alternatively, be advised to acknowledge the painful sensations but to reinterpret them in imagination as something less worrying or take a 'clinical' attitude which distances him emotionally. There have been many attempts to study the effectiveness of these strategies in laboratory experiments, but with suprisingly inconsistent results. One reason for the failure of some studies to demonstrate a positive effect may be the difficulty of ensuring that subjects follow the instructions faithfully. Those in the experimental group will sometimes reject the strategy suggested to them and substitute their own, while the control group may spontaneously employ strategies even though not instructed to do so (Scott, 1978). The very nature of the problem suggests that cognitive strategies in general play an important role in coping with pain, but it presents considerable methodological difficulties in establishing the effectiveness of a given strategy, either in absolute terms or in comparison with another strategy.

A third clearly psychological approach to pain therapy is that of hypnosis. Here the aim is to manipulate the experience directly by means of suggestion. There has been much discussion about the nature of hypnosis. Some have thought of it as a special state of consciousness or trance which is distinct from other experiences, but others have argued that it is an example of complete or almost complete absorption in a particular role and conformity with the expectations associated with this (Sarbin and Anderson, 1964). The subject has faith in the hypnotist's power to influence him, and is prepared to accept such influence to the extent that not only his outward behaviour but also his subjective experience will be modified. Hypnotic suggestion has been used for pain relief in surgery, dentistry, terminal care and obstetrics (Hilgard and Hilgard, 1975). Verbal reports of pain are affected by hypnosis, but involuntary physiological responses such as heart rate or galvanic skin responses are not generally affected. This indicates that there is still some sense in which the pain is present, and it has been suggested that the absence of the subjective experience of pain under hypnosis is a form of dissociation, with pain being processed at a preconscious, but not at a conscious, level. In one study subjects were trained to make two reports of pain simultaneously, one using a key press and another by verbal description, and the results supported the dissociation hypothesis. The key press response indicated more pain than the verbal report, although less pain than that reported verbally under comparable conditions but in a normal 'waking' state.

Hypnosis is not itself a means of preventing or alleviating pain, but a method for increasing the potency of the suggestion of analgesia made to the subject while in this state. Suggestion can have a powerful effect outside the context of hypnosis merely by creating the expectation of pain relief, and this is the basis of the well-known placebo effect. A placebo drug is a neutral substance which has a positive influence because of the expectations created by the context in which it is administered, and all treatments can be assumed to have some placebo element given that the subject is aware of their intended purpose. Substances which are known to be pharmacologically inert are thus used for comparison purposes in drug trials, rather than no treatment, in order to control for the anticipation of relief and provide a true baseline for evaluating the active and specific influence of the drug on trial. It is estimated that placebo treatments can alleviate surgical pain in about one-third of patients; laboratory studies produce lower estimates, but a significant proportion of subjects are still found to benefit. The effectiveness of a placebo will vary with the situation in which it is administered and with the status and manner of the person who administers it, since effectiveness will depend on expectations and the latter will be influenced by these factors. It will vary also with the individual to whom it is administered, and people can be grouped as either 'reactors' or 'nonreactors'; the former are not only more responsive to placebos, but are less differentially responsive to active drugs. While from a methodological viewpoint placebo effects may often be regarded as 'mock' effects for which controls must be introduced, from an applied perspective it is evident that the patient's expectations can be construed as powerful and legitimate agents of change. Their general influence will be added to that produced by the specific nature of any physical or psychological manipulation which is, with the patient's awareness, diverted at the treatment of pain, and can significantly enhance the therapeutic impact of these.

Psychological preparation for pain

The occurrence of pain may sometimes be anticipated before the event: for example, if a patient is scheduled for an unpleasant medical examination. Many of the treatments referred to earlier may be used as a form of preparation for a painful experience as distinct from an agent for relief once pain has occurred, but particular attention has recently been given to psychological preparation with an emphasis on those forms which enhance 'cognitive control'. These involve the provision of information which enables the individual to predict accurately what will happen in the situation and the nature of his experience, and instructions in strategies which may be employed to maximize the chances of successful coping. A number of laboratory studies have investigated the effect of the former, 'informational control', and have found that the stressfulness of electric shock and similarly noxious stimuli is reduced if subjects are made aware in advance of the timing and intensity of these and the fact that there is no danger of actual injury. The potential of the second kind of manipulation, 'strategic control', is demonstrated by the work of Turk (1978) who has developed a procedure for enhancing subjects' ability to control their response to painful stimuli, hence increasing their resistance to stress and tolerance for pain. The training procedure is quite complex. First, the subjects are given general instruction in the nature of pain; it is not considered essential that the explanation should be theoretically valid, but merely that it should provide a framework within which the experience may be conceptualized and the recommendations for coping presented. In the second stage of the procedure the subjects are trained to relax physically and mentally, and are provided with a selection of varied cognitive strategies with which to confront and control the pain. These strategies are similar to those described earlier, comprising methods both for redirecting attention and reinterpreting the experience. In this context, however, they are presented as a 'package' from which the subjects will select those suited to their personal needs. At this stage they will also be asked to generate feedback statements that can later be used to foster a feeling of control while in the painful situation and provide self-reinforcement. The final stage is that of rehearsal, where the subjects imagine the painful situation and their reactions, and subsequently play the role of a teacher instructing someone else in the procedure. This training has been found to increase pain endurance considerably in a cold pressor task. Subjects were able to extend the time during which they kept their hand in ice-cold water by 75 per cent, from before to after training, and this compared with a 10 per cent improvement for a 'placebo' group who had been given attention and encouragement but no instruction in specific cognitive techniques. The experimental group also showed a significant decrease in pain ratings.

It might be argued that many of the laboratory studies that have investigated informational control have involved highly structured and artificial tasks, and that the results might not be applicable to patients' experiences in clinical settings. It might also be pointed out that the cognitive training described above is highly complex; it has several components and stages and is orientated towards the particular personality and needs of each individual. It thus requires some investment of time and effort on the part of both the trainer and trainee, and such elaborate procedures might not be practicable in most naturally occurring situations. Similar, positive effects of preparation have, however, been found both under hospital conditions and in laboratory studies which have simulated these closely in terms of the nature of the painful procedures employed and the complexity of the preparation attempted.

Some of the most influential studies carried out in this area have been those conducted by Johnson and her colleagues (Johnson, 1975). In one of the first of these, male subjects were exposed to ischaemic pain in the laboratory and were either told what physical sensations they might expect as a result of the procedure, or the procedure itself was described without elaborating the sensations associated with it. It was found that the former preparation reduced distress, but the latter was ineffective in comparison with a control group. The intensity of the sensations experienced by the two information groups was the same, and the results could not be accounted for by group differences in either the degree of attention paid to these sensations or the anticipation of possible harm. It seemed, then, that this effect must have been due to the expectations held by subjects about what they were to experience, with more accurate expectations being associated with lower levels of distress. Further studies have used patients undergoing a variety of stressful medical examinations or treatments, including gastroendoscopy, cast removal and gynaecological examination. These too point to the conclusion that providing information about what to expect reduces stress and unpleasantness, especially if this focusses upon what the subject will experience rather than the objective nature of the procedure.

The effects of psychological preparation have also been extensively studied within the context of surgery. This will be a stressful experience for most patients, and the anticipation and experience of pain will contribute to this distress. The kinds of preparation attempted in these studies have varied quite widely. Most have taken a broad approach, providing information about procedures and sensations, offering reassurance and emotional support and advising on how to cope with physical discomfort and difficulty. The effects of these interventions are consistently positive, with both reductions in subjective distress and improvement in post-operative measures of recovery. Two such studies which have focussed on pain are those of Egbert, Battit, Welch and Bartlett (1964) and Hayward (1975). Wherever preparation comprises a number of different components it is difficult to determine which of these are responsible or necessary for the effectiveness of the whole. Some research has thus attempted to isolate and compare different kinds of preparation. It seems, for example, that providing instructions on how to cope with physical difficulties is not in itself very helpful, but is beneficial when presented against a background of accurate expectations (Johnson, Rice, Fuller and Endress, 1978). Only one study has attempted any detailed training in cognitive strategies and looked systematically at the impact of this training. Langer, Janis and Wolfer (1975) encouraged the development of coping devices, such as the reappraisal of threatening events, reassuring self-talk and selective attention, and showed a significant and independent effect of this instruction.

There is, then, evidence from a number of studies that the distress associated with an unpleasant procedure can be reduced by making the individual aware of what this involves from his point of view. It is, however, important to recognize that such information can only be expected to have a beneficial effect if it is presented in a reassuring way: creating an expectation of pain, whether accurate or not, can of course alarm the patient and counteract any positive effects of informational control. Instructions or training which help the individual to cope with physical or psychological stresses also have a role in the preparation for pain, and will enhance the effects of accurate expectations.

Final comments

The experience of pain depends upon a complex signalling system whose functions are determined by neurophysiological and biochemical influences which are not yet understood but are acted upon by physical and psychological factors of which we have some knowledge. These influences are many and varied, and provide a relatively broad scope for treatment. Some cases may call for one form of therapy rather than another, but for many a combination of physical and psychological approaches will present the most productive strategy.

A number of writers have called attention to the importance of the doctor-patient relationship in the treatment of pain. Szasz (1968) and Sternbach (1974) have pointed to motives which can cause the latter to resist abandoning his symptoms, and show how the physician may play a complementary role which facilitates these efforts: the patient who wishes to maintain his invalid status will have this claim effectively legitimized by the doctor who continues to treat him as though he were ill. Another common theme of doctor-patient interaction is an attempt by the patient to place responsibility for the outcome of treatment on the physician's shoulders, with the latter accepting this responsibility because of an eagerness to help and a reluctance to admit to the limitations of his professional skill. Such attitudes have been criticized as maladaptive. It has been argued that doctors should discourage passivity and helplessness, and cultivate a co-operative and problem-orientated relationship in which the patient takes an active role. This will involve confronting any undesirable attitudes he holds towards the pain, and emphasizing that the outcome of treatment will be determined as much by his own efforts as by what can be done for him. Sympathy and reassurance can reinforce pain behaviour and can foster a dependency which discourages self-help and the development of strategies for coping.

On the other hand, the total care of the pain patient should be concerned not only with the relief of pain but also with the psychological stress to which this suffering can give rise. The danger of emotionally isolating the patient is as real as that of over-protecting him. The attitude of family, friends and even professional helpers may be complex and emotionally charged, reflecting both an altruistic concern for the victim's welfare and personal fears and conflicts associated with suffering. The distress of the person in pain will in itself be distressing, particularly where it seems that there is little hope of providing immediate relief, and this can prompt either physical withdrawal or psychological distancing to prevent or defend against emotional upset. Moreover, pain is greatly feared, both for its own sake and because of its association with illness, injury and death, and contact with suffering can elicit anxiety about one's own vulnerability in this respect. This, too, can lead to avoidance or a reluctance to become practically and emotionally involved. Finally, while suffering is often unmerited, the recognition of this is disquieting, since it reminds us of the injustice of the world and our powerlessness in the face of events. Experimental studies have found that blameless victims are sometimes perceived as responsible for their fate, or are derogated so that this fate appears to be less unjust. We can predict from these studies that feelings towards the pain victim in real life might sometimes have a hostile element, and bear the implication that he is in some way to blame for his situation whether or not this is the case.

Few would dispute the importance of emotional support in alleviating immediate distress, and the availability of social support is a key factor in protecting an individual under stress from long-term maladjustment. It is therefore important to adopt a balanced approach in the care and management of the person in pain, helping him to help himself while at the same time providing the sympathy and reassurance to reduce anxiety and prevent despair.

References

Chaves, J.F. and Barber, T.X. (1974)
Acupuncture analgesia: a six-factor theory.
Psychoenergetic Systems, 1, 11-21.

Egbert, L.D., Battit, G.E., Welch, C.E. and Bartlett, M.K. (1964)
Reduction of post-operative pain by encouragement and instruction of patients. New England Journal of Medicine, 270, 825-827.

Engel, G.L. (1959)
'Psychogenic pain' and the pain prone patient. American Journal of Medicine, 26, 899-918.

Festinger, L.A. (1954)
Theory of social comparison processes. Human Relations, 7, 117-140.

Fordyce, W.E., Fowler, R.S. Jr, Lehmann, J.F. and de Lateur, B.J. (1968)
Some implications of learning in problems of chronic pain. Journal of Chronic Diseases, 21, 179-190.

Fordyce, W.E., Fowler, R.S. Jr, Lehmann, J.F., de Lateur, B.J., Sand, P.L. and Trieschmann, R.B. (1973)
Operant conditioning in the treatment of chronic pain. Archives of Physical Medicine and Rehabilitation, 54, 399-408.

Pain

Hayward, J.C. (1975)
Information: A prescription against pain. London: Royal College of Nursing.

Hilgard, E.L. and Hilgard, J.R. (1975)
Hypnosis in the Relief of Pain. Los Altos: Kaufmann.

Johnson, J.E. (1975)
Stress reduction through sensation information. In I. G. Sarason and C.D. Spielberger (eds), Stress and Anxiety: Volume II. Washington, DC: Hemisphere.

Johnson, J.E., Rice, V.H., Fuller, S.S. and Endress, M.P. (1978)
Sensory information, instruction in a coping strategy, and recovery from surgery. Research in Nursing and Health, 1, 4-17.

Langer, E.L., Janis, I.J. and Wolfer, J.A. (1975)
Reduction of psychological stress in surgical patients. Journal of Experimental Social Psychology, 11, 155-165.

Mechanic, D. and Volkart, E.H. (1960)
Illness behavior and medical diagnosis. Journal of Health and Human Behavior, 1, 86-94.

Melzack, R. (1973)
The Puzzle of Pain. Harmondsworth: Penguin.

Melzack, R. and Torgerson, W.S. (1971)
On the language of pain. Anaesthesiology, 34, 50-59.

Sarbin, T.R. and Anderson, M.L. (1964)
Role-theoretical analysis of hypnotic behavior. In J. Gordon (ed.), Handbook of Hypnosis. New York: Macmillan.

Scott, D.S. (1978)
Experimenter-suggested cognitions and pain control: problem of spontaneous strategies. Psychological Reports, 43, 156-158.

Sternbach, R.A. (1974)
Pain Patients: Traits and treatment. New York: Academic Press.

Sternbach, R.A. and Tursky, B. (1965)
Ethnic differences among housewives in psychophysical and skin potential responses to electric shock. Psychophysiology, 1, 241-246.

Szasz, T.S. (1968)
The psychology of persistent pain: a portrait of l'homme douloureux. In A. Soulairac, J. Cahn and J. Charpentier (eds), Pain. New York: Academic Press.

Turk, D.C. (1978)
Application of coping-skills training to the treatment of pain. In I.G. Sarason and C.D. Spielberger (eds), Stress and Anxiety: Volume V. Washington, DC: Hemisphere.

Zborowski, M. (1969)
People in Pain. San Francisco: Jossey-Bass.

25

Communicating with the patient
John Hall

Communicating with the patient

Human communication considered as transmission of messages is complex. There are many different types of message to be communicated and several modes of transmission. Communication is often a two-way process, with one communication source affecting the nature of communication from the other source. Other chapters in this volume examine communications where the emphasis is on messages from the patient. In interviews, tests, and other assessment settings there may be some need for instructing and guiding the patient, but essentially interest lies in what the patient does and says: that is, in what the patient communicates. When patients are being counselled, or are following a behavioural treatment programme, they are being guided, advised, reinforced and corrected. But these communications are a means to an end: the end is some change in the patients' understanding of their problems or in the frequency or quality of their problems.

Giving information

A major area of communicating occurs when the people caring for patients, be they doctors, nurses, or psychologists, want to give information on a patient's medical condition, and want the patient to act on it. There may be some need to discuss with individual patients what is wrong with them, implying some degree of two-way communication, but the discussion will be clearly directed at conveying certain information TO the patient. There may well be an interest in what eventual change will be brought about in the patient's health and condition, but the immediate concern of the doctor will simply be to ensure that the patient carries out the health care routine, or takes the medication, that is being prescribed or advised. Indeed, a major part of the job of health visitors and other public health nurses is to communicate basic health care information over and over again to people with widely varying ability to understand what is communicated to them.

The patient role

Communications addressed to patients do not take place in a social or psychological vacuum, but take place in the context of pre-existing relationships between particular members of staff and patients. There is a distinction between a

346

person having a disease, such as cancer of the breast, and being a sick person or patient. A person becomes a patient, and occupies the role of patient, only when one or more significant other person(s) identify a disease and then treat that person as occupying that role.

Certain ideas about the way in which we expect sick people or patients to behave are common. A classic formulation of the 'sick role' by Talcott Parsons (1951) suggests four main components in the role:

* sick people are exempt from normal social responsibilities;
* sick people cannot be expected to take care of themselves, or to get rid of their illness unaided;
* sick people want to get well;
* sick people should seek medical advice and co-operate with medical, nursing and other experts.

The fourth component emphasizes that it is impossible to look at patients in isolation from the number of professional and lay people who may be involved with them. Communicating effectively with patients requires an understanding of relationships between patients and all those caring for patients.

Mechanic (1968) has paid particular attention to the patient-doctor relationship, which is a key relationship central to the care of the patient. The general expectation of medical and nursing staff is that they are required to demonstrate their competence in 'medical science'. They are expected to behave according to commonly accepted rules of consent and ethics, and within what is seen as some sort of pattern of inter-professional relationships. However, the success of their interactions with patients is likely to be evaluated by the patients in terms of the staff's warmth and sympathy and the degree of emotional support which is offered. Patients are not usually able to assess technical competence, except in such obvious and usually trivial procedures such as taking blood or giving an injection. Patients are, however, competent to appraise the interest shown in them by the staff, and the degree of commitment which they show.

The patient's expectations

Patients actually enter relationships with differing specific expectations, which modify their general expectations. Their view of their illness may well differ in certain respects from the view of the staff caring for them. A patient might wish for the immediate relief of a particular symptom while the doctor might prefer to see some evidence of change in the general body system which might not have immediate implications for relief of pain or discomfort by the patient. The expectations of the patients will vary according to their own previous histories of patienthood. They may have views about an individual specialist doctor, either because of a recommendation from the family doctor, or

347

because a friend has previously been seen by the same specialist. They may have particular views of about a drug because they have had it before and suffered unpleasant side effects. They may have an opinion of an individual ward, perhaps because a relative died there or because a neighbour works there in some capacity.

Attitudes and relationships between patients and those caring for them provide a framework. Associated with this framework are the specific acts which will help the individual patient. Some acts require no active co-operation by the patient. Indeed, some may be carried out while the patient is unconscious (perhaps under anaesthetic), such as major abdominal surgery and electro-convulsive therapy (ECT). Most of the acts are, however, dependent on the co-operation and understanding of patients, and hence dependent on how much they understand and carry out what is communicated to them.

The process of communication

Patients are open to many sources of information (figure 1). Their information about illnesses and treatments comes not only from the people currently caring for them, but from earlier reading, experiences, and conversations. The range of potential information sources is shown in figure 1. The importance of non-professional sources of information should not be under-estimated. A documentary programme shown on British television in 1980 which questioned the medical criteria for death before organs are removed for transplant surgery led to a serious reduction in the number of relatives giving consent for organs to be used in this way. There is a growing interest in alternative approaches to medical treatment such as acupuncture and homeopathic medicine, and individual patients may previously have been treated for their present condition by such methods. In conveying to patients what is necessary in carrying out a current treatment, it may also be necessary to explain what other things they will not need to carry out. This will help to counteract any positive misconceptions arising from false information.

Ignorance among members of the public

A number of research studies have shown that apart from misinterpretation arising from local old wives' tales and obsolete medical textbooks, many people are ignorant about even elementary medical knowledge.

Boyle (1970) found that 54 per cent of a sample of lay people did not know the location of the kidneys, 50 per cent the location of the stomach, and 49 per cent the position of the lungs. Other studies have shown that, for example, 72 per cent of a sample of lay people did not know that Alka Seltzer contained aspirin, and about one-third of a similar group thought that lung cancer was not very serious and was easily cured.

Figure 1

Sources of information available to the patient

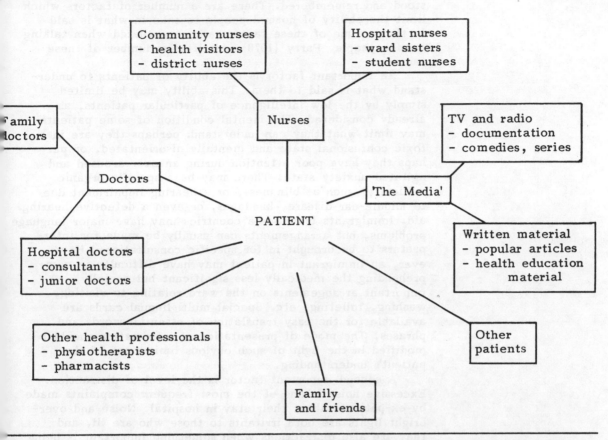

A first approach in effective communication with patients is to find out what they already know, to correct any misconceptions, and to identify topics on which they are likely to benefit from provision of basic information. Many lay people are likewise ignorant of basic medical terminology, so that in ascertaining a patient's level of knowledge it is sensible to avoid the use of jargon or unnecessary technical terms. Even then, a proportion of patients in every ward and community will still have difficulty in understanding because of relatively poor educational attainment or ability.

Depending on the catchment area of a hospital and the social make-up of a district, many patients, perhaps even the majority, may have difficulty in understanding the many commercial and government leaflets and booklets routinely available. It would be valuable to prepare material which is particularly easy to read and comprehend (as judged by an objective index of readability), so that it can be fully appreciated by people who have poor reading ability and who may be particularly at risk for some conditions.

Ensuring understanding

Having established what a patient already knows, and what needs to be known, the remaining task is to communicate information to the patient in such a way that it is understood and remembered. There are a number of factors which limit the ability of normal people to take in what is said to them: some of these factors are accentuated when talking to sick people. Parry (1970) identified a number of these factors.

An important factor is the ability of patients to understand what is said to them. This ability may be limited simply by the low intelligence of particular patients, as already considered. The mental condition of some patients may limit what they can understand: perhaps they are in a toxic confusional state and mentally disorientated, or perhaps they have poor attention during an over-aroused and agitated anxiety state. There may be a specific organic difficulty, such as blindness, or a hearing impairment due to middle-ear disease, bandages, or even a defective hearing aid. Immigrants from some countries may have major language problems, but arrangements can usually be made for interpreters to be brought in for specific consultations. However, an immigrant in-patient may have difficulty in comprehending the medically less significant but socially important arrangements on the ward relating to visiting, washing, toileting, etc. Special multi-lingual cards are available for the easy translation of essential words and phrases. The mode of presentation of information should be modified in the light of such obvious limitations of the patient's understanding.

A second important factor is the level of distraction. Excessive noise is one of the most frequent complaints made by ex-patients about their stay in hospital. Noise and over-bright lights are both irritants to those who are ill, and they are also distractions when something important is being said. Distraction arises not only from external environmental stressors, but also from pain and internal states associated with drugs. Removing or relieving distraction aids communication.

On a busy ward it is easy for the junior doctors to believe that patients may have had some medical procedure, such as a proctoscopy, explained to them. Problems occur when speakers make an assumption about prior knowledge or communication which they do not test, or make explicit. A more subtle variant of the same difficulty is when speakers have some inner framework, or scheme, which they use to organize their thinking, but which is not shared by the person to whom they are speaking. For example, a young mother may see her child's crying as a call for help to which she is honour-bound as a conscientious mother to respond, while the nursery nurse may see the same call as a symptom of an over-protected child trying to claim the attention of an indecisive parent. Unless the nurse's perception of the situation is clear to the mother, misunderstanding is likely to occur during conversation between the two.

Doctors and nurses are ordinary people living ordinary lives. For example, there are widowed nurses looking after young men who are going to die; there are doctors with alcoholic children treating alcoholic young people; and so on. Thus the presentation of information can be unwittingly slanted and altered, in ways which may not benefit the patient, but which fit the hopes and fears of the speaker. Some people working in general nursing find it very difficult to care for psychiatrically disturbed patients. Some staff may have particular religious views which affect their attitude to some patients; for example, their attitude to women who are admitted for termination of pregnancy. There are clearly many areas where, to a greater or lesser extent, what is said to the patient may be shaped by private experience and opinions of the speaker which are essentially secondary to the main needs of the patient.

A last factor to be considered here is the presentation of the communication. In everyday conversation people do not normally order their thoughts in any particular way as they talk to their friends. There are no social rules for what topic of conversation to start with, or with what topic one should finish. Yet if the express purpose of talking is to help someone to remember certain key facts, there may be ways of presenting these facts so that they are retained as well as possible. Speakers may not make clear the hard-core facts to be retained. They may make a series of qualifications or reservations to the main statement, interesting in themselves perhaps, but of no direct relevance to the particular patient in question. Some information may be better transmitted by a diagram or chart - or cartoon! - than by words or writing. A simple diagram may help to keep the patient's attention focussed, and may be remembered better in any event. Good communication does not simply require presenting the correct information: it must be presented in the right order, with the correct emphasis, and with a clear delivery.

What does the patient want to know?

Dissatisfaction with communication is the most frequent criticism made by patients following a stay in hospital. This conclusion was reached by Ley and Spelman (1967), who have provided a good general introduction to this topic. The conclusion is unlikely to result from a general negative attitude to hospital, since patients usually report satisfaction with standards of care, and with the quality of food. Ley and Spelman suggested there were several possible reasons for dissatisfaction with communications:

* insufficient time available to staff to communicate;
* patients' reticence or shyness in asking for information;
* staff believing that patients do not want to know;
* staff believing that another member of staff had already told the patient.

A considerable amount of work has been carried out to investigate the third of these reasons. Some has focussed specifically on telling patients they have cancer, and telling them they are dying. Cartwright, Hockey and Anderson (1973) produced evidence to show that not only doctors, but health visitors and the patients' relatives, thought that dying patients should not be told of their impending death. In their study, only 73 per cent of dying patients knew that they were dying. However, while the majority of doctors (69-90 per cent in a review by Feiffel, 1963) feel that patients should not be told they are dying, the majority of lay people (77-89 per cent in Feiffel's study) did want to be told when it was known that they were dying. When patients who do have cancer are told, they remain highly in favour of being told, and there may be other advantages in being told, such as a reduction in worry and an opportunity to make financial and other domestic arrangements. The results of these studies do not necessarily indicate that all patients with terminal conditions should be told, but they do suggest that giving full information about even serious conditions is appreciated by many patients and may be of benefit to them.

There are other important sources of variation in the degree to which the patients are satisfied with communications in hospital. One such source is the social background of the patients. Cartwright (1964) suggested that increased social distance between patients and doctors contributes to patients regarding doctors as in some sense superior to them. She found in her study that mothers whose husbands had manual jobs were less likely than other mothers to have received information from doctors, and were less likely to have spoken to the doctor in charge of their child. It is possible that staff may not so freely start to give information to patients from manual backgrounds since they may under-estimate the ability of such patients to understand what is said to them.

It may be the relative, not the patient, who wants to know about the condition. This is particularly relevant where the patient is a child, and the child's parents are both the best sources of information about the child's condition, and the best recipients of information about treatment and continuing care. Skipper (1966) found that mothers of children who were admitted to hospital for a tonsillectomy and who were given a lot of information about the admission and the operation were less distressed than other mothers. Relatives of adult patients may also want to obtain information directly from the responsible doctor or senior nurse, if they anticipate being heavily involved in the after-care of, for example, a spinal injury or a stroke patient. The necessity to communicate adequately with the family may be further complicated by the fact that the most accessible and convenient source of information for the family may be a social worker or district nurse who is not an expert on the patient's particular condition and who may simply be unable to provide the information requested.

The problem of compliance

While it might be desirable in principle for patients to know more about their condition, and while they might then be more satisfied with their care, would an improvement in communication lead to improved response to treatment? There is ample evidence to indicate that the compliance of patients, and the extent to which they follow instructions by health care staff, can be extremely poor. Some studies of out-patients have shown that even when patients are trying to comply, up to two-thirds may be taking the wrong dose of medicine. Ley and Spelman, for example, found that 27 out of 50 diabetic patients failed to take their insulin as prescribed.

Does improved communication increase compliance? A number of studies have found that providing patients with more information about their condition and about treatment has led to improved treatment outcome. For example, Lindemann and Van Aernam (1971) compared two groups of patients in their response to surgery, one group having pre-operation instruction on breathing, bed exercises, etc. The instructed patients left hospital on average two days earlier than the other group and were superior on some other measures of physical functioning. Wilber and Barrow (1969) looked at the effect of a public health nursing visitation programme on the rate of compliance with an anti-hypertensive regime. Those patients exposed to the programme increased from a compliance rate of 15 per cent to 80 per cent, while the control group increased only from 15 per cent to 34 per cent. For both groups there was a considerable drop in the rate of compliance in a two-year follow-up check, but the visited group was still better. It must also be said that a number of other carefully designed studies either have not shown an improvement in compliance or outcome after very positive attempts to improve communication, or have not necessarily made it clear that improvement is primarily due to better communication.

Improving communications with patients

A Ministry of Health pamphlet published in 1963 made a number of general recommendations designed to improve communications aimed at patients. The recommendations stress the value of the fullest communication between general practitioners, hospital doctors and the patient, and the need for advance information where possible: 'there should be no surprises'. The recommendations cover other detailed points, such as the value of doctors and nurses being clearly identified to patients by name, the identification to the patients of their personal doctors, and the importance of carefully considering the timing of information.

Hogue (1979) made a series of recommendations directed at nurses intended to improve compliance, particularly relevant to the care of people with chronic disease. These recommendations can be formulated as a series of rules.

Think about the treatment regime from the patient's point of view. Make the régime as comprehensible to the patient as possible, by specifying exact procedures and goals, as opposed to vague ones. Help the patient to feel competent to manage the regime: give the patient opportunities to succeed in reaching goals. Use the power of natural support systems: it has been found that social isolation is repeatedly associated with poor compliance, and conversely the support of family and friends increases compliance. Find out the key support people in the patient's life, and find out how they can help. This also suggests finding out what other professional staff are concerned with the patient, and collaborating closely with them, so that there is concordance between the professional advice the patients receive.

A more technical approach to the same problem has been taken by Ley and Spelman. They examined the extent to which patients remember what they are told; and they found that patients forgot very quickly about one-third of what they are told. Usually the most important information is retained, but even so some patients forget their diagnosis within only a few weeks. Ley and Spelman suggest a number of principles which affect the amount of information remembered by the patient.

* Patients remember best what they are told first and what they consider most important;
* Patients remember better if they are told in a logical sequence, such as (i) what is wrong with you, (ii) what we will need to do, (iii) what will then happen, (iv) what treatment you will then get, and (v) what you must do for yourself.
* Patients forget instructions and advice more than other information.
* Patients who have a good knowledge of medical facts remember better than those with a poor knowledge.
* The intelligence and age of the patient, by themselves, are not related to how much the patient remembers.
* The more information that is given to the patient, the greater the proportion that is forgotten.
* If the patient writes down what is said, it will be remembered just as well and there will later be a record to consult.

One technique sometimes used when communicating with patients is fright! People do respond to warnings; and frightening and alarming messages may change attitudes. But they may not lead to changes in behaviour. The relative level of fear provoked by the message is important. High-fear messages may be effective in changing attitudes, but in general low-fear messages are as effective in changing behaviour. It is possible that some people who have particular symptoms may fail to undergo a cervical smear, for example, if they are afraid of the surgical procedure which would then follow a positive result.

The communications which are easiest to examine are those which contain statements of fact and which are delivered intentionally. However, some communications between patients and staff are very much concerned with feelings and opinions, and occur incidentally to other communications. It is important to be aware of this parallel content of communication, some of which may well be expressed non-verbally, by eye contact, tone of voice, body posture, and in other ways (see Argyle, 1973).

The emphasis in this chapter has been communication from professional staff to the patient. There is a danger in concentrating exclusively on this one direction of communication so that undue emphasis is placed upon the value of communication for the professional staff by improving 'compliance', discharge notes, and other outcome criteria: it is as legitimate to look at communication primarily from the patient's view, to see the effect it has on them in terms of their own self-esteem and social relationships. There is also a danger in failing to pay attention to communication from patients to staff. Many interactions between staff and patients will be protracted and emotionally involved, and it can be artificial to abstract one element or component of a conversation for analysis.

It is just as possible to study communications from patients to doctors. Johnston (1976) looked at the way in which nurses in three gynaecology wards perceived the feelings of the patients in the wards. Her conclusion was that the nurses were not very aware of the patient's worries, and were therefore probably inaccurate in their assessment of the type of information the patients needed. It is useful to separate the problem of communication, as defined by the staff, from the problem of communication, as defined by patients.

Communications between patients and others take place in the context of a 'doctor-patient' or 'nurse-patient' relationship. These relationships imply certain expectations of the behaviour of the patient which, while constrained by the patient's role, will vary according to the patient's medically-relevant knowledge and prior experience of medical care.

Effective communication is dependent upon an appraisal of the patients' relevant knowledge of their current state, and of the setting. Some encounters with patients take place in conditions which are, to say the least, distracting. The car-driver trapped in the crashed vehicle; the over-excited person in the middle of a psychiatric episode opposing the GP's intentions to apply a section of the 1959 Mental Health Act; the young child in casualty suspected of swallowing laburnum pods accompanied by a distressed mother. In some circumstances action alone is required, with the words waiting until later.

Yet patients overwhelmingly want to know what is happening to them, even when that knowledge is unpleasant. The benefits of good communication are potentially considerable. 'Improving low compliance is an exciting challenge with substantial rewards for patient and provider' (Hogue, 1979).

References

Argyle, M. (1973)
Social Interaction. London: Tavistock.

Boyle, C.M. (1970)
Differences between doctors and patients interpretations of some common medical terms. British Medical Journal, 2, 286-289.

Cartwright, A. (1964)
Human Relations and Hospital Care. London: Routledge & Kegan Paul.

Cartwright, A., Hockey, L. and Anderson, J.L. (1973)
Life before Death. London: Routledge & Kegan Paul.

Feiffel, H. (1963)
Death. In N. Farberon (ed.), Taboo Topics. London: Prentice-Hall.

Hogue, C.C. (1979)
Nursing and compliance. In R.B. Haynes, D.W. Taylor and D.L. Sackett (eds), Compliance in Health Care. Baltimore, Md: Johns Hopkins Press.

Johnston, M. (1976)
Communication of patients' feelings in hospital. In A.E. Bennett (ed.), Communication between Doctors and Patients. London: Oxford University Press, for Nuffield Provincial Hospital Trust.

Ley, P. and Spelman, M.S. (1967)
Communicating with the Patient. London: Staples Press.

Lindemann, C.A. and Van Aernam, B. (1971)
Nursing intervention with the pre-surgical patients - the effects of structured and unstructured pre-operative teaching. Nursing Research, 20, 319-332.

Mechanic, D. (1968)
Medical Sociology. New York: Free Press.

Ministry of Health (1963)
Communication between Doctors, Nurses and Patients. London: HMSO.

Parry, J. (1970)
The Psychology of Human Communication. London: University of London Press.

Parsons, T. (1951)
The Social System. Chicago, Ill.: Free Press.

Skipper, J.K. (1966)
Mothers' distress over their children's hospitalization for tonsillectomy. Journal of Marriage and the Family, 18, 45.

Wilber, J.A. and Barrow, J.G. (1969)
Reducing elevated blood pressure: experience found in a community. Minnesota Medicine, 52, 1303-1305.

The psychology of illness, care and treatment: Part II questions

1. How important is the physical environment of a ward to a patient?
2. Is the size of a ward, or of a hospital, important in the care a patient receives?
3. Does it really matter whether staff wear uniform?
4. How can you 'personalize' the lives of your patients without lowering the standard of care they receive?
5. How valid is it to consider such diverse places as hospitals, public schools, monasteries, prisons, and ships as all being 'total institutions'?
6. What are the key elements of the therapeutic community approach?
7. How is it possible to involve patients more in the conduct of their treatment?
8. How independent should different wards and units be within the same hospital?
9. How important is initial staff training in creating staff attitudes?
10. What are the advantages of team nursing on a ward?
11. Is the concept of 'morale' useful in considering how hospitals work?
12. What method of leadership is likely to be most effective in producing good patient care?
13. What information will be of benefit to patients in their recovery?
14. What are the consequences of adopting the 'sick role'?
15. How can you minimize distraction to patients when you are talking to them?
16. Do patients do as they are told? If not, why not?
17. What problems can arise when someone who is not an expert on an individual's medical condition - like a social worker - is suddenly asked for advice by the family?
18. What factors limit the ability of patients to remember what they are told?
19. In what ways could you prepare an adult patient for an investigative procedure that is rather unpleasant?
20. Discuss the possible disadvantages of being 'too soft' or 'too hard' in your attitude towards the pain patient.
21. In what sense can it be said that pain is learnt?
22. What is a placebo effect? What role can it play in the treatment of pain?

23. Can pain be treated using psychological methods alone?
24. Describe the range of chemical and physical therapies available for the treatment of pain.
25. What cues do we use to identify that a person is in pain, and the degree of pain experienced?
26. Can an individual nurse change a ward?
27. What sort of events produce the greatest emotional response in patients?
28. What factors modify the expectations of patients towards particular doctors and nurses?
29. What factors modify the expectations of nurses towards working closely with members of other professions?
30. What event has given you the most personal satisfaction in your nursing career, and why?

Psychology and nursing

Abdellah, F.G. and Levine, E. (1979) Better Patient Care Through Nursing Research. New York: Macmillan Inc.

Ackerman, W.B. and Lohnes, D.R. (1981) Research Methods for Nurses. New York: McGraw-Hill.
In the same way as there are several general texts on psychology, there are several general texts on nursing research, indicating methodology, data collection and analysis, and how to write up research. These are two such books.

Anastasi, A. (1979) Fields of Applied Psychology. New York: McGraw-Hill.
This book gives a comprehensive general introduction to the fields of applied psychology, including industrial and organizational psychology, engineering and environmental psychology, consumer psychology, and clinical counselling and community psychology.

Baron, R.A. and Byrne, D. (1977) Social Psychology: Understanding human interaction. Boston: Allyn & Bacon.
Social psychology is a major field of psychological investigation, sufficiently important to generate general textbooks covering only this field such as this one.

Brown, R. and Herrnstein, R.J. (1975) Psychology. London: Methuen.

Hilgard, E.R., Atkinson, R.L. and Atkinson, R.C. (1979) Introduction to Psychology. New York: Harcourt Brace Jovanovich.
Some of the American texts are comprehensive in their coverage, and very well laid out and illustrated; these are two such examples.

Cohen, D. (1977) Psychologists on Psychology. London: Routledge & Kegan Paul.
This book looks at the subject from a highly individual point of view. It contains a series of interviews with a number of notable psychologists, including D. E. Broadbent, H. J. Eysenck, and R. D. Laing, reflecting their careers and informed opinions.

Colledge, M.M. and Jones D. (1979) Readings in Nursing. Edinburgh: Churchill Livingstone.
> Series of readings are now becoming available in nursing too; this example is a collection which covers a number of areas relevant to the practice of nursing care, presented at an advanced level.

Furnham, A. and Argyle, M. (1981) The Psychology of Social Situations: Selected readings. Oxford: Pergamon.
> General texts can often be usefully supplemented by collections of readings, or reprinted articles of particular value. This example of such a selection of readings covers 31 topics from the Polish peasant in Europe and America, to the forms of address used by members of staff in a department store.

Kratz, C.R. (1979) The Nursing Process. London: Ballière Tindall.
> Much modern research and practice in nursing refers to the 'nursing process'. An outline of the process is given here.

Roper, N., Logan, W.W. and Tierney, A.J. (1980) The Elements of Nursing. Edinburgh: Churchill Livingstone.
> Alongside ideas such as the nursing process, new approaches to a conceptualization of nursing are being tried. One particularly interesting approach is to look at nursing within a model of living and hence to create a highly psychological view of nursing. This particular approach is explored here.

Skinner, B.F. (1972) Beyond Freedom and Dignity. London: Cape.
> A classic work, by the main protagonist in the development of the 'radical behaviourist' view of human behaviour.

Understanding yourself and other people

Brown, G.W. and Harris, T. (1978) Social Origins of Depression. London: Tavistock.
> A seminal book, looking at depression, the life events which provoke it, and the factors leading to greater vulnerability.

Eysenck, H.J. (1977) You and Neurosis. London: Temple Smith.
> One of a large number of books written by this well-known and somewhat controversial figure in clinical psychology, presenting a psychologically-based theory of neurosis.

Hardy, M.E. and Conway, M.E. (eds) (1978) Role Theory: Perspectives for health professions. New York: Appleton-Century-Crofts.

Series of chapters by different authors on knowledge of self and knowledge of roles. Discussion of both theoretical constructs and practical examples.

Paterson, J.G. and Zderad, L.T. (1976) Humanistic Nursing. New York: Wiley.
An existential alternative approach to how nurses view their role.

Wilson Barnett, J. (1979) Stress in Hospital. Edinburgh: Churchill Livingstone.
An account of how people react to hospital, and of their reactions to intensive care units, medication, and malignant disease.

Yura, H. and Walsh, M.B. (eds) (1978) Human Needs and the Nursing Process. New York: Appleton-Century-Crofts.
An edited series of papers revolving around the theme of our need for activity and love.

ssessment

Comrey, A.L., Backer, T.E. and Glaser, E.M. (1973) A Source Book for Mental Health Measures. Los Angeles, Ca: Human Interaction Research Institute.
A comprehensive guide to a wide range of questionnaires, ratings, and other methods, providing a useful survey of the variety of instruments available.

Gathercole, C.E. (1968) Assessment in Clinical Psychology. Harmondsworth: Penguin.
A short account of how a clinical psychologist assesses patients, covering some of the practical aspects of assessment.

Jessup, G. (1975) Selection and Assessment at Work. London: Methuen.
One of the 'Essential Psychology' series, looking at the use of assessment procedures in an industrial setting.

Keefe, F.J., Kopel, S.A., and Gordon, S.B. (1978) A Practical Guide to Behavioral Assessment. New York: Springer.
An example of a number of recently published introductions to behavioural assessment, this one being particularly useful for nurses not familiar with this approach.

Mittler, P. (1973) The Psychological Assessment of Mental and Physical Handicaps. London: Tavistock.
The standard British reference book, covering most general types of assessment procedure, reviewing their usefulness and limitations.

Nay, W.R. (1979) Multimethod Clinical Assessment. New York: Gardner Press.
> An excellent comprehensive account of how to plan and conduct clinical assessment prior to planning intervention. Covers interview, natural observation, self-report, and psycho-physiological methods.

Oppenheim, A.N. (1966) Questionnaire Design and Attitude Measurement. London: Heinemann.
> This well-established book is still one of the best guides to questionnaire design.

Perkins, E.R. and Anderson, D.C. (1981) Self Assessment in the National Health Service. Driffield: Nafferton Books.
> Written for midwives, health visitors, and similar groups to enable them to monitor their own individual practice.

Ryback, R.S. (1974) The Problem Orientated Record in Psychiatry and Mental Health Care. New York: Grune & Stratton.
> A detailed look at the design and use of problem-orientated records, giving examples of the sort of forms used.

Wandelt, M.A. and Ager, J.W. (1974) Quality Patient Care Scale. New York: Appleton-Century-Crofts.
> An example of the development of a detailed rating scale, complete with explanatory guide.

The early years

Geraghty, P. (1981) Caring for Children. London: Ballière Tindall.
> General coverage of child development, paying particular attention to play, and children with special needs. The content of this book is designed to be especially relevant to nursery nurses.

Lamb, M.E. (ed.) (1976) The Role of the Father in Child Development. New York: Wiley.
> Discusses the function of the father in parenthood, supplementing the considerable amount of material on the mother's role.

Macy, C. and Falkner, F. (1979) Pregnancy and Birth. London: Harper & Row.
> One of the 'Life Cycle' books, giving a well-illustrated semi-popular account of pregnancy.

Melamed, B.G. (1977) Psychological preparation for hospitalization. In S. Rachman (ed.), Contributions to Medical Psychology, Volume 1. Oxford: Pergamon.
> Detailed account of four experiments, all concerned with preparation of children for entering hospital or for surgery.

Stacey, M. et al (1970) Hospitals, Children and their Families. London: Routledge & Kegan Paul.
Not a highly psychological book, but a thorough account of an attempt to implement the Platt Report to improve care in hospital.

amily life and old age

Copp, L.A. (ed.) (1981) Care of the Ageing. Edinburgh: Churchill Livingstone.
Number 2 in the Recent Advances in Nursing series: a number of contributions from an international team of expert nurses covering, for example, role stress in head nurses of nursing homes, and changing attitudes to the elderly.

Fiske, M. (1979) The Prime of Life? London: Harper & Row.
One of the 'Life Cycle' volumes covering the middle years, a period often omitted in developmental psychology.

Pattison, E.M. (1977) The Experience of Dying. Englewood Cliffs, NJ: Prentice Hall.
Twenty-nine chapters, mostly dealing with dying in relation to particular disorders and in relation to particular age groups.

Rayner, E. (1978) Human Development. London: National Institute of Social Services Library No.22, George Allen & Unwin.
Covers the entire life period from pregnancy to death.

Rosenthal, C.J., Marshall, V.W., MacPherson, A.S. and French, S.E. (1980) Nurses, Patients and Families. London: Croom Helm.
Discusses a number of issues relating to patients and their families, including the classification of problem families, and information control in nursing practice.

hanging people

Allen, H.O. and Murrell, J. (1978) Nurse Training: An enterprise in curriculum development. Plymouth: Macdonald & Evans.
A discussion of the whole process of curriculum planning.

Argyle, M. (ed.) (1981) Social Skills and Health. London: Methuen.
Series of articles on the relevance of social skills to health care, including chapters on social skills in nursing, and doctor-patient skills.

Berni, R. and Fordyce, W.E. (1977) Behavior Modification and the Nursing Process. St Louis, Mo.: C.V. Mosby.
An example of a number of books which describe the

relevance of practical behaviour modification techniques
to nursing.

Bloch, S. (ed.) (1979) An Introduction to the Psycho-
therapies. Oxford: Oxford University Press.
As the title suggests, an introduction to most of the
psychological treatments, including marital therapy,
family therapy, and crisis intervention, as well as
individual and group psychotherapy and behaviour
therapy.

Donovan, M.I. (1981) Cancer Care: A guide for patient
education. New York: Appleton Century Crofts.
Designed to help professional staff organize and implement patient education programmes, teaching them how
to cope with cancer.

Garfield, S.L. and Bergin, A.E. (eds) (1978) Handbook of
Psychotherapy and Behavior Change: An empirical analysis.
New York: Wiley.
Critical reviews of the major topics in behaviour
therapy; useful as a reference work.

Royal College of Nursing (1978) Counselling in Nursing:
Report of a Working Party. London: RCN.
A report of a 17-member working party, concerned with
the need for staff counselling and its development with
nurses.

**The psychology of illness
care and treatment**

Altman, I. (1975) The Environment and Social Behavior:
Privacy, personal space, territory, and crowding. Monterey,
Ca: Brookes Cole.
An outline of the 'social system' or 'ecological' model
of Man, viewing behaviour as being intimately entwined
with the environment.

Argyle, M. (1973) Social Interaction. London: Tavistock.
A useful introduction to ways of analysing social
introduction, written by one of the leading authorities.

Argyle, M. and Trower, P. (1979) Person to Person: Ways
of communicating. London: Harper & Row.
A 'Life Cycle' book, introducing in well-illustrated
form topics such as body language, rituals, social
conduct, and the rules of informal social interaction.

Ashworth, D. (1980) Care to Communicate. London: RCN.
A study of nurse-patient communication in intensive
care units, with a a detailed analysis of modes of
communication in that type of setting.

Boswell, D.M. and Wingrove, J.M. (1974) The Handicapped
Person in the Community. London: Tavistock.

An extremely valuable source book and reader, covering many aspects of disability, and the psychological and social consequences of handicap.

Griffiths, D. (1981) Psychology and Medicine. London: The British Psychological Society/Macmillan.
A companion volume to this one, covering some topics more suitable for doctors and medical students.

Haynes, R.B., Taylor, D.W. and Sackett, D.L. (1979) Compliance in Health Care. Baltimore, Md: Johns Hopkins University Press.
A number of essays dealing with different aspects of compliance, together forming a good review of the topic.

Hollander, E.P. (1978) Leadership Dynamics: A practical guide to effective relationships. New York: Free Press.
An examination of the nature of leadership, the function of a leader, the effectiveness of leaders, and how they bring about change.

Lamond, N. (1974) Becoming a Nurse: The registered nurse's view of general student nurse education. London: RCN.
A sociological approach to the definition of dimensions of nursing, and the adjustment to the role of being a nurse.

Ley, P. (1977) Psychological studies of doctor-patient communication. In S. Rachman (ed.), Contributions to Medical Psychology. Oxford: Pergamon Press.
A review chapter by one of the first psychologists to systematically study communications between doctors and patients.

Rachman, S. (ed.) (1977) Contributions to Medical Psychology, Volume 1. Oxford: Pergamon.

Rachman, S. (ed.) (1980) Contributions to Medical Psychology, Volume 2. Oxford: Pergamon.
Two volumes containing detailed yet significant accounts of the ways in which key topics in medical psychology have been advanced in recent years.

Rachman, S.J. and Philips, C. (1975) Psychology and Medicine. London: Temple Smith.
This easy-to-read volume covers a number of topics, such as the effectiveness of placebos and pain control, in the psychology of physical medicine.

Roberts, I. (1975) Discharged from Hospital. London: RCN Research Report Series 2, No.6.
An analysis of the effectiveness of care of 164 patients who were interviewed one week after discharge.

Annotated reading

Robinson, D. (1971) The Process of Becoming Ill. London: Routledge & Kegan Paul.
> An examination of 'illness behaviour' and decision making in illness.

Stockwell, F. (1972) The Unpopular Patient. London: RCN.
> A fascinating account of the way in which 'unpopular' patients are treated in a hospital ward, using a simple and obvious direct observation technique.

Index

Index

Index

Index

Index